AF615094

CURRENT APPROACHES TO OCCUPATIONAL MEDICINE

Current Approaches to OCCUPATIONAL MEDICINE

Edited by
A. WARD GARDNER
MD FFOM DIH

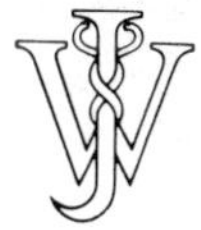

YEAR BOOK MEDICAL PUBLISHERS • INC.
35 EAST WACKER DRIVE, CHICAGO

CIP Data

Current approaches to occupational medicine.
1. Medicine, Industrial
I. Gardner, Archibald Ward
616.9'803 RC963

ISBN 0 7236 0514 9

Printed in Great Britain by
Billing & Sons Ltd., Guildford, London and Worcester.

To the memory of
ANDREW MEIKLEJOHN
Occupational physician and teacher
with affection and gratitude

Preface

The theme that runs through this book is a wish to illuminate some current problems, to give perspective, and to review progress – mainly in the field of occupational health, occupational medicine and occupational hygiene. So, the book is a *potpourri,* the flavour of which is for the most part determined by the choice both of authors and of subjects. Some readers may feel that particular subjects of interest to them have not been included. To these and like comments I can only reply that I have been extremely fortunate in being able to ask a number of busy people to devote their time to writing about topics in which each has special knowledge and authority. Their responses have been gratifying, generous and illuminating. They have written and re-written against the clock so that their topic will be up-to-date and fresh. To some extent also they have moulded their contribution into a pre-set form, both for internal consistency and for ease of reading. So that the reader's task may be pleasurable, informative and interesting I have tried to arrange related subjects together in so far as the diversity allows. In all these matters the contributors have been splendidly hard-working and uncomplaining.

It is therefore my great pleasure to thank them all most warmly for their devotion to the task, for their labours and for their tolerance and, especially in the light of their tolerance of a few editorial comments, to hope that they will continue and for long remain my friends. My colleague Archie Downie has helped by discussing a number of topics and problems with me during the preparation of the book and I am most grateful to him for his concern and interest.

A. Ward Gardner

Contributors

MICHAEL ALDERSON MD, FFCM
Professor of Epidemiology Institute of Cancer Research, Clifton Avenue, Sutton, Surrey.

P S I BARRY MRCS, LRCP, MFOM
Chief Medical Officer The Associated Octel Company Ltd.

J T CARTER MB, MSc
Medical Officer Occupational Health Unit, BP Research Centre, Sunbury-on-Thames, Middlesex.

M A COOKE MB, ChB, MFOM
Principal Medical Advisor Albright & Wilson Ltd, Honorary Visiting Reader, Department of Safety and Hygiene, University of Aston, Birmingham.

M F D'SOUZA MB, MRCGP
General Practitioner and Lecturer in the Department of Community Medicine St Thomas's Hospital and the Department of Clinical Epidemiology in General Practice, Cardio-thoracic Institute, London.

SUZETTE GAUVAIN MA, MRCP, FFCM, MFOM, DPH, DIH
Consultant Adviser in Occupational Medicine, Consultant Adviser in Medical Training Employment Medical Advisory Service, Health and Safety Executive.

MARCUS GRANT MA, DES
Director Alcohol Education Centre.

J MALCOLM HARRINGTON MD, MSc, MRCP, MFOM
Senior Lecturer in Occupational Medicine London School of Hygiene and Tropical Medicine, London.

J A HARRYMAN BSc Psychol.
Industrial Relations Manager Esso Petroleum Co Ltd, Fawley Refinery, Hants.

J W HILL MB, ChB, MFOM, DIH
Group Medical Adviser Pilkington Brothers Ltd, St Helens.

ANN HOLLINGWORTH MB, BS, LRCP, MRCS, MFOM, DIH

J L KEARNS MSc, MRCGP, FFOM

D MALCOLM MB, ChB, FFOM, DIH

G MATTHEWS MB, MRCP, MFOM

K H NICKOL FRCP, MFOM, DIH

T P OLIVER MFCM, MFOM, DPH, DIH
Surgeon Captain RN, Principal Medical Officer AM Naval Base, Portsmouth. *Consultant Adviser in Occupational Health to* Chief Executive, Royal Dockyards.
Honorary Lecturer in Occupational Medicine University of Dundee.

FRANK S PRESTON VRD, MB, ChB, MFOM, DA, FRACS
British Airways Medical Service.

DOROTHY RADWANSKI RGN, SCM, OHNC

R J G RYCROFT MRCP, DIH
St John's Hospital for Diseases of the Skin and Employment Medical Advisory Service, London.

PETER SUTTON BSc(Eng), C Eng, MIMech E, FIOA, FRSH

PETER TAYLOR MD, BSc, FRCP, FFOM, DIH
Chief Medical Officer The Post Office.

DEREK TURNER MSc, PhD, Dip Occ Hyg
The Associated Octel Company Ltd.

Contents

1. LEAD: OCCUPATIONAL AND ENVIRONMENTAL EXPOSURE

P. S. I. Barry

INTRODUCTION

It has long been known, before the advent of Christianity, that high-level exposure to lead could be a cause of ill-health. Its effects were noted and recorded by Hippocrates (BC 370) Pliny (AD 23–70) and Dioscorides (AD 100) (Hunter, 1975). The metal was much sought after by the ancients for its malleable properties and the multiple uses to which it could be put; it has been cited as a primary cause for the fall of the Roman Empire (Gilfillan, 1965), largely because of its use by the ruling classes for the preservation and sweetening of wine. In view of the multiple nefarious activities of Roman high society during the period of the decline, it would seem more probable that their other worse indulgences, resulting in cerebral dsyfunction and lunatic behaviour, were more responsible for the final collapse of the Empire than their indiscriminate use of lead.

A true appreciation of the effects of uncontrolled domestic and occupational exposure to lead became apparent during the 18th and 19th centuries AD. Ramazzini (1713) described the symptoms of lead poisoning among potters who used lead for glazing; Sir George Baker (1767) noted the effects of drinking lead-contaminated cider in Devonshire; Tanquerel Des Planches (1848) recorded a classic series of cases of lead poisoning in Paris; and Thomas Percival (1774) annotated a variety of causes of lead poisoning in England.

In his work Thomas Percival described a procedure for the preservation of wine, taken from the recommendations of the cook to his Grace the Duke of Manchester, as follows: 'To hinder wine from turning put a pound of melted lead, in fair water (soft), into your cask pretty warm, and stop it close'. No indication is given as to the state of health of his Grace, but Percival decries the practice, as follows: 'The adulteration of wine is indeed an evil so general, and so dangerous in its consequences, that it is to be hoped the legislature will interpose to prevent it'.

The legislative measures introduced since his time would probably afford Thomas Percival much satisfaction, even though less than satisfactory practices still persist in some parts of the world.

Although lead has been known to exert poisonous effects for many centuries, it was only following the publication by Kehoe et al. (1933) that it became recognized that lead was an inescapable part of all animal and vegetable life, by virtue of the ubiquitous presence of the metal on the surface of the earth. The concentrations of lead in the surface soils and rocks have been found to vary between just a few parts per million up to several hundreds of parts per million, with an overall average in the earth's crust of about 16 parts per million.

Thus all living matter contains an inevitable natural background of lead, to which must be added a quantum arising from the purposes to which the metal has been put to use by man. Patterson (1965), by an extrapolated calculation, estimated the present levels of lead in man to be about 100 times those of prehistoric eras, but this is probably a considerable overestimation, impossible of confirmation.

In his classic studies Kehoe (1961) established that the body achieves an equilibrium with the lead in the environment, whereby input is very largely balanced by excretory output in urine, faeces, bile, sweat, hair and nails. The equilibrium level will fluctuate according to the level of input and is not governed by any homeostatic mechanism.

OCCUPATIONAL EXPOSURE

Inorganic lead

Control procedures introduced during the twentieth century for the protection of lead workers have markedly reduced the incidence of lead poisoning in many countries.

Routes of absorption

Inorganic lead may be absorbed into the body by the inhalation of dusts and fume and by ingestion.

More than half the lead inhaled is usually exhaled unchanged. The amount retained in the lung will depend upon the particle size. Large particles are trapped on the muco-ciliary surfaces in the bronchi, to be returned to the naso-pharynx and swallowed. Very small particles and fume may reach the lung alveoli from where they will be absorbed.

Approximately 10 per cent of the lead ingested may be absorbed from the gastro-intestinal tract, the remainder appearing in the faeces unchanged (Kehoe, 1961). Recent studies (Chamberlain et al., 1975) suggest that the percentage uptake from the gut may be rather greater than this.

Inorganic lead is not absorbed through the skin.

Effects

High level exposure to lead may effect a number of organ systems, including the brain, the peripheral nervous system, the gastro-intestinal tract, the haemopoietic system and the renal system. Because of improved working conditions and a greater awareness of lead as a potentially toxic substance the clinical signs of encephalopathy, peripheral neuropathy, and Burtonian line are rarely seen these days. Subjective symptoms of fatigue, sleep disturbance, abdominal pain and headache may occur, but need to be differentiated from other more probable causes of psychological or pathological origin.

Control procedure

Regular medical examination and biological monitoring should be an integral part of the preventive programme, the frequency depending upon the level of potential exposure. Environmental monitoring is also a necessary adjunct for the assurance of safe working conditions.

1. *Biological monitoring* probably provides the best indication of the exposure of an individual, or groups, to the lead available for absorption at the workplace. The estimation of the lead concentration in blood is still the parameter of choice for the determination of the degree of lead absorption, but the estimation of alpha laevulinic acid and coproporphyrin in urine, both precursors of haem, are also of value.

Haemoglobin estimation should be carried out regularly, as a fall in haemoglobin may be indicative of excessive exposure to lead, or of some other disease entity, such as iron deficiency, pernicious anaemia or leukaemia, which would require investigation and be incompatible with further exposure to lead.

Urinary lead estimations are seldom used because of greater variability of results and potential for contamination, compared with blood. Punctate basophil red blood cell counts are less reliable than the other tests for the early detection of excessive lead absorption and are now seldom used for control purposes.

Lane et al. (1968) proposed a series of biochemical tests and the levels that might be expected in four arbitrary categories of lead absorption, as shown in Table 1.1.

Table 1.1 Categories of lead absorption. (1μg (microgram) = 0·00483 mole.)

Test	Normal	Acceptable	Excessive	Dangerous
Blood lead	<40μg/100ml	40–80μg/100ml	80–120μg/100ml	>120μg/100ml
Urinary lead	<80μg/l	80–150μg/l	150–250μg/l	>250μg/l
Urinary coproporphyrin	<150μg/l	150–500μg/l	500–1500μg/l	>1500μg/l
Urinary ALA	<0·6mg/100ml	0·6–2·0mg/100ml	2·0–4·0mg/100ml	>4·0mg/100ml

If the values are kept within the 'acceptable' range clinical lead poisoning will not arise. If the blood lead exceeds 80 μg/100 ml the individual concerned should be removed from further exposure to lead until values within the acceptable range are achieved. Recently government agencies have proposed a reduction in the upper levels of acceptability, although the evidence for doing so is not well substantiated.

In addition to the tests advocated by Lane et al. (1968) a recent innovation is the estimation of free erythrocyte protoporphyrins (FEP), another precursor of haem, in red blood cells. The test is simple to perform and, apart from raised FEP in blood in cases of iron deficiency, is specific to lead. Normal FEP in the blood of children has been estimated at about 65 μg/100 ml erythrocytes, to correspond with about 20 μgPb/100 ml blood (Roels et al., 1976). FEP levels in children to correspond with the 'acceptable' range of Lane et al. (1968) would lie between about 200 μg and 1000 μg/100 ml erythrocytes (Piomelli et al., 1973). Male adults, for reasons that are not clear but possibly related to iron metabolism, show a lesser response of FEP for a given blood lead level than do female adults and children, by approximately one half (Roels et al., 1976; Alessio et al., 1976; Joselow and Flores, 1977). There still remains some doubt, however, as to what represents an agreed standard figure for FEP measurement.

2. *Environmental monitoring* as a procedure for the control of lead absorption is of subsidiary importance to biological monitoring. Only when personal samplers are used can it be said to give a reasonable approximation of lead absorption. Nevertheless, regular fixed-station air monitoring at carefully chosen sites can provide useful information as to the satisfactory functioning of plant equipment and lead to the subsequent correction of faults when these arise. Present threshold limit values for lead in air vary between nations at 150 $\mu g/m^3$ and 200 $\mu g/m^3$. It has recently been proposed by the Occupational Safety and Health Agency of the USA that the value be reduced to 100 $\mu gPb/m^3$ air. The subject is under discussion and no firm decision has yet been taken to legislate for the lower figure.

Organo lead

The organo lead alkyl compounds, tetraethyl and tetramethyl lead, are manufactured solely for use as petrol additives to improve the efficiency of fuels. Approximately 0·6 g of lead alkyl (as lead) when added to one litre of petrol is sufficient to raise the octane number of a given fuel by six to eight points. This results in improved performance and a saving in crude oil and refinery equipment, which would otherwise be required to produce an equivalent effect.

Tetraethyl lead was introduced into refinery technology in 1923 and tetramethyl lead about 1959. The latter was developed because of its greater volatility which made it more suitable for use with petrol produced from a reforming process. The lead alkyl compounds convert to inorganic lead oxide when burnt with petrol vapour in the cylinder. The lead oxide prevents the spontaneous detonation of the fuel/air mixture in advance of the flame front, which leads to inefficient combustion and possible damage to the engine. The phenomenon produces an audible metallic sound, known as 'knocking' or 'pinking' – hence the term 'antiknock' as a pseudonym for lead alkyl compounds.

In order to ensure the prevention of the build-up of deposits in the combustion chamber, scavenging agents are included with the lead alkyls supplied to oil refineries. The agents used are ethylene dibromide and ethylene dichloride. These react with the lead following combustion to form lead chloro-bromides which are readily evacuated with other exhaust products.

Lead oxide is not miscible with petrol, but the lead alkyl compounds are, hence the the necessity for manufacture in this form.

Routes of absorption

Tetraethyl lead and tetramethyl lead may be absorbed by inhalation of the vapour, ingestion of the liquid or by skin absorption following liquid contact. Inhalation is the most important route of entry, followed by skin absorption and then by ingestion. Although absorption following ingestion is very rapid, ingestion rarely occurs in practice. Tetramethyl lead is less readily absorbed through the skin than is tetraethyl lead.

Effects

High level exposure to the lead alkyl compounds, which in practice is nearly always from inhalation of the vapour, affects only the brain and may give rise to a condition of toxic psychosis. Unlike inorganic lead, no other organ systems, including the peripheral nervous system, appear to be affected. The illness is always acute and the effect reversible in the event of recovery.

Early symptoms include sleep disturbance with bad dreams, agitation, tremor, loss of appetite, metallic taste, fatigue, headache and sometimes gastro-intestinal upset. The condition may not progress beyond this stage in which case the patient will recover with no residual after effects. In more severe cases the illness may progress to a state of mania with complete disorientation and the development of delusions and hallucinations. The final outcome may be death in convulsions or coma, but in the event of recovery this again will be complete with no sequelae.

Tetramethyl lead is considerably less toxic than tetraethyl lead, by four to seven times (Cremer and Callaway, 1961; Springman et al., 1963). There have been a number of reports in the literature of cases of tetraethyl lead poisoning (Cassels and Dodds, 1946; Walker and Boyd, 1952; Kitzmiller and Kehoe, 1953; Boyd et al., 1957; Beattie et al., 1972), but none of tetramethyl lead poisoning since the inception of its use in 1959. One case of high level exposure to tetramethyl lead has been reported (Gething, 1975) in which no symptom developed; had the individual experienced the same level of exposure to tetraethyl lead, symptoms would most certainly have been expected to have arisen.

Tetraethyl lead and tetramethyl lead are themselves relatively non-toxic, but they undergo breakdown in the liver to triethyl lead and trimethyl lead; it is these compounds that have been shown to be the toxic agents. Tetramethyl lead is more stable in the body and undergoes less rapid breakdown in the liver; this, together with its greater volatility allowing for exhalation of the unchanged compound, accounts to some extent for the lesser toxicity of tetramethyl lead. In addition it has been shown that trimethyl lead is less toxic then triethyl lead (Cremer and Callaway, 1961; Springman et al., 1963).

The trialkyl lead compounds exert a specific effect on brain cells, resulting in a reduced cellular capacity to utilize oxygen. The concentrations found in brain are relatively small, compared with liver and kidney, but it is the specificity of action which is the phenomenon responsible for the illness.

Control procedures

Regular medical examination is necessary to ensure the early detection of excessive exposure, or of other incipient disease, particularly of a psychiatric nature, which would be incompatible with exposure to lead alkyl compounds.

Some strange ideas sometimes develop in the minds of workers, like the individual who some years ago was being examined by me and in the course of examination complained of fatigue in his lower limbs for which he had, to him, a perfectly plausible explanation. As he put it: 'It stands to reason, Doc, because after all, that lead, it's heavy stuff and is bound to sink into your legs and feet, isn't it?' In the light of such basic logic it seemed almost unkind to disillusion him.

The frequency of examination will depend upon the level of potential exposure, as also will the necessity for biological monitoring.

1. *Biological monitoring* provides the best indication of exposure but the parameters that can be used are limited. Unlike inorganic lead, no changes have been shown to occur in haem precursors and there is no development of anaemia in cases of lead alkyl poisoning. The concentration of lead in blood shows only a small elevation because the lead alkyl compounds have but little affinity for red blood cells, which accumulate 95 per cent of the inorganic lead in whole blood. It has been shown (Beattie et al., 1972) that organo lead may appear in plasma, but the amount is not sufficient to cause a marked elevation in whole blood. Recent unpublished studies suggest that the lead alkyl compounds may have a greater affinity for red blood cells than was previously thought probable (Chamberlain, 1977).

Thus the estimation of lead content in urine has to be the biological parameter of choice. Provided the pitfalls are recognized and adequate safeguards are taken, urinary lead estimations can provide a satisfactory means for the control of the exposure of lead alkyl workers. Spot samples of urine in excess of 50 millilitres and of specific gravity between 1·010 and 1·030 are suitable for analysis, provided that samples are collected in lead-free containers and care is taken to prevent contamination during collection and at the time of analysis.

Table 1.2 shows the criteria recommended for the biological control of lead alkyl workers.

Table 1.2 Categories of urinary lead concentrations for lead alkyl workers. (1μg (microgram) = 0·00483 mole.)

	Urinary lead (μg/l)
Normal	<80
Acceptable	80–120
Close observance	120–150
Unacceptable	>150

Values between 120 and 150 μgPb/l urine require to be checked at weekly intervals. If 150 μgPb/l urine is exceeded the individual should be withdrawn from further exposure to lead alkyl compounds until results of less than 80 μgPb/l urine are obtained.

2. *Environmental monitoring* provides essential information for the adequate control of emissions from operating plant machinery, but, as with inorganic lead, is of no direct value as a measure of the exposure and absorption of lead among plant employees.

The threshold limit value for tetraethyl lead is 100 $\mu gPb/m^3$ air and for tetramethyl lead 150 $\mu gPb/m^3$ air. Where both compounds are manufactured together in the same building the lower value should be taken as the standard to be applied.

Hygiene requirements

For both organo lead and inorganic lead strict attention should be paid to plant hygiene relative to cleanliness and safe operational conditions. In particular the following should be observed:

1. Employees should be provided with complete sets of works clothing which should be laundered on site and never taken home.
2. Separate lockers for works and street clothing should be provided.
3. Adequate washing and bathing facilities are essential.
4. No eating or smoking permitted, other than in specific areas set aside for the purpose. Such precautions are necessary both for the protection of the individual and of his family.

Special protective clothing and appropriate respiratory equipment may be required for some jobs of particular hazard, but plants should be so designed as to minimize the necessity for such measures.

ENVIRONMENTAL EXPOSURE

Because lead is ubiquitous, background environmental exposure has always been an inevitable consequence of life and all living creatures contain lead to varying degrees. Although it has not yet been shown to be an essential element, the presence of lead at low level concentration has been demonstrated as a constant feature in the tissues of populations from a wide variety of geographical locations. It would not be surprising, therefore, if at some time in the future its essentiality was confirmed, as in the case of some other metals, such as cobalt, copper, zinc and selenium, which at one time were considered to be alien to human health.

Post-mortem studies of populations in various parts of the world have shown variable concentrations of lead in different types of tissue, but little variation between tissues of the same type. The highest concentrations of lead are found in bones, particularly in the dense cortical bones; about 95 per cent of the total lead in the body is in the skeleton of adults and 50–70 per cent in the skeleton of children (Horiuchi et al., 1959; Barry and Mossman, 1970; Barry, 1975). Male adults have about 30 per cent more lead in their tissues than female adults. Children show no sex difference, but their tissue lead concentrations increase up to early adulthood, after which the soft tissues show no further increase. Bone lead concentrations, on the other hand, continue to increase with age.

A typical mature male adult of about 60 years of age, with no known occupational exposure to lead, may have 25–35 ppm lead (wet weight) in the dense bones, over 1 ppm in the liver and 0·7 ppm in the kidneys. Other soft tissue concentrations of lead for the most part vary between less than 0·1 ppm and less than 0·5 ppm (wet weight), with the exception of the aorta which exceeds 1 ppm and shows evidence of increase in lead concentration with age. The concentrations of lead in teeth, nails and hair approximate to the higher levels found in bone, but do not show evidence of increasing concentration with age. The total burden of lead in an average mature male adult has been estimated at about 160 mg, and in a female adult about 120 mg (Barry, 1975).

It has been suggested that metabolic or febrile illness may cause the sudden release of lead from bone into the blood in sufficient concentration to give rise to symptomatic lead poisoning. There is no evidence to support such conjecture and in my opinion it is unlikely that such an event could occur. Lead in dense bone is so firmly bound that its release by metabolic activity into the physiologically active soft tissue pool, in sufficient concentration to cause lead poisoning, must be highly improbable.

Sources of lead exposure and their relative contribution in the body

The principal sources of environmental exposure may be categorized as follows:

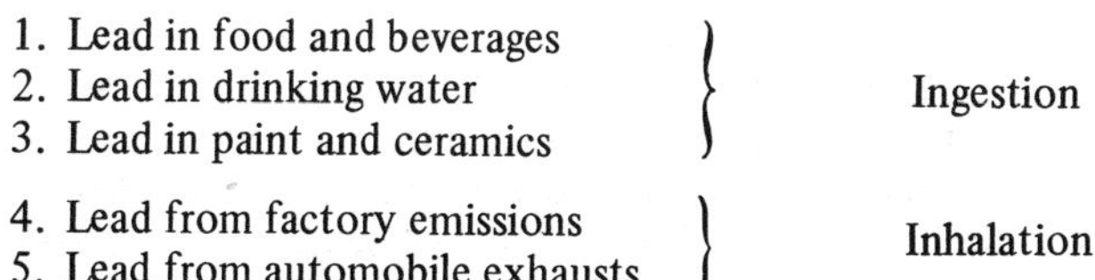
1. Lead in food and beverages
2. Lead in drinking water
3. Lead in paint and ceramics

} Ingestion

4. Lead from factory emissions
5. Lead from automobile exhausts

} Inhalation

An assessment of the contribution of lead uptake from different sources is shown in Table 1.3.

Table 1.3 Probable average daily lead absorption in micrograms. (1 μg (microgram) = 0·00483 mole.)

Source	Minimum (μg)	Percentage contribution	Maximum (μg)	Percentage contribution
Food and beverages	20	77	45	81·1
Water (0·03 ppm Pb)	3	11·5	4·5	8·1
Air (1μg Pb/m³	3	11·5	6	10·8
Total	26	–	55·5	–

The average daily intake of lead in food and beverages has been estimated at about 200–300 μg per day, of which about 10 per cent is absorbed and the remainder excreted in the faeces (Kehoe, 1961; Thompson, 1971). More recent estimates suggest that absorption may be nearer 15 per cent (Chamberlain et al., 1975). Thus between 20 and 45 μg of lead may be absorbed daily from the diet.

The World Health Organisation has recommended a limit in potable water supplies of 0·1 ppm lead, which may be reduced to 0·05 ppm in the near future. Acidic or soft waters may dissolve lead from lead pipe conduits and thus result in lead concentrations in excess of the W.H.O. recommended limit. Alkaline or hard waters do not dissolve lead and so do not take up the metal from pipework. Most potable water supplies contain lead concentrations well within the W.H.O. recommended standard and might be averaged reasonably at 0·03 ppm or less. The average adult consumes about one litre of water as tap water per day and about a further half to one litre incorporated in food. If 10–15 per cent of the lead in drinking water is absorbed, at a concentration of lead in water of 0·03 ppm, then 3 to 4·5 μg may be retained per day, equivalent to one-tenth of other dietary sources.

Most of the lead in the air of cities is derived from motor vehicle exhaust emissions, with some contribution from coal burning, industry, and garbage disposal. Studies in various parts of the world have shown average annual lead concentrations in most cities with large numbers of cars to range between less than 1 μgPb/m^3 air and 1·5 μgPb/m^3 air; in very few cities have average concentrations exceeded 2 μgPb/m^3 air. Although the results of several large scale epidemiological studies have failed to show a relationship between such low air lead concentrations and blood lead levels, a correlation has been calculated, from the results of some detailed laboratory work involving the exposure of human subjects to known air lead concentrations. These studies show that male adult exposure to a continuous concentration of 1 μgPb/m^3 air can be expected to contribute 1 to 1·5 μgPb/100 ml blood (Chamberlain et al., 1975; Griffin et al., 1975; Rabinowitz et al., 1975).

The average male adult probably inhales 15 m^3 of air in 24 hours and absorbs 20–40 per cent of the lead inhaled (Muir and Davies, 1967; Chamberlain et al., 1975) which, at a concentration of 1 μgPb/m^3 air, would mean a retention of 3–6 μg of lead per day. The blood lead concentration found in most city dwellers is between 18 and 20 μgPb/100 ml blood in male adults and between 14 and 16 μgPb/100ml blood in female adults. The difference between the sexes is probably due in the main to a larger intake by males of food and beverages. The contribution of air lead at low level exposure can be estimated as 10–15 per cent of the total blood lead, equivalent to 2–3 μg per 20 μgPb/100ml blood.

A considerable number of studies have shown that the deposition of lead from automobile exhausts is limited to a relatively narrow band which does not extend beyond about 50 metres from the side of the roadway. Very fine particles are dispersed by airborne spread much further afield, and, by dilution, become indistinguishable from background levels. Air lead concentrations close to busy highways may approximate to 10 μg/m^3, but rapidly decline within a short distance of the highway. A small proportion of the lead in the air derived from motor vehicles may be in the form of organo lead, due to evaporative losses from the carburettor and at petrol filling stations. Estimates of the percentage of organo lead of the total lead in the air have varied between 1 per cent in city streets and 10 per cent in the forecourts of filling stations (Harrison et al., 1974). These low concentrations are not considered to be of significance to health.

Another source of environmental lead exposure of particular concern for children is the presence of lead in paint. In recent years the use of lead in paint for household purposes has been limited to a content of less than 1 per cent, but in earlier times this may have exceeded 20 per cent. Paediatric lead poisoning remains a problem among the less fortunate socio-economic sections of populations in the western world, where poorly maintained old housing can give rise to a greater exposure potential from peeling flecks of old lead-containing paint and plaster. Young children with abnormal appetite for non-food items (a condition known as pica) are at particular risk. The problem is prevalent in the USA, but is not uncommon in parts of Europe.

The lead in the glaze of ceramic tableware and pottery may be released by the action of acidic beverages if the glaze has been improperly fixed by too low a firing temperature. Fruit juices and wines stored in such vessels have caused excessive lead absorption and clinical poisoning in both children and adults.

The use of solder for sealing metal food containers has been a cause of excess lead intake in the past. This practice is less prevalent at the present time so that canned foods contain less lead than before. Also lead arsenate is much less used as an insecticide than hitherto and contamination of fruit has reduced in consequence.

Emissions from lead factories, smelters in particular, have caused contamination of surrounding areas sufficient to result in increased absorption of lead by the local population. Several studies have shown elevated blood lead levels in children living adjacent to such factories (Lansdown et al., 1974; McNiel and Ptasnik, 1974; Fugas et al., 1975; Landrigan et al., 1975; Yankel et al., 1977), but none confirmed that the exposure was sufficient to cause lead poisoning. A further source of contamination of the home may be from the clothing and shoes of lead workers. The exposure potential from many lead factories has been reduced in recent years by the successful application of emission reduction measures and hygiene control procedures.

Controversial implications of low level exposure to lead

Since the publication by Patterson (1965), in which it was claimed that modern man's exposure to lead was 100 times that of his prehistoric forebears, largely because of the increased utilization of lead, there has been much speculation on unrecognized adverse effects at low levels of exposure, referred to as subclinical.

Bryce-Smith (1972) drew attention to the cerebral effects of lead and, on the basis of a publication by Lob and Desbaumes (1971) in which it was alleged that a group of criminals in a Swiss gaol had a higher concentration of lead in their blood than a control group of non-criminals, suggested that the root cause of criminal behaviour might be due to lead. A subsequent report by Lob and Desbaumes (1976), in which their earlier findings were negated by reasons of analytical error, failed to confirm the view that criminality might be associated with elevated blood lead levels.

Children are regarded as the population group most at risk, largely because of a supposed greater sensitivity to lead due to their rapid metabolic rates and to their accelerated growth, relative to adults. There is no evidence that children are more sensitive to lead than adults, but in the age range 1–6 years they may be regarded as more susceptible by virtue of greater opportunity for ingestion of lead contained in non-food items. Paint has been shown to be a cardinal source of excess lead intake in children of the 1–6 year age group (Chisolm, 1971; Barltrop, 1972; Guinee, 1972; Sachs, 1974). Dietary imbalance may also contribute to increased lead absorption; iron and calcium deficiency and excess fat in the diet have been shown to cause increased absorption of lead from the gastrointestinal tract (Barltrop and Khoo, 1975).

Subclinical effects in children have been ascribed primarily to the central nervous system. Some investigators have reported hyperactivity (David et al., 1972) and reduction of learning ability and cognitive response (Landrigan et al., 1975) at blood lead concentrations of about 25 μg/100 ml, but others (Lansdown et al., 1974; McNiel and Ptasnik, 1974) have not noted any adverse change at blood lead concentrations considerably in excess of this figure. The reduction of peripheral nerve conduction velocity has been reported in adults (Catton et al., 1970; Seppalainen and Hernberg, 1972) but only at blood lead concentrations in excess of 50 μg/100 ml, an unacceptably high figure if derived solely from environmental sources. Milburn et al. (1976), on the other hand, failed to find any alteration in nerve conduction velocity at similar blood lead concentrations.

In a soft water area, where the W.H.O. recommended standard of 0·1 ppm was greatly exceeded, Beattie et al. (1975) found mentally retarded children aged 2–6 years had been exposed to a higher water lead concentration than a group of non-retarded matched controls. The blood lead was also higher in the retarded group. There was a significant excess of retarded children coming from homes with water lead in excess of 0·8 ppm; none of the control group were exposed to water lead in excess of 0·8 ppm, whereas 17 per cent of the retarded group were exposed to lead in water concentrations ranging between 0·8 and 2·0 ppm. However, since 83 per cent of the retarded children were exposed to similar water lead concentrations as the controls, i.e. less than 0·8 ppm, and 56 per cent to water lead of less than 0·2 ppm, compared with 61 per cent of the controls, there is strong probability that some cause other than lead may have been responsible for the mental retardation, at least for water lead concentration of less than 0·8 ppm.

The activity in blood of alpha laevulinic acid dehydratase (ALAD) (an enzyme which takes part in the conversion of alpha laevulinic acid (ALA) to porphobilinogen and a step in the haem synthesis pathway) is reduced by low level concentration of lead in blood, that is, 15–20 μgPb/100 ml. ALAD appears particularly sensitive to lead, but is also sensitive to alcohol. In whole blood, where no haem synthesis takes place, it has no function to perform, but it is present in considerable excess. As there is no increase of ALA at blood lead concentrations below 40 μg/100 ml, it is highly improbable that reduced activity of ALAD at ambient blood lead levels is of any health consequence.

It has been shown that protoporphyrin, formed in the course of haem synthesis, increases with increasing blood lead concentration (Piomelli et al., 1973; Chisolm et al., 1975; Alessio et al., 1976; Roels et al., 1976; Joselow and Flores, 1977). Increase in protoporphyrin beyond a normal background in children of 60–80 μg/100 ml erythrocytes is considered by some to be evidence of a subclinical effect. The relationship of protoporphyrin to blood lead, however, is not precise. It has been suggested that protoporphyrin may begin to increase at blood lead concentrations as low as 15 μg/100 ml (Piomelli et al., 1977), but others have indicated no change up to 20–25 μgPb/100 ml blood (Roels et al., 1976) or up to 40 μgPb/100 ml blood (Piomelli et al., 1973; Chisolm et al., 1975). It is improbable that accumulation of protoporphyrin in blood is of any significance at blood lead concentrations of less than 40 μg/100 ml, but it has been shown that it may represent an earlier exposure to lead, as the protoporphyrin remains elevated after blood lead levels have reduced (Alessio et al., 1976). In addition to effect from lead, protoporphyrin is influenced by iron and shows an increase in the blood in cases of iron deficiency. It has also been shown that children and women have higher concentrations of protoporphyrin in their blood than do male adults (Roels et al., 1976). This suggests a difference in iron metabolism rather than a lead effect, particularly since male adults have higher concentrations of lead in their tissues than do female adults and children (Horiuchi et al., 1959; Barry, 1975).

In the past 13 years much attention has been paid to the emission of lead from motor vehicles and fears have been expressed that this source may be of great significance for health. Many of the arguments put forward have been emotive in content and lacking in objectivity. Most of the concern has been related to children, although the evidence has not shown that lead from motor vehicles has caused ill health among any section of the population. There is no question that the lead in motor vehicle exhausts has contributed to the body burden, but the level of contribution has often been grossly exaggerated.

Apart from lead in the air, lead in dust derived from motor vehicles has been indicted as a particular cause for concern for children in the 1–6 year age group. This may be so in children with pica, but it is doubtful that even in these, whose major risk would be from leaded paint, the lead absorbed from ingested dust would be substantial. Barltrop et al. (1975) showed that 1000 ppm lead in soil might be expected to contribute about 0·6 μgPb/100 ml blood and observed no difference in the blood lead of children with and without pica living in areas of high soil lead. The content of lead in busy city streets immediately adjacent to heavy traffic may range between 1000 and 2000 ppm, but it is doubtful that this would be available to very young children as it is inconceivable that they would be permitted to play in such close proximity to unrestricted heavy traffic.

Governments in various parts of the world have introduced measures to reduce the content of lead in petrol as a means towards the reduction of lead in exhaust emissions and so in air and dust. The European Economic Commission (EEC) has proposed an ambient air quality for lead of 2 $\mu g/m^3$, which has yet to be agreed by the nine member countries, and the

Environmental Protection Agency (EPA) of the USA has proposed an even lower standard of 1·5 μg/m^3. Close examination of the EPA data suggests that this is an unnecessarily cautious figure; a standard of around 5 μgPb/m^3 air would have been more logical, and in my view would have given a more than adequate safety margin.

The reduction or elimination of lead in petrol will result inevitably in increased costs of production, by reason of an additional crude oil requirement, and also of refinery equipment that would be necessary if the efficiency of modern fuels is to be maintained. If, for whatever reason, it is considered desirable to reduce the lead in exhaust emissions, an alternative to the reduction of lead in petrol would be its reduction at the point of emission.

An inexpensive filter device has been developed which has been shown to be effective in reducing lead emissions and other particulates by 50–90 per cent, depending on the mode of operation of the vehicle. As it is also an effective silencer the device has been designed to replace the conventional silencer at the same position on existing exhaust systems. The effective operational life of the filter is about 50 000 miles. Since most exhaust systems fail and require replacement before the completion of such mileage, this would offer no problem. The arrangements for disposal of old filters could be the same as apply for worn-out silencers.

Exhaust filter devices are at present under trial in a number of countries. As an alternative to the reduction of lead in petrol they could provide an effective and practical solution for the control of lead emissions from motor vehicles. Their application should receive serious consideration for reasons of economy and the conservation of existing oil supplies, although the evidence does not suggest that present ambient air lead concentrations derived from motor vehicle exhausts require further control or are a cause for concern relative to the health of any section of the population in any part of the world. A possible exception could be Los Angeles in the USA where the number of cars far exceeds that of any other city in the world and where atmospheric inversion problems are particularly severe.

Summary

Lead in Man's environment has been studied extensively. Because of its ubiquitous presence on the surface of the earth, lead has always been present in body tissues where it is in equilibrium, input being very largely balanced by output. Lead accumulates in bones with age, but not in the soft tissues.

A W.H.O. criteria document on lead reviews the subject at length (*Environmental Health Criteria 3 – Lead*). It confirms that the principal source of lead absorption is from food and beverages with a lesser contribution from air and water.

Children in the age range 1–6 years are considered to be at greater risk than other sections of the population because of greater potential for exposure to non-food items, in particular leaded-paint in old dilapidated housing.

It has been suggested that undetected subclinical effects may arise from low level exposure to lead. The evidence for this is tenuous at best and of very doubtful health significance.

Urban air lead emanates largely from motor vehicle exhausts. Its contribution to the total body burden is considered to be small. Practical measures are described for the reduction of lead in the air, without the necessity to reduce lead in petrol.

Emission control and other measures taken in recent years for the reduction of man-made sources of environmental exposure have ensured no increase in lead absorption and a probable reduction. Although localized foci of excess exposure still exist, the general levels of lead in the environment are not considered to be a cause for concern in relation to the public health.

REFERENCES

Alessio L., Bertazzi P. A., Monelli O. et al. (1976) Free erythrocyte protoporphyrin as an indicator of the biological effect of lead in adult males. *Int. Arch. Occup. Environ. Health* **38**, 77–86.

Baker G. (1767) *An Essay Concerning the Cause of the Endemial Colic of Devonshire.* London, Cadell.

Barltrop D. (1972) Children and environmental lead. In: *Conference on Lead in the Environment.* London, The Zoological Society.

Barltrop D. and Khoo H. E. (1975) The influence of nutritional factors on lead absorption. *Postgrad. Med. J.* **51**, 795.

Barltrop D., Strehlow C. D., Thornton I. et al. (1975) Absorption of lead from dust and soil. *Postgrad. Med. J.* **51**, 801–804.

Barry P. S. I. and Mossman D. B. (1970) Lead concentrations in human tissues. *Br. J. Ind. Med.* **27**, 339–351.

Barry P. S. I. (1975) A comparison of concentrations of lead in human tissues. *Br. J. Ind. Med.* **32**, 119–139.

Beattie A. D., Moore M. R., Goldberg A. et al. (1975) Role of chronic low-level lead exposure in the aetiology of mental retardation. *Lancet* **1**, 589–592.

Boyd P. R., Walker G. and Henderson I. M. (1957) The treatment of tetraethyl lead poisoning. *Lancet* **1**, 181–185.

Bryce-Smith D. (1972) Behavioural effects of lead and other heavy metal pollutants. *Chem. Br.* **8**, 240–243.

Cassels D. A. K. and Dodds E. C. (1946) Tetraethyl lead poisoning. *Br. Med. J.* **2**, 681.

Catton M. J., Harrison M. J. G., Fullerton P. M. et al. (1970) Subclinical neuropathy in lead workers. *Br. Med. J.* **2**, 80–82.

Chamberlain A. C. (1977) Personal communication.

Chamberlain A. C., Clough W. S., Heard M. J. et al. (1975) Uptake of lead by inhalation of motor exhaust. *Proc. R. Soc. Lond. (Biol.)* **192**, 77–110.

Chisolm J. J. (1971) Lead poisoning. *Sci. Am.* **2**, 15–23.

Chisolm J. J., Barrett M. B. and Mellits E. D. (1975) Dose-effect and dose-response relationships for lead in children. *J. Pediatr.* **87**, No. 6, Part 2, 1152–1160.

Cremer J. E. and Callaway S. (1961) Further studies on the toxicity of some tetra and trialkyl lead compounds. *Br. J. Ind. Med.* **18**, 277.

David O., Clark J. and Voeller K. (1972) Lead and hyperactivity. *Lancet* **2**, 900–903.

Fugas M., Markicevic A., Prpic-Majic D. et al. (1975) Health study of a lead exposed population. *Arh. Hig. Rada. Toksikol.* **26**, Supplement 119–137.

Gething J. (1975) Tetramethyl lead absorption: A report of human exposure to a high level of tetramethyl lead. *Br. J. Ind. Med.* **32,** 329–333.

Gilfillan S. C. (1965) Lead poisoning and the fall of Rome. *J. Occup. Med.* **7,** 53–60.

Griffin T. B., Coulston F., Goldberg L. et al. (1975) Clinical studies on men continuously exposed to airborne particulate lead. In: Griffin T. B. and Knelson J. H. (ed.), *Lead.* Stuttgart, Thieme, pp. 221–240.

Guinee V. F. (1972) Epidemiologic studies of lead exposure in New York City. *International Symposium on Environmental Health Aspects of Lead,* Amsterdam.

Harrison R. M., Perry R. and Slater D. H. (1974) An adsorption technique for the determination of organic lead in street air. *Atmos. Environ.* **8,** 1187–1194.

Horiuchi K., Horiguchi S. and Suekane M. (1959) Studies on the industrial lead poisoning. *Osaka City Med. J.* **5,** 41–70.

Hunter D. (1975) *The Diseases of Occupations,* 5th ed. London, English Universities Press, p. 240.

Joselow M. M. and Flores J. (1977) Application of the zinc protoporphyrin (ZP) test as a monitor of occupational exposure to lead. *Am. Ind. Hyg. Assoc. J.* **38,** 63–66.

Kehoe R. A., Thamann F. and Cholak J. (1933) On the normal absorption and excretion of lead. *J. Ind. Hyg.* **15,** 257–272.

Kehoe R. A. (1961) The Harben lectures, 1960. The metabolism of lead in man in health and disease. *J. R. Inst. Publ. Health* **24,** 81–95, 101–120, 129–143, 177–203.

Kitzmiller K. V. and Kehoe R. A. (1953) *Tetraethyl Lead Poisoning – A Recent Occurrence in Panama.* Kettering Laboratory, College of Medicine, University of Cincinnati.

Landrigan P. J., Whitworth R. H., Baloh R. W. et al. (1975) Neuropsychological dysfunction in children with chronic low-level lead absorption. *Lancet* **1,** 708–712.

Lane R. E. et al. (1968) Diagnosis of inorganic lead poisoning: a statement. *Br. Med. J.* **4,** 501.

Lansdown R. G., Shepherd J., Clayton B. E. et al. (1974) Blood lead levels, behaviour and intelligence – a population study. *Lancet* **1,** 538–541.

Lob M. and Desbaumes P. (1971) Étude de la plombémie et de la plomburie chez deux groupes de détenus, les uns internés à la campagne, les autres à proximité immediate d'une autoroute. *Schweiz. Med. Wochenschr.* **101,** 357–361.

Lob M. and Desbaumes P. (1976) Lead and criminality. *Br. J. Ind. Med.* **33,** No. 2, 125–127.

McNeil J. L. and Ptasnik J. A. (1974) Evaluation of long-term effects of elevated blood lead concentrations in asymptomatic children. In: *Proceedings of International Symposium on Recent Advances in the Assessment of the Health Effects of Environmental Pollution,* Paris.

Milburn H., Mitran E. and Crockford G. W. (1976) An investigation of lead workers for subclinical effects of lead using three performance tests. *Ann. Occup. Hyg.* **19,** 239–249.

Muir D. C. F. and Davies C. N. (1967) The deposition of 0·5 μ diameter aerosols in the lungs of man. *Ann. Occup. Hyg.* **10,** 161–174.

Patterson C. C. (1965) Contaminated and natural lead environments of man. *Arch. Environ. Hlth.* **11,** 344–360.

Percival T. (1774) *Observations and Experiments on the Poison of Lead.* London, Johnson.

Piomelli S., Davidow B., Guinee V. F. et al. (1973) The FEP (free erythrocyte porphyrins) Test: a screening micromethod for lead poisoning. *Pediatrics* **51,** 254–259.

Piomelli S., Seaman C., Zullow D. et al. (1977) Metabolic evidence of lead toxicity in 'normal' urban children. *Clin. Chem.* **25,** 459A.

Rabinowitz M., Wetherill G. and Kopple J. (1975) Absorption, storage and excretion of lead by normal humans. Presented at *The 9th Annual Conference on Trace Substances in Environmental Health,* University of Missouri, Columbia.

Ramazzini B. (1713) *De Morbis Artificum Bernardini Ramazzini, Diatriba (Diseases of Workers).* The Latin text of 1713. Revised (1940) with translation and notes by Wright W. C. Chicago, University of Chicago Press.

Roels H., Buchet J. P., Lauwerys R. et al. (1976) Impact of air pollution by lead on the heme biosynthetic pathway in school-age children. *Arch. Environ. Health* **31,** 6, 310–315.

Sachs H. K. (1974) Effect of a screening program on changing patterns of lead poisoning. *Environ. Health Perspect.,* Exp. Issue No. 7, 41–47.

Seppalainen A. M. and Hernberg S. (1972) Sensitive technique for detecting subclinical lead neuropathy. *Br. J. Ind. Med.* **29,** 443–449.

Springman F., Bingham E. and Stemmer K. L. (1963) The acute effects of lead alkyls. *Arch. Environ. Health* **6,** 469–472.

Tanquerel des Planches (1848) *Lead Diseases – A Treatise.* Translated by Dana S. L. Massachusetts, Daniel Bixby Lowell, pp. 31–36, 43–45.

Thompson J. A. (1971) Balance between intake and output of lead in normal individuals. *Br. J. Ind. Med.* **28,** 189–194.

Walker G. and Boyd P. R. (1952) Tetraethyl lead poisoning – report of a non-fatal case. *Lancet* **2,** 467.

World Health Organisation (1977) *Environmental Health Criteria 3 – Lead.* Geneva, W.H.O.

Yankel A. J., von Lindern I. H. and Walter S. D. (1977) The silver valley lead study: the relationship between childhood blood lead levels and environmental exposure. *J. Air Pollut. Control Assoc.* **27,** No. 8, 764–767.

2. TOXICOLOGY OF METALS OTHER THAN LEAD

D. Malcolm

INTRODUCTION

It is not appropriate in a book of this size to try to deal with the toxicology of all metals, so the subject will be covered by dealing with those which are significantly toxic and most likely to be encountered in industrial use. Whether a metal is likely to be toxic in industrial use depends on the form in which it is used as well as the conditions under which it is used. A large number of metals are present as trace elements in food and drink. Some of these are essential elements but may also be toxic in excessive dose or in certain chemical forms, for instance cobalt or chromium. Thus traces of many metals will be a normal constituent of body tissues whether there is industrial exposure or not.

Industrial absorption is primarily via the respiratory tract. Particles below a mean diameter of about 7 μm are capable of penetrating the alveolae where they diffuse onto the alveolae walls and if soluble in body fluids will be absorbed into the bloodstream. Particles larger than 7 μm are selectively deposited in the upper respiratory tract and down as far as the terminal bronchioles. While some compounds may be absorbed via the bronchiole walls our knowledge of this route of absorption is very inadequate. It has however been calculated that particles deposited in the bronchial tree are cleared by the muco-ciliary mechanism from the lung and may be swallowed with the possibility of intestinal absorption, or expectorated. The danger to health depends on whether or not the substance in use is likely to be absorbed via the lungs or intestinal tract, unless like beryllium it has a local toxic action.

Ingestion is not a normal method of absorption in industry but can occur either accidentally or because of bad hygienic habits such as eating in workshops, eating with unwashed hands or from smoking with contaminated hands, as well as from swallowing sputum as indicated above. Certain metals such as mercury and some of the alkyl and other organic or solvent compounds may be absorbed through the skin.

Our aim should be to prevent absorption by controlling working methods so that the dose is less than that which would adversely affect the health and well-being of the whole organism. There is a view today that any measurable biological change is not acceptable. Such views are largely expressed by academic researchers who have no clinical responsibility for the care of workers exposed to the toxic substances concerned. In *Effects and Dose Response Relationships of Toxic Metals* (Nordberg, 1976) the following concepts are described:

Critical concentration for a cell is that concentration at which adverse functional changes, reversible or irreversible, occur in the cell. *Critical organ concentration* is defined as the mean concentration in the organ at the time any of the cells reaches critical concentration. *Critical organ* is defined as that particular organ which attains the critical concentration. We can in most cases recognize the critical organ or organs, and these may vary according to routes of absorption, type of compound and whether effects are related to acute or chronic absorption. In most cases we have little or no knowledge of organ or cell concentrations, and normally only blood and urine are easily available for analysis. The electron microscope microanalyser (EMMA) is capable of analysing many metals even in cellular organelles, but biopsy specimens or post-mortem material are necessary.

These concepts can to some extent be applied to lead and cadmium, but with many metals little is known about changes at cellular level. For instance, do either arsenic or mercury cause slowing of nerve conduction velocity at levels at present regarded as acceptable for the health control of workers exposed to these metals?

The decision to regard a decrease in δ-aminoleavulinic acid dehydrase activity as a subcritical effect (acceptable), but an increase in erythrocyte protoporphyrin as a critical effect where there is no measurable reduction in haemoglobin formation seems to me to be arbitrary as neither has any effect on the health and well-being of the individual. I do not believe we know enough about the implications of such effects and in the case of most metals we do not even know if similar effects occur. Setting standards on this basis and not on measurable clinical effects on health may be very safe but we have not proved that it is necessary.

We still know far too little about the dose response curves in human beings of most metals in spite of the fact that some of them have been used since early historic times. This results in standards for those metals which have been most extensively researched being much stricter than those about which we know comparatively little. Our aim should be to have good dose response curves for all potentially toxic metals. Too often dose response curves are based on academic models and not on measurements of what happens to people in the factory. Too many of us in industry have failed to use the data we have collected in practice for drawing up soundly based dose response curves. For the future we also need to know more precisely whether dose response relationships are linear or logarithmic in form.

Although individual response to a given dose level varies considerably, levels of metal in the blood should usually give the best available indication of total body burden. The possibility of using such methods however depends on how the metal is distributed in body tissues. If measurement of blood levels is not practicable, urinary output can be a useful indicator of intake but it suffers from a number of problems. *First,* great care needs to be taken to avoid contamination of specimens, and *second,* since urinary output may depend on variable intake and on variable loss of fluid via routes other than the kidney, the actual concentration of metals in the urine will vary even if intake could be kept constant. In other cases excretion may be independent of urinary volume. In practice 24-hour samples are very difficult to collect outside a hospital so it is usual to relate concentrations to specific gravity or to creatinine levels. In many cases, such as cadmium, results are so variable that only the mean level in working groups is useful as a guide to the range of absorption.

Dust in air concentrations

Our knowledge in this field is not good. Threshold Limit Values, TLVs, can be very useful as guidelines to the adequacy of control of working conditions. They are, however, nothing like as precise as many people believe. Too many are based on inadequate data and here again this is partly the fault of doctors and hygienists in industry who have not collected and analysed their data in order to add to our knowledge of the control of potentially harmful substances. TLVs would be more useful if methods of measurement were standardized. Assumptions have been made about the amount of air breathed in a normal working day and at one time this was assumed to be approximately 10 m^3. Today, models are being based on ranges from about 10–20 m^3 and it can be seen that what we really need is a more accurate knowledge of the total ranges of air breathed by any group of workers exposed to toxic metals.

Table 2.1 shows the principal target organs of the metals discussed.

ANTIMONY

Uses

The principal use is in alloys with lead, tin and copper. The trisulphide and pentasulphide are used as rubber additives. In the textile industry antimony trioxide is used for flameproofing fabrics. The trichloride is used as a dye. Antimony oxides are used in glass and enamels as opacifiers and may also be used as a decolourizing agent in glass. The trioxide is used as a fire retardant paint additive. 'Naples yellow' pigment contains lead antimonate.

Industrial poisoning

There is little evidence of health effects in the normal industrial use of antimony. The fact that it is commonly associated with arsenic may be the reason for a suspicion of a link with lung cancer, but the evidence is doubtful. Skin irritation is generally mentioned but in my experience is rare.

Table 2.1 Metals liable to cause health hazards in industry.

Metal	Biologically essential	Target Organs									TLV
		Gastro-intestinal tract	Respiratory	CNS	Heart and vessels	Liver	Kidney	Blood	Skin	Other	mg/M³
Antimony	–	+	+		+	+		SbH	+		0·50
Arsenic	–	+	+	+		+	+	+		Endocrine	0·5
Beryllium	–		+						+	Bone	0·002
Boron	–	+		+							10·0
Boranes			+			+	+		+		1·0
Cadmium	–	+	+				+			Bone	0·2
Chrome	Trivalent										0·05 as fume
											0·5
Manganese	+		+	+							5·0
Mercury	–		+	+			+				0·05 Alkyl 10·01
Nickel	–		+	Ni carbonyl					+		0·01
Platinum	–		+						+		0·002 sol.
Selenium	+	+		+		+			+		0·02
Thallium	–	+	+	+		+	+			Endocrine	0·1
Tin (Organic)	–	+		+							0·1
Vanadium	–		+	+			+		+		0·5
Zirconium	–		+						+		5
Uranium	–		+				+				0·2

The chief danger is from stibine (SbH_3), a gas with haemolytic properties and an unpleasant smell, which may be formed by the action of water on stibides which antimony forms with calcium and aluminium or by the action of acids on other antimony compounds. The effects, which are identical, are described under arsine.

The TLV is 0·5 mg/m^3 Stibine 0·1 ppm or 0·5 mg/m^3

There is some interesting detective work described in one of James Herriot's vet books when butter of antimony (anhydrous antimony-chloride) is used to remove the horn buds on calves and produces the classic fatal gastro-intestinal symptoms of antimony ingestion.

Control

There is no real need of medical supervision in the normal use of antimony. When there is any risk of stibine, clear guidelines for safe working practices should be laid down and understood by all persons likely to be involved. Where regular exposure to low concentrations is likely, for instance in some type of rapid charging of lead-acid batteries, tests for anaemia should be considered if the TLV is regularly exceeded. In acute cases, onset of symptoms is normally delayed for several hours so that first aid treatment is not required. Since exposure is usually accidental it is useful for persons who may be accidentally exposed to be provided with a card to alert any doctor to the possibility of stibine or arsine poisoning, should symptoms occur. Where the possibility of stibine evolution in toxic amounts exists, suitable breathing equipment should be readily available at the site.

ARSENIC

Occurrence and production

Arsenic exists in several allotropic forms, in a semi-metallic form which is grey and crystalline and also commonly as yellow crystalline or black amorphous arsenic. The most common source of arsenic is from arsenical pyrites FeAsS. Arsenic is also found in many other ores such as gold, copper, tin, lead, tungsten and zinc. Because it sublimes at 218 °C at normal atmospheric pressure it is normally found in the flue dust filters chiefly as the trioxide.

Uses

It is used in alloys, particularly lead and copper, to increase hardness. In glass manufacture it is used to decolourize, or in larger amounts to produce a bronze colouration and also to make opaque glass and enamels. It has been used in the manufacture of insecticides, weed killers and as a wood preservative, but is now largely replaced by more modern preparations. Its use for medical and veterinary therapeutic purposes is also being replaced, except for cattle and sheep dips. A variety of organic arsenical compounds were developed as war gases. The aromatic arsines being more poisonous than the aliphatic compounds. One of these, chlorovinyl dichlorarsine, was also known as Lewisite and the search for an antidote resulted in the discovery of British Anti-Lewisite (BAL).

Metabolism and toxicity

Being commonly distributed in the earth's surface, small quantities are continuously absorbed. It is distributed throughout the body with a tendency to concentrate in the liver, abdominal viscera, bone and skin. Its concentration in the hair and nails has been used to detect arsenical poisoning in forensic cases.

Industrial absorption is principally by inhalation, with the possibility of ingestion where hygienic practices are unsatisfactory. In the case of organic arsenicals skin absorption is also a serious risk.

Industrial poisoning is usually of a chronic nature. Acute symptoms were described by Genkin (1932). Onset consisted of respiratory irritation with cough, chest pain and dyspnoea. This was followed by giddiness, headache, general weakness and later by nausea, vomiting, colic and diarrhoea and limb pains. Chronic poisoning is chiefly related both to skin irritation, particularly in areas of skin folds and moisture, and to hyperkeratosis, sometimes with pigmentation. Skin cancer has been rare in industry. Such changes may also be accompanied by a polyneuritis which, unlike lead, primarily affects the sensory nerves. There are also numerous reports of an excess of bronchial carcinomas; for instance, cases cited by Braun (1958) among workers who sprayed vines with arsenical insecticides in the Moselle wine growing area.

Arsine

When arsenic combines with calcium, magnesium or aluminium it forms arsenides. The action of water on an arsenide liberates arsine, AsH_3, a colourless gas with a slight odour of garlic. Acids which react with arsenic-containing compounds and liberate hydrogen will also form arsine.

Arsine absorbed by inhalation causes haemolysis which may be rapidly fatal. Industrial cases usually occur due to the accidental formation of arsine. Haemolysis usually occurs after about 6 hours, and is accompanied by the symptoms of shock, together with haemoglobinuria and albuminuria, with haemolytic jaundice developing later. The antimony compound stibine SbH_3 has virtually identical properties to arsine, causing haemolysis.

Organic arsenicals

The organic arsenical compounds are primarily skin and mucous membrane irritants. A small amount on the skin or contact with vapour can result in the rapid development of erythema and later vesical formation which may spread to other areas of the body. Inhalation of arsenical gases, smokes or vapours will produce pulmonary oedema rapidly.

Prevention and treatment of toxic effects

When contact with inorganic arsenic compounds is likely, careful control of dust and fume is essential, particularly for people handling flue dusts which may contain arsenic.

Where there is any risk of arsine formation, written guidelines for safe working practices are essential.

Manufacture or handling of organic arsenicals also require very strict hygiene precautions and suitable protective clothing.

Early work on the toxic effects of arsenic show that it has an affinity for sulphydryl group. BAL was developed on the basis of simple dithiol compounds forming relatively stable compounds with Lewisite. BAL is very effective in ointment form against organic arsenical skin lesions. The preferred method of treatment of all types of arsenic poisoning is now by early intramuscular injection of adequate doses of BAL to ensure an adequate reserve of dithiol groups to take up any arsenic.

In the case of arsine or stibine poisoning massive blood transfusions may also be necessary to replace any blood lost by haemolysis. In some cases where haemolysis is severe, renal dialysis may be required to avoid overloading the kidneys.

BERYLLIUM

Sources and extraction

Beryllium is found in the form of beryl ($3BeO,Al_2O_3,6SiO_2$). Emeralds are a form of beryl, owing their green colour to traces of chromium oxide. Aquamarines, which are greenish blue, and yellow chrysoberyl are also varieties of beryl. Beryl-containing ores are usually found in feldspar.

Exposure to beryllium-containing dusts may occur during the extraction of the metal. The ore is first powdered in a dry crusher and is then treated by wet milling. Briquettes are made when the wet powder is mixed with both soda ash and sodium fluorosilicate. Sodium beryllium fluoride is formed in a high-temperature furnace. The sodium beryllium fluoride is dissolved in water and then precipitated with caustic soda. Further heating in a furnace converts the hydroxide to beryllium oxide.

Uses

The principal use today is to make hard alloys with high tensile strength. Most of these are based on copper and can be used where the good electrical and heat transfer properties of copper are needed and pure copper is too soft. Non-sparking tools are made for use in areas where there are explosion risks. Alloys are also made with aluminium, nickel, magnesium and iron.

Formerly beryllium was used extensively as a fluorescent coating on the inside of lighting tubes. This use gave rise to health problems and considerable difficulty in disposing of old tubes. Since suitable safe alternatives are available this use of beryllium has been abandoned.

Because of beryllium's low neutron capture properties it was being used to make cans for uranium fuels as well as other accessories for atomic reactors. Because of the difficulty of safe manufacture there has been a tendency to change to magnesium alloys.

Toxicity

Beryllium is not normally well absorbed by any route, and when inhaled it tends to accumulate in the lungs.

Three principal effects have been described in industrial use. *First*, an acute chemical pneumonitis develops, with continued low level inhalation. *Second*, a chronic granulomatous lesion of the lung occurs. *Third*, skin effects include both dermatitis, which may be severe, and sensitization which once it occurs is permanent. Beryllium compounds entering cuts give rise to chronic granulomatous lesions which heal only when all the beryllium has been removed.

Symptoms of acute pneumonitis are severe cough, often with blood stained sputum, retro-sternal pain, dyspnoea, cyanosis and loss of weight. van Ordstraand et al. (1943) reported 5 deaths in 38 cases.

The chronic chest disease may not be seen for some years after first exposure and has occurred up to 6 years after leaving the industry. Most cases have been reported from the fluorescent lamp industry. Symptoms start with anorexia and weakness and progressive weight loss. A cough with little sputum is usual. Severe dyspnoea is present and is sometimes the presenting symptom. *Cor pulmonale* may develop and about one-third of the patients die. Another third remain permanently disabled and the rest become free from symptoms although the lung changes do not completely resolve.

The clinical signs and X-ray changes are indistinguishable from sarcoidosis. A toolmaker who had occasionally carried out dry grinding of a 2 per cent beryllium alloy was seen at an industrial diseases clinic with symptoms and signs of sarcoidosis. This man also had Marfan's syndrome, so it was not clear whether his exposure to beryllium was the cause of his illness.

Animal experiments with beryllium have shown varying results. Kay and Skill (1934) reported the development of rickets, Upsets in calcium-phosphorous metabolism have been described. Schepers et al. (1957) reported some lung neoplasms in animals inhaling beryllium sulphate aerosol. Osteosarcomas have also been reported in animals following intravenous injections of various beryllium compounds.

Neither osteomalacia nor neoplasms have been described in human cases. This may be due to the very low levels of systemic absorption which occurs in industrial exposure.

Treatment of toxic effects

Chronic granulomas of the skin should be treated by excision of the beryllium. Acute respiratory effects should not now occur, but cases of accidental inhalation of high concentrations of dust or fume should be sent to hospital and retained for observation and symptomatic treatment. Chronic chest cases have been treated with BAL without much success. Kennedy et al. (1950) reported considerable relief of symptoms with cortisone.

BORON

Boron is not really a metal but belongs to group III A metals in the periodic table. Boron seems to be an essential element concerned with carbohydrate metabolism in plants, but there is no evidence that it is essential to animal life. In spite of its widespread industrial use poisoning has not been reported except from boranes.

Uses

Boron has been used for many years as boracic acid as a mild antiseptic particularly for treating eye conditions. It may however result in allergic reactions. Its uses include neutron absorption and shielding in atomic energy power plants, deoxidation of copper and brass, hardening steel and as a constituent of glass and enamels. It is used as a mordant for dyeing in the textile industry and also for fireproofing. Boron carbide is used as an abrasive. A relatively recent use is in the form of hydrides, diborane (B_2H_6), decaborane ($B_{10}H_{14}$) and pentaborane (B_5H_9). Their principal uses are as high energy fuels in rockets, although decaborane is also used in vulcanizing rubber in place of sulphur.

Toxicology

All of these boranes are highly toxic, particularly pentaborane. Diborane is a gas and is highly irritant to the lungs and kidneys, while decaborane and pentaborane are central nervous system poisons in the same way as boric acid but probably about 250 times as toxic. Cases of acute poisoning were reported by Rozendaal (1951) suffering from muscular cramps, convulsive attacks, disorientation and memory loss. In another case exposed first to diborane, the symptoms were dyspnoea, rigors, exhaustion and later, after exposure to pentaborane and solid boron compounds, the symptoms were spasmodic seizures and mental confusion. In more prolonged exposure diborane caused primarily severe pulmonary irritation, which was followed by symptoms of central nervous system effects, including headache, dizziness, fatigue and muscular weakness accompanied by feeling cold. Severe prolonged poisoning is also likely to affect the liver and kidneys. According to Browning (1961) the mechanism of borane toxicology is not yet understood. The routes of absorption are primarily inhalation, but it is probable that pentaborane is absorbed through the skin.

Protection

Suitable protective clothing and respirators with a silica gel type of cartridge where vapours or fumes may exceed threshold limit values. The TLVs of boranes are:

diborane (a gas)	0·1 mg/m^3
decaborane (a crystalline solid)	0·5 mg/m^3
pentaborane (a volatile liquid)	0·1 mg/m^3

Medical supervision

This should include lung function tests and tests for renal damage. It would probably be wise to assess whether any long-term central nervous system damage occurs. Anyone having responsibility for the safe use of boranes would be well advised to consult colleagues with practical experience of their use. Treatment would most likely be of emergencies. Hospitalization with suitable symptomatic treatment for respiratory distress would be necessary.

CADMIUM

Source and recovery

Cadmium is found in lead zinc ores. It is a by-product of recovery of these metals and is reclaimed from the flue dust in zinc smelters by leaching or by precipitation and distillation.

Acute cadmium poisoning

There does not appear to be any record of acute industrial poisoning due to the ingestion of cadmium compounds. Acid-containing drinks which have been stored in cadmium plated containers or enamel containers with leachable cadmium in the enamel have caused acute gastro-intestinal irritation in those drinking such preparations. High concentrations of cadmium fume which may occur due to the heating of cadmium plated metal, or the smelting of cadmium, or the reclaiming of scrap by distillation process have caused acute pulmonary oedema leading to marked dyspnoea in 12–48 hours after exposure. Such cases have had about a 30 per cent fatality rate. If the patient does not die from pulmonary oedema then chemical pneumonitis may lead to peribronchial and perivascular fibrosis. Some cases are reported to have made a good recovery while others have suffered permanent lung damage. I would only be convinced that recovery was satisfactory if lung function was within normal limits 20 or more years after the episode.

Chronic industrial poisoning

This was first clearly described by Friberg in 1948 when he investigated a group of men making nickel-cadmium alkaline batteries. The men had complained of undue fatigue and breathlessness. Friberg (1948) found emphysema in a number of these men who showed increased residual capacity in relation to their total lung capacity. Cadmium in air levels ranged from 3 to 15 mg/m^3. He also found a low molecular weight proteinuria which did not appear to cause any clinical symptoms. Subsequently Adams and Crabtree (1969) have described soreness of the nose and anosmia in a group of cadmium battery workers. Detailed work on the proteinuria suggests that this is due to the accumulation of cadmium in the proximal renal tubules. Cadmium interferes with the ability of the proximal tubules to reabsorb low molecular weight protein. According to studies by Ahlmark et al. (1961) and Adams et al. (1969), decreased glomerular filtration rates occur, but these are a late finding and possibly secondary to tubular dysfunction. In my experience there have been no long-term effects on the kidney which produce any symptoms directly related to renal disease. However some cases of renal failure were described in a group of cases studied by Bonnell (1955). Additional effects of the tubular damage are loss of calcium, while the blood calcium level remains constant. A probable excess of renal calculi may occur in those with renal tubular damage. Adams et al. (1969) also describe the excretion of lysozyme and ribonuclease in the urine of cadmium workers with proteinuria.

Nicaud et al. in 1942 described the association between exposure to cadmium and possibly low calcium diet leading to osteomalacia. Similar effects amongst a farming community in Japan gave rise to the epidemic of itai-itai disease, which included marked skeletal deformity and bone pain. A possible mechanism for the effect may be the suppression of 25-hydroxy-calciferol which has a potent effect on calcium metabolism, and is manufactured in the kidney tubules.

In 1965 Potts reported deaths among men who had been exposed to cadmium in the manufacture of alkaline batteries. Three had died of carcinoma of the prostate. A further follow up by Kipling and Waterhouse (1967) showed that four men exposed to cadmium and nickel had died from carcinoma of the prostate compared with an expected incidence of 0·4. Animal studies of rats and mice over a two to three year period did not reveal any incidence of prostatic carcinoma although relatively high doses were used. Levy et al. (1973), Pavirek and Zahor (1956) have shown that single large doses of cadmium cause testicular atrophy and later result in Leydig cell tumours of the testes. Recently Chandler (1977) has shown that cadmium replaces zinc in prostatic cells and can interfere with normal cell development in tissue cell cultures. At present the situation remains unresolved and no further cases have occurred in the group studied by Kipling and Waterhouse.

Prevention

The British Occupational Hygiene Society published a British Standard for cadmium in January 1978. This describes the nature of cadmium poisoning and the methods appropriate to its prevention. They recommend that the TLV for cadmium should be 0·2 mg/m^3 of soluble cadmium compounds, and that cadmium fume should be limited to 0·05/m^3. The reason for the lower figure for fume is the much higher rate of emphysema found amongst men making copper cadmium alloys where these men are exposed to newly formed cadmium fume. Whether or not this is more active in causing lung damage or whether the lung damage is due to much higher concentrations of cadmium reaching the alveolae is not clear.

Clinical supervision

Most of the cadmium absorbed is concentrated in the liver and kidneys. Since cadmium, unlike lead, does not have an affinity for the red cells high concentrations do not develop in the blood. It is only recently that analytical methods for cadmium in blood have been developed to a state of accuracy which can distinguish between normal blood cadmium levels, usually below 1 μg/100 ml and that of cadmium workers which is in the range of 1–5 μg/100 ml.

Cadmium in urine

The excretion of cadmium is so variable from one individual to another that spot samples, or even 24-hour samples, have not been a good indication of individual exposure or absorption. However they are at present the best biological test in determining an individual's level of absorption. Every attempt should be made to keep individual cadmium in urine levels below 20 μg/1. The average level of a working group provides additional information on whether exposure of the group is increasing or decreasing or being maintained at a satisfactory level as an additional quality control procedure.

Medical examination

A thorough clinical examination should be carried out at least once per year. This should include estimation of low molecular weight protein in the urine, an examination of the nose for inflammation or atrophy of the mucous membrane, and a simple test of comparative sensitivity of the sense of smell. This can be done with dilutions of phenol in liquid paraffin as described by Adams and Crabtree (1961). Lung function tests should also be included to see whether or not there is any emphysema, although it is recognized that this condition is difficult to diagnose. It is normal to remove men who develop proteinuria from further exposure to cadmium at work. Adams (1972) has shown that heavy smokers tend to have higher cadmium in urine levels than non-smokers. In older workers and retired workers with proteinuria a watch should be kept for bone pain and any signs of developing osteomalacia.

Treatment of cadmium poisoning

Anyone who has been exposed to large or unknown amount of cadmium fumes should be under observation in hospital. Treatment is largely symptomatic and supportive. As the chronic effects on the kidney are normally symptomless the only action required is removal from further exposure of men who develop proteinuria. Treatment with EDTA or penicillinamine is not advised (Lyle, 1972) as it may cause more severe kidney damage.

CHROMIUM

Sources and production

Chromium is produced mostly from the chromite ore ($FeOCr_2O_3$). The metal is prepared by reduction of the sesquioxide with powdered aluminium and magnesium or with carbon in a vacuum electric furnace. The purest form is obtained by electrolysis of chromic acid.

Absorption excretion

Trivalent chromium is an essential element for glucose and lipid metabolism. The main source of chromium is from food, particularly in raw sugar and animal fats. Hexavalent compounds which are the toxic forms of chromium can be converted to trivalent compounds in the body but the converse process does not apply.

Uses

Chrome is frequently used in alloys with nickel molybdenum and vanadium to produce stainless steel, steels of high elasticity and tensile strength, and heat and corrosion resistance. Cobalt-chrome molybdenum alloys are used in jet engines. Chrome salts are also used in plating, tanning leather, lithography, and as heat stable pigments, reds, yellows, blue and greens. It is from its ability to form colours that chromium gets its name. Chromium compounds are also used as catalysts in the manufacture of high octane fuels.

Industrial toxicology

Toxic effects occur from exposure to the hexavalent compounds principally in the chrome plating industry, but may also occur when dusts or mists of these chrome compounds are created in the working atmosphere. Irritation of the skin causes dermatitis but not usually until after six months' or more exposure. In addition if a chrome solution or compound enters a cut in the skin a punched-out type of ulcer known as a chrome hole occurs. These are usually slow to heal especially if contact with chrome is continued. Treatment with an ointment containing 10 per cent calcium EDTA is very effective. The same chrome compounds may also attack the mucous membrane of the nasal septum. This results in perforation of the septum which surprisingly is a painless process. Here again EDTA ointment will give a degree of protection.

Lung cancer has occurred in Germany, the United States and the United Kingdom in workers exposed to chromate and bichromate dusts in the refining industry. According to Hunter (1975) the evidence is that one or more of the furnace products in the form of an intermediate chromate may be responsible. No increased incidence of lung cancer has been reported among other users, but this possibility should be carefully studied.

Prevention and treatment of toxic effects

Suppression of chromate mists by anti-misting agents or good lip ventilation on chromium plating tanks should prevent the occurrence of nasal perforation and most of the dermatitis in the chrome plating industry. Adequate protective clothing is important. This should include good quality rubber gloves free from pin holes. It should also be remembered that accidental contamination of gloves on the inside is a common source of skin troubles. Adequate control of dust and fumes on chrome furnaces and any other producer of chromate and dichromate dusts or chromic acid mists is essential in view of the increased risk of lung cancer. The 1977 TLV is:

Chromate ore processing	$0{\cdot}1\ mg/m^3$
Chromic acid and chromates	$0{\cdot}1\ mg/m^3$
Chromium, soluble chromic or chromous salts	$0{\cdot}5\ mg/m^3$

Statutory medical inspection of persons in the manufacture of chromate or bichromate of potassium or sodium are required (Chemical Works Regulation, 1922).

MANGANESE

Uses

The main source of manganese is pyrolusite (MnO_2). The metal is used for making steel alloys, dry batteries, electrical coils, ceramic glazes, in· matches, dyes, fertilizers, welding rods, and as oxidizing agents. At one time potassium permanganate was commonly used as an antiseptic.

Toxicology

Manganese is an essential element and takes part in a number of enzyme reactions related to potassium metabolism. Under normal conditions of life, the body burden of manganese is kept very stable. While ingested manganese is not particularly toxic, large doses cause diarrhoea and so are quickly eliminated.

Industrial poisoning is due to inhalation. Large doses will result in acute irritation of the lungs, causing a chemical pneumonitis. Men employed in the manufacture of potassium permanganate breathing air containing high concentrations of fine manganese particles have shown up to 30 times the normal incidence of pneumonia with an excess of pharyngitis and bronchitis (Lloyd Davies, 1946). In 1923 an electrical plant for smelting manganese was erected in Sanda in Norway. Smoke, containing fine particles of manganese, caused a tenfold increase in the incidence of pneumonia in the area (Riddervold and Halvorsen, 1943). No cases of manganese-related disease have been reported in the dry battery industry in Britain.

Another form of manganese poisoning due to continued inhalation usually of fine manganese dioxide dust over a period of years affects the central nervous system producing an effect not unlike Parkinson's disease. There is usually irritability, difficulty in walking, monotonous slurred speech, lack of facial expression and a tendency to compulsive behaviour. Such cases tend to recover slowly when removed from exposure. Manganese poisoning of the nervous system has occurred in mining and refining, manufacture of alloys and grinding manganese dioxide. Pneumonia has been described around a smelter, in miners, and in men manufacturing potassium permanganate.

Treatment of toxic effects

Metal chelating drugs such as BAL and calcium EDTA have not been very helpful in treating cases of manganese poisoning. However L-dopa has been more useful than it is in Parkinson's disease.

Prognosis

In mild cases of manganese effects on the central nervous system, removal from further exposure usually leads to a slow recovery. Men more severely affected may not improve following cessation of exposure.

Prevention of poisoning

This involves good hygienic practices and control of manganese dust levels in the atmosphere. The recommended TLV is 5 mg/m^3. The wearing of suitable dust respirators has been found helpful in mining the ore.

Supervision

The control of finely divided dust is of primary importance. There does not appear to be much information on dose response relationships. Increased knowledge of biological tests for absorption is required.

MERCURY

Sources and recovery

Mercury exists in the free state, but most mercury for industrial use is obtained by roasting cinnabar (HgS) in air when SO_2 is driven off and the mercury vapour is condensed.

Properties

At normal room temperature mercury has a vapour pressure of 1·3 μg/Hg which is equivalent to 10 mg/m^3 of mercury in air. The vapour pressure doubles with a 10 °C rise in temperature. This means that the concentration of mercury vapour at room temperature could be 100 times the TLV. This property together with the way in which spilled mercury breaks up into very small droplets and its persistence on most normal surfaces or in tiny cracks or crevices is one of the chief dangers in the use of metallic mercury.

Uses

Mercury was known to the Greeks and Romans and they also recognized its toxic effects. The ability of mercury to form amalgams with gold and silver was used to extract these metals from their ores.

1. Mercury has been used in scientific instruments such as thermometers and barometers for many years. In the electrical industry it is used for mercury arc rectifiers, automatic switches, various electric meters and at one time mercury vapour signs and street lamps were common. The use in mirror-making was abandoned after Liebig invented the process of depositing silver from an ammoniacal solution of silver nitrate by adding an aldehyde (Hunter, 1975).

2. Mercury amalgams of tin, silver and gold are still used particularly in fire gilding where the mercury is driven off by heating. Dentists still use mercury–silver, tin amalgams for fillings, and the exposure of dentists and their assistants is currently being investigated (FDI Recommendations, 1978).

3. One of the biggest uses of metallic mercury is the electrolysis of brine, when chlorine is given off at the anode and a mercury–sodium amalgam is formed. This amalgam is reacted with water to form sodium hydroxide and hydrogen, the mercury being returned to the electrolytic cells.

4. Acid mercury nitrate was used for felting rabbit fur to make fur hats and the resulting central nervous system poisoning was the basis for the Mad Hatter in *Alice in Wonderland.*

5. Mercury fulminate ($HgC_2N_2O_2$) is used in explosive detonators.

6. Organic mercurial compounds are used as antifungal seed dressings. Although these preparations are manufactured in fully enclosed plant, their use has caused a good deal of illness and a number of deaths.

Absorption, distribution and excretion

Mercury vapours and dusts are chiefly absorbed via the lungs. Skin absorption of metallic mercury and compounds can take place. Ingestion in an industrial context is only likely due to eating in workshops or bad hygienic practices. Ramazzini (1700) describes how painters were in the habit of pointing their brushes with their lips. Most ingested inorganic mercury is excreted in the faeces. Mercury absorbed by other routes is mostly excreted in the urine.

Inorganic mercury is widely distributed in the tissues, the highest concentrations being in the kidneys and the liver.

Organic mercury shows higher concentrations in the blood and central nervous systems, with lower kidney concentrations. Methyl mercury is more slowly excreted than phenyl mercury and inorganic forms. About half of a dose of methyl mercury is excreted in the faeces in inorganic form following partial detoxification by the liver.

Signs and symptoms of inorganic mercury poisoning

Acute poisoning

Acute poisoning is rare but may occur due either to ingestion of mercury compounds or to the inhalation of high concentrations of mercury vapour. In the latter case acute irritation of the skin and mucous membranes may occur, together with an acute chemical pneumonitis leading to possible death from pulmonary oedema. In animals, massive experimental dosage leads to severe haemorrhage in the kidneys, brain, heart, lungs and colon.

Chronic effects

Industrial mercurialism is usually of a chronic nature. Symptoms often start with excessive salivation. Later the mouth and gums become painful and swollen and teeth may be lost. Tremor develops and writing may become illegible. Loss of weight, nausea, vomiting and diarrhoea occur. Finally effects on the central nervous system follow, which include being easily upset, timid and a general depression. The individual may become quarrelsome and neglects his work and his family. In more severe cases drowsiness may occur with loss of memory, hallucinations or mania. These effects on the central nervous system are referred to as erythrism. Albuminuria may also occur and may develop into the nephrotic syndrome.

Minamata disease

In 1953 an unusual type of nervous disease affected both people and cats in the area of Minamata Bay in Japan. This was found to be due to organic mercury compounds. A local factory making polyvinyl chloride used mercuric chloride as a catalyst. Some mercury appears to have been discharged in the effluent. Bacterial action is thought to have formed methyl mercury compounds which tend to concentrate in fish and these were subsequently absorbed by man and cats eating the fish. This episode illustrates the importance of safe disposal of all potentially toxic waste.

Prevention and control of mercury poisoning

Hygienic measures must be carefully planned. Account should be taken of the manner in which mercury if spilled can break up into small droplets and become hidden in tiny crevices. This, together with its ability to form toxic amounts of vapour at room temperature, requires special attention.

Organic mercury, particularly methyl mercury, is normally manufactured in enclosed processes, and special equipment is used to coat seeds with the powder. Most of the tragedies have occurred due to eating treated seed and special education and warning procedures are required to prevent this type of accident.

The handling of mercury fulminate requires suitable protective clothing to prevent any skin contact. Mixing requires good ventilation and suitable respirators.

Medical supervision should ensure adequate environmental control to prevent any symptoms of mercury poisoning. At present mercury tests in urine are normally used to control absorption, but there are always difficulties associated with variations in specific gravity and a full understanding of whether mercury is filtered out by the glomeruli and then concentrated or whether there is excretion or absorption via the tubules is needed.

Tests for albuminuria are normally carried out, but adequate control measures should ensure that no increase in protein excretion occurs.

Removal from further exposure should be instituted when absorption is regarded as excessive before any symptoms arise.

Guidance Note EH17 (1977) recommends that mercury in urine levels should be kept within or below the range 15–30 micromoles/l. Bidstrup (1964) recommended keeping urinary concentrations below 15 micromoles/l. Excretion of organic mercurials should be kept below 1·5 micromoles/l.

Treatment

Alstead and Girdwood (1974) recommend BAL in acute cases of mercury poisoning provided that it is given early. Bidstrup (1964) reported that *N*-acetylpenicillinamine was the most effective treatment in chronic cases. Drug treatment of established cases of organic mercurial poisoning has not proved very successful.

NICKEL

Sources and recovery

The principal nickel ores are found in association with iron and copper, particularly in Ontario, Canada. In the United Kingdom the largest production of nickel is carried out by the Mond process. This involves roasting the concentrated ore to remove sulphur. From the mixture of copper and nickel oxide the copper is removed by treating with sulphuric acid. The nickel is treated with carbon monoxide forming nickel carbonyl $Ni(CO)_4$. Passing this gas over moving nickel pellets deposits the nickel and the carbon monoxide is returned to the process.

An alternative method is the Orford system which removes the copper by fusing it with sodium sulphide. On cooling the copper floats on the nickel and the nickel is then recovered by electrolysis.

Uses

Nickel is often used for plating or as a base for chrome plating because of its resistance to corrosion. It is used in electronic equipment, nickel–cadmium batteries, coins, food processing equipment and is an important component of stainless steel. It is also used as a catalyst in the hydrogenation of oils.

Toxicity

The commonest problem in handling nickel is the development of an allergic dermatitis. This ability to produce sensitivity has resulted in nickel plating being largely replaced by plastics for brassière strap clips and watch cases.

Nickel is not absorbed very effectively from the gut and not at all through the skin. It is absorbed through the lungs although nearly 40 per cent appears to be retained in the lungs. According to Hunter (1975) when nickel carbonyl enters the lung it splits into nickel, which is deposited, and carbon dioxide, some of which is absorbed into the blood. The toxicity of inhaled nickel carbonyl is at least 5 times that of carbon monoxide (Amor, 1932). A number of deaths have occurred from inhaling nickel carbonyl. The symptoms are giddiness, some dyspnoea, nausea and vomiting. These pass off rapidly in the open air. After 12 to 36 hours dyspnoea occurs with cyanosis, cough and increased temperature. Blood stained sputum may occur. Abnormal physical signs are usually absent. The usual cause of death is pulmonary oedema and this would seem to be a form of chemical pneumonitis not unlike exposure to cadmium fume.

In 1933 Bridge drew attention to a considerable excess of cancer of the nasal sinuses and the lung occurring in the Mond nickel plant at Clydach. Similar reports have come from Canada (Sutherland, 1959) and Norway (Pederson et al., 1973) as well as from other countries. Considerable improvements made in 1925 at Clydach, particularly in reducing the dust in the treatment of the concentrated ore (matte), would appear to have eliminated nasal cancer. The excess of lung cancers, although reduced, has persisted in men first exposed after 1925 and even in the most recent report the incidence of lung cancer is still excessive in men first exposed in the 1930–44 period (Doll et al., 1977). Although nickel carbonyl and metallic nickel can, under certain experimental circumstances, produce cancers it would seem from an epidemiological point of view that most of the men affected had been exposed to the dusty process of matte handling and copper separation. The problem is further complicated by the fact that the matte as well as the sulphuric acid used to extract copper both contained arsenic, although as Doll has pointed out arsenic has not been associated with nasal cancers. Undoubtedly improvements would also have been made over the years to the containment of nickel carbonyl because of its highly toxic properties. A more detailed job history study is now taking place on the group described in the paper by Doll et al. (1977).

Prevention and treatment of toxic effects

The prevention of nickel dust or compounds coming in contact with the skin, particularly under conditions of high humidity is desirable. At present the precise cause of the excess of lung cancer is not known, but reduction of dust, good housekeeping and the total enclosure of the nickel carbonyl process is clearly necessary. This latter requirement should also prevent nickel carbonyl exposure, but special precautions will need to be enforced for maintenance or possible breakdown. Medical supervision should include early detection of lung cancer by periodic X-ray as surgical removal in the early stages is now generally very successful.

PLATINUM

Source and recovery

Platinum is normally found alloyed with other metals of the group such as palladium, osmium, iridium, ruthenium and rhodium and also with gold and iron.

Uses

This precious metal is principally used in industry as a catalyst. Its corrosion resistance is also useful in pure or alloy forms for electrical contacts and as dies for the production of fibre glass. Other uses include electroplating, use in laboratory apparatus and as a sensitizing agent in photography. It has also been used in the manufacture of some types of fuel cells. It has the same coefficient of expansion as glass.

Toxicity

Some people show an allergic response to platinum compounds. Symptoms include nasal and upper respiratory tract irritation with sneezing, running of the eyes and a cough. These symptoms last for about an hour after leaving work. Later an asthmatic type of reaction occurs with cough, wheezing, and shortness of breath and tends to become progressively worse as exposure continues. Skin reactions are also fairly common with redness, dryness, scaling and itching. Sometimes wheals of urticaria are produced.

Prevention of toxic effects

This depends on very careful dust control and good housekeeping and ventilation. Suitable protective clothing should be provided where required. People who become sensitized will normally have to be kept away from further contact. Hunter (1975) advises that the double salts of platinum should not be used dry unless absolutely necessary. Persons with a history of allergies should be excluded from work with platinum compounds.

SELENIUM

Sources

The chief source of selenium is as a by-product in electrolitic copper refining where it is found in the mud at the anode. Selenium is not really a metal but it has certain metallic properties and belongs to the periodic group VI like sulphur.

Uses

There are a wide range of uses for this metalloid which has many properties similar to sulphur, including a number of allotropic forms. The metallic form is used in the manufacture of electrical rectifiers. It has been suggested that accidental burning out of rectifiers might produce toxic amounts of fume, but this does not appear to have happened in practice. Selenium is used in glass, as a red colouring agent, and in ceramics manufacture and also to make pigments and dyes and paints. It may be used to vulcanize rubber and as a catalyst in manufacturing vitamin C. The best known use is probably in photoelectric cells, although cadmium seems to be gaining ground in this field. Compounds have been used as insecticides and the oxychloride as a solvent and plasticizer.

Metabolism and toxicity

Traces of selenium are essential to animal life, but excessive amounts may give rise to 'alkali' disease in animals. This leads to muscle weakness and impairment of vision which in severe poisoning gives rise to paralysis and abdominal pain; death occurs from respiratory failure. Liver damage is found in rat experiments as well as in fetal toxicity. Teratogenic effects also occur. Arsenic will counteract some of the effects of selenium.

Industrial effects

According to Browning (1961) the chief industrial effect is dermatitis. Selenium oxychloride is highly vesicant. Selenium dioxide has also been recorded as causing skin burns and severe corneal injury. Acute fume exposure has caused irritation to the eyes and upper respiratory tract together with severe headache. Alice Hamilton (1925) reported chronic industrial poisoning among copper refiners. Symptoms include upper respiratory irritation, gastro-intestinal upset, a metallic taste in the mouth and the well-known garlic odour of the breath. Levander and Argrett (1969), cited by Cassarett and Doull (1975), describe some interesting synergistic effects when combined with mercury, thallium or arsenic. Hunter (1975) suggests that selenium in the diet could be a cause of a high rate of dental caries in Clatsop, in Oregon. Irritation of the nasal passages may also lead to anosmia.

Hydrogen selenide H_2Se has a foul odour and is more toxic than hydrogen sulphide. Symptoms include a metallic taste in the mouth, nausea, vomiting, dizziness and extreme lassitude. This compound together with methyl and ethyl selenides are probably the most toxic selenium compounds used in industry.

Prevention and treatment

This primarily involves avoiding skin contact, particularly with solvent compounds such as the oxychloride, and controlling any dust or fume which might be produced. Most selenium is fairly rapidly excreted in the urine and selenium in urine testing would seem to be appropriate where excessive absorption is suspected. Selenium in blood analysis is worth investigating. In view of reported possible teratogenic effects the employment of women of childbearing potential is probably best avoided where significant absorption is likely. The present TLV of selenium (1977) is 0·2 mg/m^3.

No specific treatments are at present available although Hunter (1975) advises 10 mg of ascorbic acid per kilogram of body weight per day.

The disposal of waste, particularly of soluble compounds, needs to be carefully controlled to prevent selenium getting into water supplies.

THALLIUM

Sources and extraction

Thallium is found as cookerite which is a mixture of selenides of thallium, copper and silver. It is recovered in Canada as a by-product of zinc ore treatment.

Uses

Thallium is used in insecticides and also commonly as a rat poison. It is also used in optical glass to which it gives a high refractive index, as a stainless alloy with silver, in the manufacture of fireworks, in dyes and pigments, with mercury in low temperature thermometers, and as a catalyst in organic chemistry. It is also the basis of some hair removers. Cassarett and Doull (1975) draw attention to the particular industrial risk of manufacturing the fused halides for the production of lenses.

My first experience of the use of thallium was at the time an ex-Broadmoor patient decided to poison some work colleagues with thallium.

The Unions became very concerned when thallium was being used to make an alloy with magnesium because the billets when left for any length of time corroded on the surface producing a white deposit, which was cut off on a lathe. This produced a fair amount of dust with a relatively high thallium content. The coating of the billets with a suitable oil prevented the corrosion and reduced airborne thallium.

Control

Dust should be controlled within the recommended TLV of 0·1 mg/m^3 and skin contact avoided. Protective clothing should include gloves. According to Lockett (1957) the use of thallium acetate as a depilatory was frequently followed by mild symptoms of toxicity. Urinary testing for thallium should be carried out. Medical supervision is advisable if risk of excessive absorption is suspected. The difficulties of diagnosis are largely related to lack of information about possible exposure. The value of thallium in blood and urine estimations requires careful study. It is important to remember that thallium is a cumulative poison due to its slow excretion.

Toxicology and symptoms

Thallium is not an essential element. It can be absorbed via the gastro-intestinal tract and by inhalation of dust and also through the skin. Excretion is slow, mainly via the urine, but also in the faeces. Gastro-intestinal irritation and central nervous symptoms of a psychic type may develop. In chronic cases ascending paralysis may occur. Industrial poisoning is rare and has generally taken the form of fatigue, pain in the limbs and loss of hair, and sometimes albuminuria. Optic atrophy and retrobulbar neuritis along with cloudiness of the lens have been described. Effects on the eyes tend to be permanent. Abnormal white cell patterns with lymphocytosis and eosinophilia have been reported (Carrozie, 1934). No fatal industrial cases have been reported.

Treatment

Treatment of symptomatic cases should respond to versene, but there is little knowledge of its use at present.

TIN

Uses

Alkyl tin compounds are used as stabilizers in polyvinyl chloride plastics and in chlorinated rubber paints, insecticides and anthelmintics for poultry.

Toxicity

Tin is not normally regarded as toxic but tin compounds or dusts if inhaled produce dense X-ray shadows without interfering with the function of the lungs.

Dibutyl and tributyl tin compounds can produce severe skin burns and are especially dangerous to the eyes.

Trialkyl tin compounds predominantly affect the central nervous sytem in a similar way to triethyl lead, causing a form of encephalopathy. They may also affect the normal functioning of liver cell mitochondria. Although central nervous system effects have not been reported from industrial use of trialkyl tin compounds, they will certainly be absorbed via the skin, so that very strict precautions are required to avoid both skin contact and inhalation of vapours. Barnes and Stoner (1958) showed that the effects of trialkyl tin on the central nervous system was very similar to that of trialkyl lead. There was a tragic occurrence in France where trialkyl tin was ingested as a remedy for boils and resulted in the death of over 100 people.

URANIUM

Source and recovery

Uranium ore is known as 'pitchblende' on account of its black pitch-like appearance. It exists in several isotopes with atomic weights of 234, 235, 238 and 239.

Uses

The principal use of uranium is in atomic reactors as a fuel for generation of electricity, or for the production of plutonium for atomic weapons. It has also been used to colour ceramic glazes.

Toxicity

Uranium is not particularly toxic except in soluble form. All soluble compounds can be absorbed through the skin and a single dose is lethal to rabbits. The primary target is the kidney and death may result from renal failure either rapidly or within a few weeks. In cases of survival, recovery appears to be complete. Uranium is fairly rapidly excreted and does not accumulate in the kidneys like cadmium. About 25 per cent of absorbed uranium is deposited in the bones. Patty's description of uranium mining in the United States with over 1000 mines suggests that hygiene and ventilation were often inadequate.

The second risk from uranium exposure is radiation, particularly from enriched uranium. These risks are normally very well controlled within the various atomic energy agencies and safety procedures have been so strict that few accidents have occurred.

ZIRCONIUM

Source

The principal source of zirconium is zircon sand ($ZrSiO_2$).

Uses

Zirconium is used in nuclear shielding and metal alloys. It is also used as a catalyst in organic chemistry, dyes and ceramic pigments as well as abrasives.

Toxicity

Zirconium is generally regarded as non-toxic. However, in the form of zirconium oxychloride it has been used in antiperspirant compounds both as sticks and later as sprays. A few people appear to be sensitive to the sticks and axillary granulomas have occurred. These normally disappear some time after the use of the stick has stopped. In the USA the food and the drugs administration raised the question of whether antiperspirant sprays containing zirconium might cause granulomas of the lung.

I investigated the health of men taking various zirconium compounds including potassium zirconium fluoride, zirconium oxide and zirconium carbonate. Some of the processes were dusty while others were wet chemical processes which did not give rise to dust. Out of 72 men examined, 11 had 0/1 or 1/1 category small round or irregular lung shadows which correlated with the time of exposure to dusts containing zirconium. There was no obvious deterioration of lung function tests related to zirconium exposure, but there was a clear relationship between poor lung function tests and smoking. This confirms the paper by McCallum (1975) that exposure to zirconium compounds can produce a benign pneumoconiosis.

Zirconium (ZrO) is now being produced in fibre form. If the fibres are less than 3 μm in diameter and more than 10 μm in length they will need to be investigated as potentially capable of causing fibrosis and possibly mesotheliomas. I believe that the potential risk of mesotheliomas also depends on the durability of the fibres if they are inhaled.

Control

Although the pneumoconiosis is benign it is advisable to control the concentrations of dust below the TLV of 5 mg/m^3 and probably lower particularly when the particle size is below 7 μm diameter.

REFERENCES AND FURTHER READING

Adams R. G. and Crabtree W. (1961) *Br. J. Ind. Med.* **18,** 216.

Adams R. G., Harrison J. F. and Scott P. (1969) The development of cadmium induced proteinuria and osteomalacia in alkaline battery workers. *Q. J. Med.* **38,** 425.

Ahlmark A., Axelson B. and Friberg L. (1961) Further investigations into kidney function and proteinuria in chronic cadmium poisoning. *Int. Congr. Occup. Health* **13,** 201.

Alstead S. and Girdwood R. H. (1974) *Textbook of Medical Treatment.* Edinburgh, Churchill Livingstone.

Amor A. J. (1932) Toxicology of the carbonyls. *J. Ind. Hyg.* **14,** 216.

Barnes J. M. and Stoner H. B. (1958) Toxic properties of some dialkyl and trialkyl tin salts. *Br. J. Ind. Med.* **15,** 15.

Bidstrup P. L. (1964) *Toxicity of Mercury and its Compounds.* Amsterdam, Elsevier.

Bonnel J. H. (1955) Emphysema and proteinuria in men casting copper cadmium alloys. *Br. J. Ind. Med.* **12,** 385.

Braun W. (1958) Krebs an Haut und inneren Organen, hervorgerufen durch Arsen. *Dtsch. Med. Wochenschr.* **83,** 870.

Bridge J. C. (1933) *Annual Report of the Chief Inspector of Factories, 1932.* London, H.M.S.O.

Browning E. (1961) *Toxicology of Industrial Metals.* London, Butterworth.

Carrozie L. (1934) *Occup. Health* **2,** 1038.

Cassarett J. D. and Doull J. (1975) *Toxicology.* New York, Macmillan.

Chandler J. (1977) Personal communication.

Doll R., Mathews J. D. and Morgan L. G. (1977) Cancer of the lung and nasal sinuses in nickel workers: a reassessment of the period of risk. *Br. J. Ind. Med.* **34,** 102.

Durkan T. M., Delahant A. B. and Creedon F. T. (1957) The biological action of inhaled beryllium sulphate. *Arch. Ind. Health* **15,** 32.

F.D.I. Recommendations on Dental Mercury Hygiene 1978. *Br. Dent J.* **144,** 87.

Friberg L. (1948) Proteinuria and kidney injury among workmen exposed to cadmium and nickel dust. *J. Ind. Hyg. Toxicol.* **30,** 32.

Genkin S. (1932) Zur Klinik der akuten Arsenvergiftung durch Einatmung der arsenhaltigen Staube. *Arch. Gewerbepath. Gewerbe hyg.* **3,** 770.

Grandjean P. (1977) *Standards Setting.* Copenhagen, Arbejdsmiljofφndet Vesterbrograde 69.

Hamilton A. (1925) *Industrial Poisons in the U.S.* New York, Macmillan.

Herriot J. (1976) *That Vets Might Fly.* London, Pan Books.

Hunter D. (1975) *The Diseases of Occupations*, 5th ed. London, English Universities Press.

Kay H. D. and Skill D. I. (1934) Beryllium Rickets. *Biochem. J.* **28**, 1232.

Kennedy B. J., Pare J. H. P., Pump K. K. et al. (1950), The effect of A.C.T.H. on beryllium granulomatosis, *Can. Med. Assoc. J.* **62**, 426.

Kipling M. D. and Waterhouse J. A. H. (1967) *Lancet* **1**, 730.

Leeman R. A., Lee J. S. and Wagoner J. K. (1977) *Cancer Mortality among Cadmium Production Workers.* Cincinnati, Ohio. NIOSH Centre for Disease Control, Dept. Hlth Educn. and Welfare.

Levander O. A. and Argrett L. C. (1969) Effects of arsenic, mercury, thallium and lead on selenium metabolism in rats. *Toxicol. Appl. Pharmacol.* **14**, 308. Cited by Cassarett J. D. and Doull J. (1975).

Levy L. S. and Clack J. (1975) Further studies on the effect of cadmium on the prostate gland. *Ann. Occup. Hyg.* **17**, 205.

Levy L. S., Clack J. and Roe F. J. C. (1975) Further studies on the effect of cadmium on the prostate gland. *Ann. Occup. Hyg. II.* **17**, 213.

Levy L. S., Roe F. J. C., Malcolm D. et al. (1973) Absence of prostatic changes in rats exposed to cadmium. *Ann. Occup. Hyg.* **16**, 111.

Lloyd Davies T. A. (1946) Manganese pneumonitis. *Br. J. Ind. Med.* **3**, 111.

Lockets S. (1957) *Clinical Toxicology.* London, Kimpton, p. 596.

Lyle H. (1972) Personal communication.

McCallum I. (1975) Personal communication.

Nicaud P., Lafitte, A. and Gros A. (1942) Les troubles de l'intoxication chronique par le cadmium. *J. Cell. Biol.* **23**, 519.

Nordberg G. F. (1976) *Effects and Dose Response Relationships of Toxic Metals.* Amsterdam, Elsevier.

Patty A. F. (1962) *Industrial Hygiene and Toxicology*. New York, Interscience.

Pavirek J. and Zahor Z. (1956) *Nature* **177**, 1036.

Pederson E., Hogeveit A. C. and Anderson A. (1973) Cancer of the respiratory organs among workers at a nickel refinery in Norway. *Int. J. Cancer* **12**, 32.

Potts C. (1965) *Ann. Occup. Hyg.*

Ramazzini B. (1700) *De Morbis Artificum Diatriba.* Geneva.

Riddervold J. and Halvorsen K. (1943) Bacteriological investigations on pneumonia and pneumonia carriers in Sanda, an isolated industrial community in Norway. *Acta Path Microbiol. Scand. [A]* **20**, 272.

Rosendaal H. M. (1951) Clinical observations on the toxicology of boron hydrides. *Arch. Indust. Hyg.* **4**, 257.

Schepers G. W. H., Ourkan T. M., Delahout A. B. et al. (1957) The biological action of inhaled beryllium sulphate. *Arch. Indust. Hlth.* **19**, 16.

Sutherland R. B. (1959) Respiratory cancer mortality in workers employed in an Ontario nickel refinery. Cited by Doll et al. (1977).

van Ordstrand H. S., Hughes R. and Carmody M. G. (1943) *Cleve. Clin. Q.* **10**, 10.

3. GASES, VAPOURS AND FUMES

G. Matthews

Gases, vapours and fumes are among the most potentially dangerous forms of matter and are particularly hazardous because of their physical state. They may cause acute lung damage. They may be absorbed into the body through the lungs and cause acute and chronic systemic disorders. They may cause chronic inflammatory changes in the lungs, either following upon acute damage, or by slow degrees, leading to later disturbances of function. They may act as sensitizers causing an allergic response. Any of these actions may cause death or disability. In addition, they may have the potential to cause catastrophic explosions in factories, plants, ships, aircraft, streets or homes.

DEFINITIONS

Gas

A gas is a state of matter in which the molecules move freely causing the matter to expand indefinitely (e.g., air).

Vapour

A gas which is at a temperature below its critical temperature and can therefore be liquefied by a suitable increase in pressure (e.g., steam).

Fume

A cloud of airborne particles, generally visible, of low volatility and less than a micrometre in size, arising from a condensation of vapours or from a chemical reaction (e.g., smoke).

Vapour pressure (VP)

Vapour pressure is defined as the pressure exerted by a vapour either by itself or as a mixture of gases: it is customarily expressed in millimetres of mercury at normal temperature and pressure (NTP). Liquids and solids also possess vapour pressures which will increase proportionately with increase in temperature. The higher the VP the more volatile the substance. These definitions are taken from *Chamber's Dictionary of Science and Technology*, 1971.

General effects

The inhalation of gases and vapours often represents the most urgent problem of resuscitation and treatment. This is because of two essential characteristics of the lung. It constitutes a vast absorptive area and its lining epithelium responds to irritation by rapidly producing an inflammatory exudate. Through the alveoli molecules of gas or vapour can enter the circulation extremely rapidly. The rate of absorption depends upon the concentration of the gas or vapour, its solubility in water, and upon the rate of circulation of the blood. A subject at rest in a given concentration will absorb less gas in a given time than a subject performing hard physical work.

LUNG IRRITANT EFFECTS

When a gas or vapour is irritant the rate of exudate production depends upon the concentration of the irritant and upon its instrinsic chemical characteristics. Highly irritant gases, for example chlorine, can cause death rapidly from pulmonary congestion and oedema. It should be remembered that in these circumstances pulmonary oedema represents a loss of fluid to the circulation (in the same way as burns of the skin). Unlike pulmonary oedema due to cardiac causes, in which diuretics are used to rid the body of excess fluid, the blood itself has lost water and so the blood volume is reduced. This represents the need for fine judgement in the intensive therapy required. An additional hazard to the victim is the possibility of damage to the eyes which can be severe with most irritant gases and fumes – ammonia, the halogens, and the strongly acidic fumes and vapours. It should never be forgotten that the immediate treatment of the victim at the place of injury is often crucial. Basic issues are the rapid removal of the victim from contact with the irritant, the application of oxygen, and the flooding with plain water of affected tissues, especially the eyes.

SYSTEMIC EFFECTS

Systemic damage may occur with gases normally considered quite harmless. Oxygen, the supporter of life, and nitrogen, the inert diluent, are good examples. When men move into situations for which they are biologically unadapted the biophysical activity of oxygen changes. Air at sea level consists largely of about 21 per cent oxygen, 78 per cent nitrogen with argon, carbon dioxide and the rare gases making up a further 1 per cent. The partial pressure of oxygen is 160 mmHg and that of nitrogen 600 mmHg. Both in diving beneath the sea and rising into the sky, the partial pressures change, altering the environment drastically. It will be remembered that a gas will be compressed or expand depending upon the pressure. To maintain a constant volume in conditions of high pressure, a gas will itself be under equivalently high pressure. Under conditions of low pressure, a gas of constant volume will be of lower pressure.

Boyle's law states:

$$\left.\begin{array}{lcl} \text{Pressure x Volume} & = & \text{Constant} \\ PV & = & K \end{array}\right\}$$

The following tables illustrate this.

Table 3.1 Under water (approximate figures).

Depth (metres)	Total pressure (mmHg)	Partial pressure (mmHg) Oxygen	Nitrogen
0	760	160	600
10	1520	320	1200
20	2280	480	1800

For every 10 metres increase in depth, the pressure rises by 760 mmHg or one atmosphere.

Table 3.2 Rising above the earth (approximate figures).

Height (metres)	Total pressure (mmHg)	Partial pressure (mmHg) Oxygen	Nitrogen
0	760	160	600
1500	630	130	500
3000	525	110	415
6000	350	75	275
9000	230	50	180

Under conditions of increased pressure the physiological significance of both oxygen and nitrogen changes. It is now clear that nitrogen is a narcotic agent at high pressures. Cousteau (1954) uses the words 'l'ivresse des grands profondeurs' which certainly sounds splendid. An English translation, 'the rapture of the deeps', sounds less romantic – the rupture of the deeps is perhaps more apposite when it is recognized that the higher cerebral functions are splintered. Miles (1969) gives the symptoms at depths increasing from 30 metres to 100 metres as an increasing light-headedness, self-confidence, jollity and laughter along with a decreasing response to stimuli, depression and near unconsciousness. The mechanism involved is probably related to the lipid solubility of the gas (c.f. anaesthetics) leading to a histotoxic anoxia (Meyer, 1899), quoted by Ebert et al. (1958) and Miles (1969).

At increased pressures, oxygen also becomes hazardous. Convulsions may occur without warning. The time of onset is directly related to the pressure. Experiments by Donald (1947) also showed that individual tolerance was highly variable, and that hard work increased the risk.

Rules now exist to govern the concentrations of oxygen and nitrogen in gas mixtures for diving purposes.

Chronic exposures to pure oxygen at normal pressure has been known for some time to cause retrolental fibroplasia in very young infants. Prolonged exposure to both lower and higher than normal atmospheric concentrations of oxygen have been shown to cause damage to the lungs of young adult rats (Chvapil and Peng, 1975)

An accidental entry into an atmosphere containing little or no oxygen results in a series of symptoms which may culminate in death. Irreversible brain damage occurs when oxygen deprivation lasts between 4 and 6 minutes. No matter what the toxic effect of a gas may be, if no oxygen is present, unconsciousness occurs almost at once. Entry into a nitrogen filled space, or a chalk pit after rain which may be filled with carbon dioxide, can result in rapid death.

Exposure to low, or decreasing concentrations of oxygen produces symptoms akin to increasing drunkenness. An initial inability to think clearly becomes worse; judgement becomes increasingly faulty and control of emotions is lost. Stimuli are scarcely felt. Control of muscles fails, collapse occurs and death may result. Dangerously low concentrations lie between 6 per cent and 10 per cent.

Probably the most important industrial hazard of oxygen is its ability to accelerate combustion. In an oxygen-enriched atmosphere a smouldering cigarette may burst into flame, and a spark on oil or grease may start an inferno. Rules for oxygen storage and controls for its use exist in all industrialized countries.

ACUTE SYSTEMIC EFFECTS

Acute systemic disorder may occur with many gases with little or no direct respiratory effect. Carbon monoxide and arsine are non-irritant; hydrogen cyanide, cyanogen and cyanogen chloride, together with hydrogen sulphide are only slightly irritant; but all can cause death by their systemic action. There are specific methods for the emergency treatment of cyanide and kindred poisoning. Cyanides and related nitrile compounds produce their effect by their great affinity for cytochrome oxidase, the final enzymatic mechanism for the transfer of oxygen to the tissues. The standard treatment of acute poisoning is with amyl nitrite capsules, oxygen and the slow intravenous injection of dicobalt edetate (SHW 385, HM Factory Inspectorate, HSE, Baynards House, London W2 and Label 15, obtainable from Chemical Industries Association, Alembic House, 93 Albert Embankment, London SE1 7TU). Atkinson et al. (1974) have described the effective use of the enzyme rhodanese experimentally.

Carbon monoxide

It is an adage that common things commonly occur. A common thing that commonly occurs is carbon monoxide (CO) poisoning. CO is a gas that causes scarcely any lung irritation and is colourless and odourless. The current Threshold Limit Value (TLV) (UK and US) is 50 ppm. In any condition of incomplete combustion CO is formed and so it is encountered in steel works, foundries and in a variety of industrial furnace operations. It may also be found in more unexpected situations; in domestic circumstances where, because of the sealing of sources of ventilation in cold weather, the flame from a boiler or heater is starved of oxygen and the concentration of CO builds up. Slow combustion in old mines, pits and quarries may also give rise to lethal levels of CO. Probably the greatest actual amount is emitted from motor vehicle exhausts, and undoubtedly the amount in human blood is infinitely greater in cigarette and cigar smokers than in the rest of the population. Acute exposures to carbon monoxide are not uncommon. Its toxicity is due to the fact of its affinity for haemoglobin (Hb) being some 250 times more powerful than that of oxygen. Carbon monoxide binds with Hb to form carboxyhaemoglobin (COHb), a relatively stable compound, so blocking the uptake of oxygen by Hb. Steady exposure to a relatively small concentration of carbon monoxide therefore has a progressively severe effect. In addition oxygen dissociates from Hb less readily. These two physico-chemical effects, the reduction in oxygen-carrying capacity and the reduced oxygen dissociation produces a calamitous union. Details of oxygen dissociation curves can be found in textbooks of physiology.

The following figures are approximated from Stewart (1970):

Table 3.3 Percentage of blood CO levels at given ambient levels and periods.

Carbon monoxide	Time of exposure (minutes) percentage CO at times. 30 min	100 min	200 min	500 min
50 ppm	1·5	2·8	4·0	5·6
100 ppm	2·0	5·0	7·6	13·0
200 ppm	3·6	8·5	15·0	23·0
500 ppm	7·8	20·0	33·0	44·0

2000 ppm is dangerous after an hour's exposure and over 4000 ppm is very dangerous indeed. The symptoms of CO poisoning are of increasing breathlessness especially related to exertion and of an increasing cherry-redness of the lips, conjunctiva and nail beds. Treatment is by removal of the victim from the atmosphere, the giving of oxygen and such resuscitative procedures as are demanded. A sequel to severe CO poisoning may be the relatively rapid development of Parkinsonism due to necrosis of the globus pallidus. A review of 25 cases has been written by Schwab and England (1968). It has been difficult to evaluate the significance of chronic CO poisoning, and difficult to relate blood CO percentage to disease. Cigarette and cigar smoking produces blood levels of anything between 3·5 and 10 per cent at the end of a day's work (Jones and Walters, 1972). To this level should be added that due to occupational exposure.

The significance of carbon monoxide as a factor in the cause of ischaemic heart disease (IHD) is debatable. Heliovaara et al. (1978) consider that a prospective study is required. There is no doubt at all of the association between cigarette smoking and IHD. There is confirmatory evidence of the clinical observation that exposure to carbon monoxide in anginal patients produces exertional pain at earlier than the customary onset time (Knelson, 1972) and hypoxia at rest (Ayres et al., 1958).

Carbon dioxide

Carbon dioxide (CO_2) is released by fermentation and so is potentially a hazard in any activity in which fermentation may occur – bakeries, silage making, breweries. It may also be evolved in chalk pits, here being especially dangerous because its greater density may well displace oxygen. In heavy work in poorly ventilated confined spaces the level may rise concomitantly with the effort, the stimulation of the respiratory centre creating a vicious circle. CO_2 is mildy toxic and not simply an asphyxiant, although the process responsible for the evolution of the CO_2 may be equally responsible for a falling level of oxygen. It is a stimulant of the respiratory centre in low and a depressant in high concentrations. 5 per cent CO_2 in air increases ventilation threefold. Over 25 per cent may lead to death. Treatment of gross exposure is by resuscitation with oxygen.

Hydrogen sulphide

Some gases and vapours are so acutely toxic systemically that rigid controls are placed on their use. There are toxic gases, however, which can be produced in unexpected circumstances and consequently present a much greater hazard. Hydrogen sulphide (H_2S) occurs naturally in the decomposition of proteins (rotten egg smell) and can be encountered in marshes, underground workings, sewers and varying industrial processes, especially oil refineries and chemical works. A specific characteristic is that it can be detected by smell clearly at about 0·3 ppm but at increasing concentrations the odour does not become stronger and at concentrations over 200 ppm may appear to diminish as the sense of smell is fatigued. The gas is oxidized in the blood, but when the level rises to that at which the oxidation mechanisms are overtaken, rapid poisoning occurs. 700 ppm and over constitute a grave risk. The gas is an acute poison; removal to air and application of artificial respiration is effective if life is still present. Its acute effects are much the most important, but the gas may act as a chronic irritant in prolonged exposure to low concentrations and may affect the eyes severely. More details are given by Patty (1963). The TLV (UK and US) is 10 ppm.

Arsine

Arsine (AsH_3) poisoning still occurs unexpectedly. Arsine is evolved when nascent hydrogen comes into contact with an arsenical containing compound or when water comes into contact with a metallic arsenide (Buchanan, 1962). A great number of ores contain significant quantities of arsenic. The evolution of AsH_3 in metal and scrap yards may be quite unforeseen. A dilute acid dripping onto a heap of mixed scrap metals and waste ores can provide the hydrogen to combine with any arsenic impurity. Acute exposure results in increasing haemolysis of red cells, kidney damage and a toxic jaundice compounded by the haemolysis. The symptoms are those of increasing anoxaemia. The effects of chronic arsine poisoning are a garlic odour of the breath with a generalized malaise, attacks of nausea and vomiting and jaundice. Recovery is the rule – if the diagnosis is made. The treatment of acute arsine poisoning is well documented by Wilkinson et al. (1975). The essential matters are early diagnosis and removal to first-class hospital facilities. Exchange transfusion is the keystone of treatment.

CHRONIC SYSTEMIC EFFECTS

Chronic systemic effects from exposure to some gases, vapours and fumes are very well known and documented. The effect of lead fume needs no elaboration; chronic renal damage due to exposure to mercury vapour and severe emphysema after chronic cadmium fume exposure are well known. Cadmium also produces tubular dysfunction in which there is a loss of a low molecular weight protein which can be measured accurately electrophoretically or qualitatively by precipitation with salicyl-sulphonic acid. The tubular dysfunction is trivial compared with the lung disability. A general review is given by Kazantzis et al. (1963). Cadmium is a constituent of some soft solders, fume being released if the solder is overheated. Substitution is clearly the wisest solution. It is also used for metal coatings, pigments and alloys.

Vinyl chloride

The best known example of chronic systemic damage in recent times is that of vinyl chloride. Vinyl chloride monomer (VCM; $CH_2 = CHCl$) is a gas at normal temperatures. Under pressure at a temperature of between 40 and 70 °C it is easily polymerized to give polyvinyl chloride, the rate of polymerization slowing steadily so that the process is usually stopped at about 95 per cent polymerization. VCM is narcotic and explosive and these dangers have been well known and catered for since the early days of the industry. In 1971 Viola et al. reported carcinogenic effects at high dosages. Maltoni et al. confirmed cancer in animals at lower exposures in 1973. In 1974 three cases of angiosarcoma of the liver were identified at an American factory. Since that time further cases have arisen. In 1975 there were 32 reported cases world-wide (Lloyd, 1975). The effect is probably due to the vinyl free radical which up to a certain level is mopped up by available SH groups in the liver. When the dose received is greater the potential for damage is increased. The TLV of VCM was generally 200 ppm (UK and US) before its carcinogenic potential was realized: levels are now strictly monitored and controlled with zero exposure as the target. Compulsory medical screening is in force. A code of practice for vinyl chloride, obtainable from the Health and Safety Executive gives the British procedures.

In the United Kingdom, Fox and Collier have described the mortality experience (1977) in 7000 men. They found two angiosarcomas and two other liver cancers. They reserve judgement in this study since it is not yet possible to forecast future experience. Ott et al. (1975) found no liver cancers in a detailed study of a relatively small sample of exposed workers but did find an increase in deaths due to cancer among the most highly exposed employees, but fewer than expected among employees with low exposure to VCM. They suggest that high VCM exposure may have increased the susceptibility to cancer in workers already at risk due to other factors.

It is also known that VCM has been positively associated with scleroderma, and that the condition is an immune-complex vasculitis. Skin capillary abnormalities akin to those in scleroderma are described by Maricq et al. (1978). The scleroderma may be classic or may be partly manifest by Raynaud's phenomenon and/or acro-osteolysis. Scleroderma has also been described in association with other occupational exposures (Rowell, 1978). The tale of VCM is salutary in that, with hindsight, pointers to its dangers had been evident for some years earlier, and that it is chemically a reactive material. An excellent group of papers covering the whole story is contained in the *Proceedings of the Royal Society of Medicine* (1976) **4**, 275–310.

SENSITIZATION EFFECTS

Sensitizing substances are known to us all. House dust and pollens in allergic rhinitis, innumerable materials in contact dermatitis are everyday examples. In industrial practice, dermatitis is by far the commonest allergic condition encountered. *Bacillus subtilis,* utilized in the manufacture of biological detergents, has been responsible for cases of allergic lung disorders. The fume of complex platinum (Pt) salts is a strong irritant and sensitizer. Skin sensitization to the metal itself is probably not uncommon. Upper and lower respiratory symptoms due to high Pt salt fume exposures are well documented (Patty, 1963). Acute rhinitis followed by asthma and accompanied by urticaria is the most severe manifestation. Milder examples show nose and throat irritation, conjunctivitis and dermatitis. In common with many equivalent disorders the fair-skinned are more susceptible. Recovery is the rule when exposure ceases.

More recently, the vapour of the isocyanates has become widely recognized as being a sensitizer. Unlike platinum, the allergic manifestations appear in the small percentage of atopic individuals. In moderately high exposures toluene diisocyanate (TDI), which is the reference material for the group of isocyanates, is an eye, skin and gut irritant. The predominant symptom is upper respiratory tract irritation. These effects occur universally given sufficient exposure. In a few, asthma develops and those affected should not be further exposed. Since atopy appears to be a predetermining characteristic, such people should be advised not to work with TDI. Recommendations have been made for full medical control: a review of the isocyanates and recommendations for control are given in the NIOSH document, *Occupational Exposure to Toluene Diisocyanate.*

SOLVENT VAPOURS

The cleansing of metals is an integral part of modern manufacturing. In all the processes involved, gases and vapours, more or less toxic, may be evolved. Acid pickling may release toxic gases by reacting with trace impurities; the acid vapours themselves are acutely irritant. Alkali baths do not usually give rise to fume or vapour. Solvent degreasing is a ubiquitous process and may be simple, the solvent being applied by brush or the part being soaked in a cold tank. Low flash-point solvent spraying (with adequate ventilation) is also employed. Other methods include vapour degreasing, the vapour being released from the surface of a hot solvent, and immersion in or spraying with a hot solvent. The vapours of most solvents in common use are toxic in some degree: they will almost invariably give rise to unconsciousness if inhaled in sufficient quantity – this usually occurs unwittingly in relatively confined spaces when, for example, an exhaust system is faulty or a can is left open near a source of heat. Most solvents are hydrocarbons. Many hydrocarbons, whether gaseous or liquid, are narcotic to some extent, a property which is probaby related to lipid solubility (c.f. nitrogen). In addition to unconsciousness, which if undiscovered can lead to death, some solvents have more specific toxic actions.

Some solvents used widely in the past are now rarely employed. Carbon tetrachloride for example, as well as being an acute narcotic, may severely damage the liver and kidneys. This is perhaps more likely to occur in low dose chronic exposures.

Benzene

Benzene has been widely used as a solvent, but with decreasing frequency in the last 20 years. Its lingering use has been in small leather workshops, printing works and the like, more especially in remoter parts of partially industrialized countries. It is an acute narcotic in high concentrations but the effect of chronic exposure on the haemopoietic system is far more important and has been known for many years.

Benzene may be absorbed through the skin, but the most important route is by inhalation. It is distributed in the body primarily to tissues high in fat. The bone marrow especially contains high levels. Benzene is very soluble in lipids. Almost half is excreted unchanged through the lungs and the remainder is metabolized through reactive benzene epoxide (probably the myelotoxic agent) to phenylmercapturic acid. Other oxidation products may occur. Exposure can be estimated by measurement of the concentration of benzene in expired air, of the urinary phenol (Sherwood, 1972a) and of the ratio of inorganic to total urinary sulphate. The ratio of inorganic sulphate to total sulphate decreases with increasing exposure to benzene (Yant et al., 1936). Sherwood (1972b) also shows that alcohol enhances the elimination of benzene. Benzene exposure has been associated causally with blood dyscrasias, chromosomal abnormality and an excess risk of leukaemia. It is probably true to say that blood dyscrasias and leukaemias are associated with high levels of exposure usually for some years: there may be a gradient from anaemia to leukaemia depending on time and dose. There is a mass of literature on the subject: a good general review has been made by Browning (1965) and Henschler and his committee (1975) have gathered an impressive body of material. NIOSH published a criteria document in the USA in 1976 providing copious references and recommending a TLV (time weighted average, TWA) of 1 ppm. The current TLV in other countries varies up to 25 ppm. Whatever TLV may be finally agreed upon, it is quite clear that benzene should not be used except under strictly controlled conditions. There is simply no place for it as a solvent in the usual sense; there are adequate substitutes. As a chemical feed-stock it is invaluable and in these large-scale operations exposure is carefully controlled.

Industrial solvents

The commoner solvents now employed are trichloroethylene (current TLV: US and UK = 100 ppm; in Sweden = 30 ppm), perchloroethylene (tetrachloroethylene) (current TLV: US and UK = 100 ppm) and 1, 1, 1, trichloroethane (methyl chloroform) (current TLV: US and UK = 350 ppm). They all decompose when overheated to form hydrochloric acid and variable amounts of phosgene. The chlorinated hydrocarbon solvents, with the exception of perchloroethylene, have been incriminated rarely in cases of sudden death, possibly due to cardiac arrythmias. Given sufficient exposure, they are all narcotic and all have the propensity to cause liver damage. 1,1,1, trichloroethane is the least hepatotoxic of the common solvents and probably the most inert, 98 per cent being excreted in the breath (Hake et al., 1960). Its metabolic pathway produces CO which of course compounds any narcotic effect. There are innumerable studies of behavioural effects during exposure to chlorinated hydrocarbon solvents. In brief, these effects are of a steadily increasing incompetence of mental and physical ability culminating in unconsciousness at extremely high levels of exposure.

Trichloroethylene

Trichloroethylene (Tric - Trilene - TRI) is probably the most widely used and studied solvent. It is easily absorbed through the skin, but most commonly through the lungs. Recently Astrand and Ovrum (1976) have described the uptake and distribution in the body. They found that the arteriolar concentration increases linearly with the concentration in alveolar air. The uptake is about 55 per cent of that supplied at rest, but the higher the work rate the lower percentage uptake occurs, probably due to the relatively low solubility of TRI in blood and tissue.

TRI is metabolized in the body to chloral hydrate and then to trichloroethanol (TCE) and trichloroacetic acid (TCA). Vesterberg et al. (1976) have investigated the metabolites in a study involving 15 subjects. TCE is mostly converted to the corresponding gluconuride, while TCA is excreted directly. The relationship between TCA in urine and TRI levels in the air has been used widely to estimate TRI exposure: commonly 100 mg/litre TCA is said to equate with 100 ppm TRI in air. Vesterberg et al. (1976) show that TCA accumulates with continued exposure over several days and does not therefore accurately reflect recent exposure. They consider TCE the most important metabolite because of its effect on the CNS. They find that the concentration of TCE in blood after the beginning of exposure and for at least two hours is maintained at a constant level. Droz and Fernandez (1978) argue cogently for a method of biological monitoring by measuring TCE in the urine or TRI in the alveolar air before and after exposure.

Gamberale et al. (1976) tested subjects individually on three separate occasions during exposure for 70 minutes to 100 and 200 ppm levels of TRI and under control conditions. Alveolar air samples were also taken. Reaction time or short-term memory tests were not affected. Numerical ability tests were significantly reduced.

Testing for carcinogenicity has been performed by the National Cancer Institute, US Department of Health and Welfare (NCA, 1976). Commercial TRI was given orally to rats and mice, five times a week for 78 weeks, average doses being about 550 mg/kg and 110 mg/kg for two sets of male and female rats and 1170 and 2340, and 870 and 1740 mg/kg for sets of male and female mice respectively. Signs of toxicity became clear in the rats. Neoplasms were observed but no significant difference between those occurring in TRI-treated and control animals were established. Hepatocellular carcinomas were found in male and female TRI-treated mice. The differences between these and controls were highly significant especially among male mice. (Carbon tetrachloride, used as a positive control, produced hepatocellular carcinomas in virtually all mice.) This study therefore shows that large doses of TRI given orally daily will produce a significant number of liver cancers in specific strains of mice. A long-term inhalation study is currently proceeding in the US; the results are awaited with interest.

WELDING

Process considerations

In modern industrial practice welding is a basic process, as important to the fabrication of metal structures as stitching is to cloth. In welding, heat is applied to the edges of two pieces of metal with or without pressure, in order to join them (plastics can be similarly welded). Cutting is the reverse process. Sister processes include brazing and soldering. In brazing, a join is made between two pieces of metal, a filler metal with a melting point (m.p.) below that of the pieces, but over 500 °C, being drawn into the join by capillary action. Soldering is similar, but the filler has a m.p. below 500 °C. The commonest heat sources are a fuel gas plus oxygen or an electric arc struck between an electrode and the work piece. Most welding is carried out by the electric arc process. In order to prevent oxidation of the molten weld, the arc is shielded by an inert gas (CO_2 or argon) either supplied directly, or produced by a flux which covers the filler electrode itself, releasing CO_2 and forming a shielding slag. Welding electrodes are either consumable (they melt and play an integral part in the welding process) or non-consumable (when a filler rod is additionally used to help produce the weld).

There are many welding and allied processes for specific applications: hot metal spraying, stud welding, plasma-arc welding (rapid flow ionized gas giving very high temperatures and producing high levels of noise), methods which utilize electrical resistance, electron beams, thermit welding (heat produced by exothermic reaction of aluminium powder and a metal oxide). A description of these and others is provided by Challen (1965).

The metals melt, vapourize and condense to produce metallic oxide fume; gases are evolved by chemical change in the immediate atmosphere. The work piece may be coated with a pigment or resin. Steel (1964) has reviewed the hazards resulting from thermal decomposition of coatings and compared laboratory results with field investigations. The hazardous pigments are those containing cadmium, chromium and lead. Zinc is well known to cause metal fume fever in high concentrations but there are no lasting sequelae. Cadmium fume has certainly been an acute cause of death (*see* Ch. 2). Resins (PVC, epoxy, acrylic, polyurethane, polystyrene and others) produce a variety of toxic decomposition products including hydrochloric acid, phosgene, hydrogen cyanide and diisocyanate. Electrodes themselves may contain fluorides and manganese; special electrodes for stainless and other special steels may contain nickel and/or chromium; copper, zinc and vanadium may also be present.

General hazards

The major risks in welding are the simple and obvious ones – fire, explosion and electrocution – and safety measures to minimize these should be understood. Details of safety measures are given by Challen (1965) and in detail in the American Welding Society booklet, *Safety in Welding and Cutting* (1975). Hazards apart from those due to gas and fume are given briefly here. The heat source may produce skin pigmentation and metal droplets may give rise to burns. Infra-red and ultraviolet radiation is produced. Infra-red radiation has not been shown to be a factor in the production of cataracts in welders. Ultraviolet radiation causes a painful and disabling kerato-conjunctivitis in the unprotected eye which is happily short-lived. Arc welding provides the highest risk. UV light is reflected easily and non-reflective UV-absorbent screens should be placed around welding bays to avoid eye injury to other workers. Protective filters must be used; various countries produce their own specifications: in the United Kingdom these are given in British Standard 679. BS 1542 gives dimensions for goggles, helmets and handshields. Someren and Rollason (1948) conclude in a detailed study that protective filters have a considerable safety margin.

Solvent vapours can break down in the presence of heat and UV light, chlorinated hydrocarbons producing the highly dangerous gas phosgene. Preventive measures are clear – no vapours should be present where welding is carried out.

A survey in British shipyards (DEP, 1970) showed that in open workshop conditions, ventilation was needed when zinc-coated metal was worked and in order to reduce ozone levels in argon arc welding of aluminium. In semi-confined spaces, extract ventilation was needed. In closely confined spaces, self-contained breathing apparatus was necessary. Steel (1968) has comprehensively reviewed the respiratory hazards in shipbuilding and assessed the severity of health risks and discussed methods of hazard control. Oliver and Molyneux (1975) have described methods of evaluating risk in detail, including epidemiological data and biological monitoring. They emphasize the need to define clearly both the limits of risk and the ventilation requirements for a given situation. They cite the example shown by Oliver and Sanderson (1973) of the very high rate of extraction needed in air-arc gouging.

Hazardous gases

The fuel gas and oxygen flame process yields CO_2 with normal combustion, CO (TLV: US and UK = 50 ppm) with reduced combustion and nitrogen oxides (TLV: US and UK = 5 ppm) with excess oxygen. CO can also be produced in the CO_2 shielded arc processes. Some nitrogen oxides are also evolved in arc welding. Ozone (TLV: US and UK = 0·1 ppm) is produced by the interaction of UV with oxygen. The argon-shielded processes give rise to more ozone than others.

The logical method of preventing generation of ozone is to shield the arc from the surrounding atmosphere with material opaque to UV; this is not, however, always practical. Lunau (1967) has found levels of ozone of 0·47 ppm in welders' breathing zones during bare-wire argon shielded welding of aluminium and considers methods of protection and exhaust ventilation. In particular he finds that general horizontal ventilation is a less effective remedy than general upward or downward ventilation. He has also found that ozone levels diminish with time, given a constant arc, and that the ozone concentration rapidly decreases as the distance from the arc increases; the variables are too great for a mathematical formula to be reached.

Ozone and the nitrogen oxides are lung irritants and can cause an acute, often somewhat delayed pulmonary oedema if inhaled in sufficient quantity. Ozone is lethal at a few ppm in a few hours (Stokinger, 1957) and produces chronic bronchitis in animals exposed for 6 hours daily for a year to just over 1 ppm (Stokinger et al., 1957). Scheel et al. (1959) and several other investigators have shown that exposure to 2–4 ppm ozone for several hours results in pulmonary oedema, damage to alveoli, and depression of enzyme activity in the lung. Pulmonary congestion was found by Challen et al. (1958) in welders exposed to under 2 ppm which vanished at levels of 0·2 ppm.

Mustafa and Lee (1976) suggest that low concentrations of ozone (below 0·8 ppm) cause metabolic lung disturbances and that vitamin E, a natural antioxidant, offers some protection. Pierce et al. (1976) have shown that the increased glucose–6–phosphate dehydrogenase (G6PD) activity due to cigarette smoke exposure in rats is decreased by exposure to ozone; G6PD activity in non-exposed rats is depressed. All this work indicates that ozone has a profound effect on the lung homeostatic systems. It is interesting that vitamin E, so long considered to be of no great importance, is here shown to play a specific role.

Chronic lung effects

Prolonged exposure to welding fume leads to changes in X-ray films due to deposits of iron in the lungs. Doig and McLaughlin (1938, 1948) considered these deposits inert. Doig and Challen (1964) still believed this to be largely the case but noted the findings of Harding et al. (1958) of pathological fibrotic changes in three of five welders.

150 welders with matched controls were the subject of a comprehensive investigation in Denmark (*Welding in the World,* 1972). A clinical examination was supported by estimations of Hb, ESR, blood lead and blood CO. The eyes were examined in detail and chest films and lung function tests were performed. There was no statistically significant difference in lung function test results. Symptoms of bronchitis were increased in welders who smoked, compared both with non-smoking welders and with smoking controls. Lange et al. (1977) examined a total of 183 arc welders. Serum electrophoretic fractions and immunoglobulin levels were compared between groups of arc welders with long and short occupational exposures as well as between groups with an without pulmonary lesions. No significant difference between mean values of IgG and IgM were found. Welders with years of occupational exposure had, by and large, significantly higher IgA levels than those found both in welders with shorter occupational experience and in controls. Lower IgA levels were found in welders with

silicosiderosis and lung function impairment. Lange et al. (1977) suggest that the higher levels of IgA reflect adaptation to chronic irritation of the bronchial linings. Kagan et al. (1975) had previously described lower IgA levels in patients with recurrent chest infections than among normal subjects.

Current research

Refined methods of tracing the fate of fume particulates are now being used: Hewitt et al. (1975) have introduced radioactively labelled fume into the lungs of experimental animals and have described the distribution and fate of the particles. Electron micro probe analysis of particulate material found in lung biopsy tissue of two welders, one with severe, the other with moderate lung fibrosis, was compared by Stettler et al. (1977) with air samples from the working environment. The composition of the majority of the particles found in the lung tissue was akin to that of the samples. The authors conclude that the source of most of the particles was in the working environment.

There is increasing interest in the role of metals within fume and especially whether chromium and nickel have carcinogenic effects in this form. There is of course a wealth of data on the hazards of nickel and hexavalent chromium, but studies have so far concentrated on workers engaged in specific industries.

There is also the problem of whether sensitivity to elements in the fume can develop. It has been demonstrated that in sensitized animals, exposure to fume containing the allergen results in an explosive hypersensitivity reaction (Hewitt, 1977). In man, however, it seems that acute hypersensitivity reactions to fume do not occur, otherwise they would have been reported. It is uncertain whether or not chronic allergic reactions take place.

The chemistry and kinetics of fume production and reaction are far more complex than would seem at first sight. In the conditions of the welding process, the boiling points, vapour pressures and physical and chemical characteristics of metals in what amount to fluid mixtures are affected by the components of the mixture. Intermediate reactions occur which may not be forecast theoretically. The time scale for reactions in these small infernos is measured in milliseconds and so the techniques of analysis are complicated. Work is currently being undertaken to provide models for these reactions under different conditions (Hewitt, 1977).

Occupational risk

Gas and electric welders, cutters and braziers form Unit 3b of the occupation groups in the Registrar-General's periodical mortality surveys for England and Wales. The standardized mortality ratio (SMR) for this group was high at 122 for the years 1970–72 (Registrar-General, 1978). Pneumonia has been a prominent diagnosis in the past and the SMR for this condition based on deaths in 1949–53 was 226, in 1959–63 was 184 and in 1970–72 was 157. The comment is made that the group as a whole may be exposed to variable fumes. The SMR for cancer of the lung is 151: other groups with high SMR's for this condition are sheet metal workers, metal plate workers, foundry moulders, other metal and electrical process workers, food processors, bricklayers, plasterers, construction workers, paint sprayers, boiler firemen, drivers, stevedores, delivery roundsmen; there is a pattern in some but not so clearly in others. Mortality figures, of course, deal with the past and one would dearly like to have accurately projected figures for the future – an obvious impossibility. Welders are clearly at some risk, but acute injury is probably now quite rare. As in many cases today, it is the chronic hazard that causes concern. There is no doubt that in the next two decades the mechanisms of lung damage, occurring perhaps in only a small number of susceptible subjects, will be made plain. Hopefully, the subjects of clinical investigations will become rapidly fewer in number as better control of fume and gas levels is achieved in the workplace. If the causes are removed, then nobody needs examining, because there is nothing to find.

The future looks hopeful. The directions in which advances are already being made include:

1. Detailed physio-chemical work on the production of fume constituents.
2. Further elaboration of elemental and compound particulate absorption, distribution and excretion.
3. Genetic, immunological and biochemical studies linked with clinical and epidemiological investigations.

It is likely that a combination of epidemiological and biophysical data will reveal damaging effects to life that we had not suspected. In an age when butter and hard water are considered by many to be factors in the genesis of one of the greatest epidemics of history – the coronary disasters affecting the middle-aged industrialized male – who knows what factor may lurk in the factories of industry all over the world? Acute events are understood. Unexpected disasters will occasionally occur. Further long-term risks will unfold themselves. We can prevent some of those risks even if we do not know them by substituting a potentially damaging material for one less harmful, and by sound engineering and ventilation practice. We cannot, unfortunately, prevent the progress of damage which may already have taken place; we must be wary of over-reacting to evidence of chronic harm done to people in circumstances which no longer apply. If drinking water may be a factor in an early death, then an adjustment to the water supply will only prove itself in 20 years. We must encourage the creation of a decent environment in which to work so that anyone can say, 'It's OK. It's a good place to work.'

REFERENCES

Atkinson A., Rutter D. A. and Sargeant K. (1974) *Lancet* **2,** 1446.

American Welding Society (1973) *Safety in Welding and Cutting.* Miami, Florida, American Welding Society.

Astrand I. and Ovrum P. (1976) *Scand. J. Work Environ. Health* **4,** 199–221.

Ayres S. M., Mueller H. S., Gregory J. J. et al. (1969) *Arch. Environ. Health* **18,** 699–704.

Best C. H. and Taylor N. B. (1966) *The Physiological Basis of Medical Practice,* 8th ed. Baltimore, Williams & Wilkins.

Browning E. (1965) *Toxicology and Metabolism of Industrial Solvents.* Amsterdam, Elsevier.

Buchanan W. D. (1962) *Toxicity of Arsenic Compounds.* Amsterdam, Elsevier.

Challen P. J. R., Hickish D. E. and Bedford J. (1958) *Br. J. Ind. Med.* **15,** 276.

Challen P. J. R. (1965) *Health and Safety in Welding and Allied Processes.* Cambridge, England, The Institute of Welding.

Chvapil M. and Peng Y. M. (1975) *Arch. Environ. Health* **30,** 528.

Coffin D. L. and Gardner D. E. (1972) *Ann. Occup. Hyg.* **15,** 219–234.

Coffin D. L., Blommer E. J., Gardner D. E. et al. (1967) *Proceedings of 3rd Annual Conference on Atmospheric Contamination in Confined Space,* Dayton, Ohio. 71–80.

Cousteau J. Y. (1954) *The Silent World.* London, Hamish Hamilton.

Cordier J. M., Fievez C., Lefevre M. J. et al. (1966) *Cah. Med. Travail* **4,** 6.

DEP (1970) *Fumes from Welding and Flame Cutting.* London, H.M.S.O.

Donald K. W. (1947) *Br. Med. J.* **1,** 172.

Droz P. O. and Fernandez J. G. (1978) *Br. J. Ind. Med.* **35,** 35–42.

Ducatman A., Hirchhorn K. and Selikoff I. J. (1975) *Mutat. Res.* **31,** 163.

Ebert M., Hornsey S. and Howard A. (1958) *Nature* **181,** 613.

Ehrlich R. (1966) *Bacteriol. Rev.* **30,** 610–614.

Fairchild G. A., Roan J. and McCarroll J. (1972) *Arch. Environ. Health* **25,** 174–182.

Fox A. J. and Collier P. F. (1977) *Br. J. Ind. Med.* **34,** 1–10.

Funes-Crairoto F., Lambert B., Linsten J. et al. (1975) *Lancet* **1,** 459.

Gamberale F., Annwall G. and Olson B. A. (1976) *Scand. J. Work Environ. Health* **4,** 220–224.

Hake C. L., Waggoner T. B., Robertson D. N. et al. (1960) *Arch. Environ. Health* **1,** 101.

Heliovaraa M., Karvonen M. J. Vilkunen R. et al. (1978) *Br. Med. J.* **1,** 268–272.

Henschler D. (1975) *Considerations bearing on the question of safe concentrations of benzene in the work environment* (Mak-Wert) – Communication of the Working Group. Boppard, Bolt.

Hewitt P. J. (1975) Personal communication.

Hewitt P. J. (1977) Personal communication.

Jones J. G. and Walters D. H. (1962) *Ann. Occup. Hyg.* **5,** 221–230.

Kagan E., Soskolne C. L., Zvi S. et al. (1975) *Am. Rev. Respir. Dis.* **111,** 441–451.

Kazantzis G. (1963) *Q. J. Med.* **32,** 126.

Knelson J. H. (1972) *Cardiovascular Effects during Low Level CO Exposure,* Paper presented to the Committee on Motor Vehicle Emission, NAS-NRC, Washington, D.C.

Lange A., Smolik R., Zatonski W. et al. (1977) *Int. Arch. Occup. Environ. Health* **38,** 189–196.

Lloyd J. W. (1975) *J. Occup. Med.* **17,** 333–334.

Maltoni C., Crespi M. and Burch P. L. R. (1973) *Excerpta Med. Int. Congr. Ser.* 275.

Maricq H. R., Darke C. S., Archibald R. Mcl. et al. (1978) *Br. J. Ind. Med.* **35,** 1–7.

Meyer H. H. (1899) Zur Theorie der Alkoholnarkose, *Arch. Exp. Pathol. J. Pharmakol.* **12,** 109.

Miles S. (1969) *Underwater Medicine.* London, Staples.

Mustafa M. G. and Lee St Duk (1976) *Ann. Occup. Hyg.* **19**, 17–26.

National Cancer Institute, *Technical Report Series No: 2,* February 1976. *Carcinogenesis Bioassay of Trichloroethylene.*

NIOSH (1973) *Occupational Exposure to Toluene Diisocyanate.* US Department of Health, Education and Welfare.

Oliver T. P. and Molyneux M. K. B. (1975) *Ann. Occup. Hyg.* **17**, 293–302.

Ott M. G., Langner R. R. and Holder B. B. (1975) *Arch. Environ. Health* **30**, 333–339.

Patty F. F. (1963) *Industrial Hygiene and Toxicology: 2, Toxicology.* New York, Interscience.

Pierce T. H., York G. K., Franti C. E. et al. (1976) *Arch. Environ. Health* **31**, 290–2.

Purchase I. F. H., Richardson C. R. and Anderson D. (1975) *Lancet* **2**, 410.

Purchase I. F. H., Richardson C. R. and Anderson D. (1976) *Proc. R. Soc. Med.* **69**, 290–292.

Registrar-General (1978) *Occupational Mortality, Decennial Supplement 1970–72,* London, H.M.S.O.

Report on a Danish Investigation into the Health and Working Environment of Arc Welders (1972) *Welding in the World.* vol 10, 100–112.

Rowell N. (1977) *Practitioner* **219**, 824.

Scheel L. D., Dobrogorski O. J., Mountain J. T. et al. (1959) *J. Appl. Physiol.* **14**, 67–80.

Schwab R. S. and England A. C. (1968) *Diseases of the Basal Ganglia, Handbook of Clinical Neurology,* **6**, New York, Wiley, pp. 225–247.

Sherwood R. J. (1972) *Br. J. Ind. Med.* **29**, 65.

Sollman T. (1944) *A Manual of Pharmacology,* 6th ed. Philadelphia, Saunders.

Spurgash A., Ehrlich R. and Petzold R. (1968) *Arch. Environ. Health* **16**, 385–391.

Steel J. (1964) *Ann. Occup. Hyg.* **7**, 247–252.

Steel J. (1968) *Ann. Occup. Hyg.* **11**, 115–121.

Stettler L. E., Groth D. H. and MacKay G. R. (1977) *Am. Ind. Hyg. Assoc. J.* **38**, 76–82.

Stewart R. D. et al. (1970) *Arch. Environ. Hlth.* **21**, 154–164.

Stokinger H. E. (1957) *Arch. Ind. Health* **15**, 181.

Stokinger H. E. (1965) *Arch. Environ. Health* **10**, 719.

Stokinger H. E., Wagner W. D. and Dobrogorski O. J. (1957) *Arch. Ind. Health* **16**, 514.

Van Somern E. and Rollason E. C. (1948) *Trans. Inst. Welding,* June issue.

Vesterberg O., Gorczak J. and Krasts M. (1976) *Scand. J. Work Environ. Health* **4**, 212–219.

Viola P. L., Bigotti A. and Caputo A. (1971) *Cancer Res.* **31**, 516.

Wilkinson S. P., McHugh P., Horsley S. et al. (1975) *Br. Med. J.* **3**, 559–563.

Williamson K. S. (1976) *Proc. R. Soc. Med* **69**, 281–303.

Wilson R. H., McCormick W. E., Tatum C. F. et al. (1967) *J. Am. Med. Assoc.* **201**, 577.

Yant W. P., Schrenk H. H. and Patty F. A. (1936) *J. Ind. Hyg.* **18**, 349.

4. CLINICAL AND BIOCHEMICAL MONITORING OF BENZENE WORKERS

J. T. Carter

The investigation of clinical and biochemical changes in workers exposed to benzene can provide valuable information about benzene exposure levels and their biological consequences. Clinical techniques may also be used in an attempt to ensure that individuals at excess risk from the effects of benzene are not exposed.

EVALUATION OF EXPOSURE

A valid technique for estimating the exposure of an individual or groups of individuals to benzene must be sensitive enough to detect changes at the level of exposure under investigation. In addition the changes must be specific to benzene exposure and not caused by other agents. For a method to be suitable for regular use it should be acceptable to those tested; that is, free from uncomfortable or embarrassing procedures and economically feasible.

Analytical methods must be reproducible, unbiased and precise. Clearly, no method can meet all these requirements and different methods may be appropriate under differing conditions of exposure.

URINARY PHENOL

Benzene is partially metabolized to phenol which is excreted conjugated to sulphates or glucuronates in the urine (Hunter, 1972). The phenol concentration can be estimated by gas chromatography (Van Haaften, 1965) after hydrolysis of the conjugates. Phenol conjugates are excreted in declining quantities for about 48 hours after an episode of benzene exposure (Docter, 1967).

Validity

The analytical technique is sensitive enough to detect low concentrations (*circa* 1 ppm) of phenol in urine. Its use is limited by lack of specificity.

There are sources of phenol in the diet and a number of medications may break down to phenol. Hence a variable amount of phenol is found in the urine of non-benzene-exposed individuals (Fishbeck, 1975). Attempts to minimize interference by subtraction of a baseline value have been made but the marked fluctuations on non-occupational phenol excretion limit the value of a pre-exposure estimate. One recent study indicated that correlation with exposure is not improved by baseline subtraction (Roush, 1977). In practice exposure levels of less than 10 ppm – 8-hour time weighted average (TWA) – do not show up clearly in individual samples.

Acceptability

There are few problems in obtaining single untimed urine samples at the start and at the end of a period of exposure. The rate of urine production will affect urinary phenol concentrations and a number of correction factors have been applied. The most widely used are a correction to a standard urine specific gravity or a correction expressing phenol excretion per gram of creatinine excreted.

Estimation of phenol excretion over a timed interval of up to 24 hours could increase the accuracy of the estimate of excretion rate but this presents problems in an industrial setting as sample bottles must be taken home and returned the following day.

Exposure/concentration relationships

There is a linear relationship between exposure and phenol concentration (Van Haaften, 1965). Background concentrations are variable, but average less than 10 mg/1.

Discussion

Urinary phenol measurements are an effective method of estimating exposure to benzene at ambient concentrations in excess of 10 ppm 8-hour TWA. They may be of some use when results from large groups of employees are analysed at lower ambient concentrations as a measure of the efficiency with which contamination is controlled. Individual high results are difficult to interpret as they may not be occupational in origin.

To be an effective monitoring tool group mean values must be regularly produced and time trends used as a measure of group exposure.

Individual high results will require investigation to establish whether they are attributable to benzene exposure. A scheme of sampling at regular intervals may fail to detect short periods of high exposure. Effort could usefully be directed at the detailed biological monitoring of specific operations and occupations. Where several shifts perform similar operations, sampling one shift each week can be used to provide early information on failures in environmental control.

The validity of urinary phenol measurement is limited by non-occupational sources of phenol and by variables affecting the renal handling of phenol conjugates. Detailed investigation of these factors might allow some marginal improvements in the method, particularly by defining the optimum interval between paired samples and examining the best methods of correction for urinary flow. It is unlikely that the method can be developed to be of use in estimating individual exposures much below 10 ppm.

EXPIRED AIR BENZENE CONCENTRATIONS

Some 12 per cent of absorbed benzene is expired unchanged (Hunter, 1972). Excretion of benzene by this route is rapid, with a two phased exponential decline in excretion, with half times of 2·5 hours for the major component and 1 day for a smaller part (Sherwood, 1972). For this reason expired air benzene concentration will predominantly reflect exposure in the few hours prior to sampling.

Sensitivity

Benzene may be detected in breath at concentrations as low as 0·0025 ppm (Gayl, 1977.)

Specificity

Occupational exposure to benzene is likely to be the major contribution to the expired air benzene concentrations but the widespread occurrence of low concentrations of benzene in and around cars, particularly during fuelling, could seriously bias results collected to estimate exposures on the previous work shift. Sampling several hours after the last exposure would be the preferred method of examination, in the absence of non-occupational exposure, as a sample taken immediately after the end of a shift will reflect exposure in the last few hours of the exposure period rather than the average throughout the shift.

Acceptability

There should be few problems in collecting expired air benzene samples provided employees are assured that breath alcohol levels are not being measured.

Discussion

Improved techniques of analysis have increased the sensitivity of expired air benzene monitoring. Drawbacks to its widespread use are a lack of experience with the method, other than as a research tool, and the bias to very recent exposure caused by the rapid decline in expired air benzene concentrations. As a periodic investigation in exposed workers pre-shift samples reflecting exposure in the previous shift are likely to be the preferred method. These could be used in conjunction with an end of shift screen to identify those with any significant exposure in need of follow-up.

Expired air measurement would be well suited to the investigations of exposure during specific operating procedures. The high sensitivity and short duration of effect could be used to great advantage.

A programme of further development of this method at a production site is required.

BLOOD BENZENE CONCENTRATION

Methods are available for estimating benzene levels in tissues (Snyder, 1977). Their use on blood or other tissue samples is unlikely to offer any advantages compared with expired air estimation and will be far less acceptable in an industrial setting. It will not be considered in any detail.

FUTURE DEVELOPMENTS

Further refinement of urinary phenol estimation as a measure of benzene exposure does not seem likely. The use of expired air measurement could be developed for use at levels of exposure of the order of 1 ppm, but a trial of the method at an industrial location will be needed before the technique can be endorsed.

Scope for the development of other monitoring techniques is limited by the common metabolic pathways of benzene and other compounds present in the diet. Further investigation of the quantitative excretion rates of metabolites could be undertaken.

EVALUATION OF BIOLOGICAL RESPONSES

Exposure to high concentrations of benzene causes toxic effects. If sufficiently sensitive methods are available, biological responses to benzene exposure may be measured and used either as means for estimating exposure or as screening tests for subclinical disease.

When used for estimating exposure the criteria for a valid method will be similar to those already noted. When used for screening for early disease a number of additional problems arise.

If the change detected is reversible on cessation of exposure, the test may be used to indicate the need to remove the individual from exposure or to control exposure more effectively. If the change indicates the presence of the early stages of a treatable disease then appropriate treatment can be instituted. If, however, it is not possible to alter the natural history of the disease process, the use of a screening process cannot be justified, except as part of a scientific study. The consequences for the individual must always be considered before any investigation is undertaken which may detect abnormalities which are of uncertain significance or not amenable to treatment.

BLOOD COUNTS

The most important long-term effect of exposure to high levels of benzene is damage to the bone marrow, usually presenting as an aplastic anaemia or leukopenia, which may often be reversed by removal from exposure. Lower levels of exposure could be expected to produce less severe effects which could be used both to monitor exposure and to detect individuals at risk of serious haematological effects (Jandle, 1977).

Validity

Both the sensitivity and specificity of this method of surveillance are limited by the marked temporal fluctuations in blood cell counts induced by infection, nutrition and blood loss (Sanders, 1968). For this reason it is unlikely that blood counts could be of any use for monitoring exposures of less than 20 ppm 8-hour TWA and even at this level a considerable number of false positives would require follow-up.

The value of blood counts as a screening test for early disease is less readily evaluated. The detection of bone marrow depression – a reversible change – at an early stage would be valuable. The detection of acute myelogenous leukaemia less so, as the prognosis cannot be significantly improved by treatment. The screening value of the test might be further evaluated by the analyses of a large body of test data. As there are no reports of severe bone marrow depression at concentrations of benzene similar to current operating levels it is unlikely to be of great value.

Acceptability

A blood sample, either capillary or venous must be taken. This requires co-operation, but provided the frequency of examination is not excessive it is usually accepted by employees, if the need for the test can be demonstrated.

Discussion

The regular examination of blood counts using the standard criteria of abnormality is of limited value in the surveillance of benzene workers. A better case could be made for an initial examination prior to employment, as a means of ensuring that there are no gross abnormalities, which could later be attributed to benzene exposure. Any initial sample should not be considered as a static pre-exposure value to be used in subsequent comparisons because of the inherent variability with time.

A recent report (Reuvers, 1977) has suggested that examination of the lymphocyte/neutrophil ratio may be of use in monitoring the early effects of benzene exposure, with a relative lymphocytosis as evidence of exposure. Unfortunately viral lymphocytosis and bacterial neutrophil leucocytosis will render the changes non-specific. This method requires nevertheless further evaluation.

CHROMOSOME DAMAGE

A number of reports (Wolman, 1977) have shown an excess of chromosomal abnormalities in benzene-exposed workers. The changes seen have not been specific to benzene exposure and it is not possible to assess their significance in terms of disease causation. All have included individuals with relatively high levels of exposure.

Validity

Chromosome abnormalities vary greatly in frequency between individuals, hence studies of groups of exposed workers would be required to use this method for exposure evaluation. Uncertainty about the significance of any changes found makes the technique useless for clinical screening.

There is insufficient evidence available to allow the dose response relationship of this technique to be derived.

Acceptability
Chromosome examination requires a venous blood sample. Preparation and examination of a single sample takes approximately one man/day.

Discussion
This technique requires further evaluation of both dose response relationships and the significance of observed changes, before it can be of any use in surveillance. The method is unlikely to become anything other than a research tool unless the examination of preparations can be made less labour intensive.

CLINICAL STUDIES

There are no methods of clinical investigation, other than blood examination which will be of value in detecting the long-term effects of benzene exposure at an early stage. Hence it is not possible to justify any routine clinical examination procedures or investigations over and above those provided for non-exposed employees.

Nevertheless mechanisms should be available to ensure that any benzene-exposed worker who develops anaemia or other blood disease is fully investigated to ascertain whether benzene exposure could have been responsible for his illness. For current employees this information could be obtained by a continuing review of absences, at periodic medical examinations performed for other reasons, or by informing employees and local practitioners of the need for this information. None of these methods is likely to provide full data.

FUTURE DEVELOPMENTS

Further evaluation of the use of differential white cell counts in the monitoring of exposure and as a means of screening for reversible disease is required. Chromosome studies offer little immediate promise as a routine screening method.

It is possible that fundamental studies of the effects of benzene on the bone marrow may indicate biochemical or cytological changes which occur at low exposure levels. The value of clinical studies as measures of exposure must be compared with the biological monitoring and environmental assessments of exposure. It is most unlikely that they will provide such an accurate assessment because of the variation in individual response to both benzene and other unrelated environmental factors.

Clinical studies will be of value in disease screening if exposures are high enough to cause reversible disease or pre-disease states. There is no evidence that current exposure levels cause detectable changes, hence the benefits from screening are unlikely to be great and considerable anxiety may be caused to individuals who require further investigation after false positive results.

THE SELECTION OF EMPLOYEES FOR WORK WITH BENZENE

The prime aim of medical selection prior to employment is the identification of those individuals who may be considered at excess risk from exposure to benzene.

There is no published evidence indicating that any group of individuals are at excess risk from benzene exposure and with increasing concern about the discriminatory effects of pre-employment medical examination, it may be difficult to justify exclusion on any grounds other than a history of bone marrow disease. At some stage in the recruitment procedure an assessment of the individual's ability and willingness to work within a defined code of operating instructions designed to minimize exposure should, however, be made.

The examination should follow current practice at the employing location with specific questioning about any history of blood disease and in addition a full blood count may be included to detect any gross abnormalities which should be investigated prior to employment. It is important to ensure that employees are aware of the hazards of benzene and the precautions required for safe handling. Some aspects of this training may take place during the medical examination.

For administrative purposes a defined group of 'Benzene workers' will be required. All transfers to this group, both by recruitment externally and internal movement, should pass through a similar medical selection process.

THE REGULAR SURVEILLANCE OF BENZENE WORKERS

The nature and frequency of surveillance will depend on the pattern of exposure. Information on exposure may be obtained from environmental and biological monitoring results (*Table* 4.1).

There are no indications for any specific clinical examinations. Periodic blood counts may have some value in detecting early changes in those who are exposed to levels above currently accepted standards but will yield little useful information at 10 ppm TWA unless the value of differential counts is confirmed and the interference produced by infection is shown not to be a problem.

Urinary phenol monitoring reaches its useful limit at between 5 and 10 ppm TWA and so will remain useful at currently acceptable concentrations. The method is unlikely to be of use if TWA concentrations are below 5 ppm, although examination of results from large groups of uniformly exposed employees may be used to estimate lower exposures. It is of interest that German legislation uses a group mean urinary phenol value as one of the criteria for defining benzene exposure. 'No exposure is deemed to exist where the urine of at least 95 per cent of the workers exposed contains less phenol than 20 mg/l'.

The use of expired air benzene concentrations as a monitoring tool at low concentrations requires further investigation. It may be particularly valuable as a way of evaluating short-term exposures during operating and maintenance procedures.

The frequency of any blood count examinations should be governed by the time taken for severe marrow depression to develop. This may occur in

Table 4.1 Suggested routine for biological monitoring.

1. Estimate 8-hour time weighted average exposure by personal sampling for each occupational group.

Exposure		
	> 10 ppm	–2, 3
< 10 ppm	> 5 ppm	–2, 3 optional 4 optional
< 5 ppm	> 1 ppm	–2 optional 4 optional
	< 1 ppm	–4 optional

2. Monthly urinary phenol estimations. Detailed investigation of values in excess of 50mg/l. Maintain records of individual and group time trends.

3. Six monthly blood counts with investigation of abnormalities. Removal of those with significant abnormalities from exposure.

4. Monthly breath benzene levels (after validity of technique has been investigated) performed 16 hours after last occupational exposure. Maintain records of individual and group time trends.

the course of one to two weeks and sampling with this frequency is rarely practicable.

In practice blood counts are done at longer intervals – often every 6 months – although some authorities have suggested a greater frequency for new employees (Jandle, 1977). The prime motive behind testing at current exposure levels would appear to be the reassurance given by repeated values in the normal range. Hence any decision to initiate a programme of regular blood counts should only be taken after considering the very low probability of detecting benzene related disease at currently accepted levels of exposure.

Urinary phenol examinations are used to estimate individual or group exposure to benzene. The frequency of examination required to estimate exposure will depend on the number of exposed persons, the variability of exposure levels and the change in exposure which needs to be detected for medical or environmental control action to be taken.

In practice the frequency is often determined by the rota of shift work and rest days and monthly examinations are commonly used. As exposure in the 48 hours prior to sampling is reflected in the results every episode of over-exposure will not be recorded.

THE INVESTIGATION OF SUSPECTED EPISODES OF OVER-EXPOSURE

When an episode of over-exposure is reported, biological monitoring techniques may play a vital part in estimating the severity of the incident. Significant over-exposure should be detectable as an increased phenol excretion rate for at least 48 hours. Urine samples should be collected as soon as possible after the incident and again at 24 and 48 hours. Where levels in excess of 50 mg/l are detected blood counts should be performed within a few days of the incident and again after 3 weeks. Any abnormality should be further investigated.

Individuals accidentally exposed to high levels of benzene vapour would be a priority group for chromosome studies if this method is available. The problems of interpretation must be considered prior to any such study.

Employees should be aware that additional monitoring is advisable after episodes of over-exposure.

THE FOLLOW-UP OF WORKERS AFTER CESSATION OF EXPOSURE

No specific monitoring routines are indicated. Where chromosome studies are in use the examination of a population of ex-employees within known exposure histories would be of interest.

SUMMARY

Both environmental and biological monitoring aim to estimate benzene exposure. The evidence linking specific exposure levels with a defined frequency or severity of adverse effect is scanty and hence these estimates will not provide a reliable estimate of risk, although they may enable compliance with a standard to be determined.

Estimates of individual exposure may be useful as indications of which employees or operations are most at risk. Unfortunately their value diminishes with reduced levels of exposure. The counting of blood cells is not likely to be useful as a measure of compliance with a 10 ppm TWA standard, although it may detect idiosyncrasy. Urinary phenol estimates will be of little use if the ambient concentration is less than 5 ppm TWA. Group means may allow an on-going check on the quality of environmental control to be maintained at lower levels. The decision on the relative merits of environmental and biological monitoring for this purpose will depend on the pattern of exposure in the work place.

Expired air benzene may provide sensitivity down to exposures of 1 ppm TWA but requires further evaluation. The rapid decline in excretion makes the method unreliable for fluctuating concentrations unless samples 16 hours after exposure are taken. These may be biased by trivial non-occupational exposures.

Increased effort is now being directed at the monitoring of benzene exposure. Much of the emphasis is on an adminstrative need to comply with standards. This should not hide the fundamental aim of all monitoring activity – the estimation of exposure to, and absorption of, potentially hazardous agents. It is only by adequate recording of exposure and absorption now that we shall be able to make better estimates of the risks from benzene and other substances in the future.

REFERENCES

Docter H. J. and Zelhuis R. L. (1967) Phenol excretion as a measure of benzene exposure. *Ann. Occup. Hyg.* **10**, 317–326.

Fishbeck W. A., Langner R. R. and Kociba R. J. (1975) Elevated urinary phenol levels not related to benzene exposure. *Am. Ind. Hyg. Assoc. J.* **36**, 820–824.

Gayl J. C., Lagesson V. and Tunek A. (1977) A method for the determination of low concentration of organic vapours in air and exhaled breath. *Ann. Occup. Hyg.* **20**, 127–134.

Hunter C. G. and Blair D. (1972) Benzene pharmacokinetics. *Ann. Occup. Hyg.* **15**, 193–199.

Jandle J. H. (1977) *Benzene Toxicity: A Review of the Subject.* Submission to OSHA hearings on proposed permanent standard for occupational exposure to benzene.

Reuvers J. (1977) *Surveillance of Benzene Exposure in a Dutch Petrochemical Plant.* Medichem Conference, San Francisco.

Roush G. J. and Ott M. G. (1977) A study of benzene exposure versus urinary phenol levels. *Am. Ind. Hyg. Assoc. J.* **38**, 67–75.

Sanders C., Orr R. G. and Evans R. J. (1968) *Blood Counts on Radiation Employees, U.K.A.E.A. Harwell.* AERE R5766. London, HMSO.

Sherwood R. J. (1972) Benzene: the interpretation of monitoring results. *Ann. Occup. Hyg.* **15**, 409–421.

Sherwood R. J. and Carter F. W. G. (1970) The measurement of occupational exposure to benzene vapour. *Ann. Occup. Hyg.* **13**, 125–140.

Snyder C. A., Erlichman M. N., Goldstein B. D. et al. (1977) An extraction method for determination of benzene in tissue by gas chromatography. *Am. Ind. Hyg. Assoc. J.* **38**, 272–276.

Van Haaften A. B. and Sie S. T. (1965) The measurement of phenol in urine by gas chromatography as a check on benzene exposure. *Am. Ind. Hyg. Assoc. J.* **26**, 52–58.

Wolman S. R. (1977) In: *A Critical Evaluation of Benzene Toxicity.* New York University Medical Center, Institute of Environmental Medicine.

5. ASBESTOS IN USE

T. P. Oliver

INTRODUCTION

The occupational health problems arising from the use of asbestos have been the focus of increased attention from the medical profession in the past 20 years. Coupled, not surprisingly, with this has been the publicity given to the problems in the news media. While some of the articles and programmes have been factual and informed, others have been shallow, factually incorrect, biased towards a particular management, union or political viewpoint, or positively alarmist. This media treatment has brought a backlash to all engaged in the field of occupational health and safety. 'All dust is dangerous' is becoming a common trade union or even ecological viewpoint, with indiscriminate extrapolation of the problems in the use of asbestos into other fields.

The early background

A better perspective of the present asbestos profile can be obtained by looking into the past and seeing the time scale both in the use of the material and the recognition of its effect on the health of those exposed to its dust.

Asbestos was used as long ago as 2500 BC. It was mined and used by the Romans who appreciated its dusty nature. However, it was not until the late nineteenth century that the modern asbestos industry was born from the mining of large deposits in Canada and Russia. It is important to realize that the world production of asbestos in 1880 was a mere 500 tons a year. Thus the number of people potentially exposed to its dust was small and its use extremely circumscribed. The advent of steam turbines and the greatly increased working temperatures of such machinery, bringing with it the need to contain the heat produced, was undoubtedly a major early factor in the increasing use of the material.

Types of asbestos

Asbestos is a name applied to a variety of silicate materials which differ in their chemical and physical properties. Two main types of asbestos are recognized mineralogically. By far the most important of these is the serpentine form, chrysotile. This is a hydrated magnesium silicate and the main centres of production are Canada, the USSR and Southern Africa. The world production of chrysotile in 1973 approached 4·5 million tons.

Chrysotile is the softest asbestos type and has therefore been particularly amenable to spinning and weaving to produce cloth products.

The other main type of asbestos is the group known collectively as 'amphiboles'. Of these the three most important are amosite – a magnesium iron silicate which is mined in the Transvaal, crocidolite – again mainly from South Africa, and anthophyllite from Scandinavia. They are harsher and more brittle. The world production of these amphiboles totalled some 440 000 tons in 1973, less than 10 per cent of the total mined. All in this group are extremely stable chemically and particularly resistant to acids and heat.

Thus in the last 100 years the amount of asbestos used has increased by nearly 10 000 fold, the majority in the last 35 years. This, by itself, has meant that far more of the world's population have been exposed to its dust and, not suprisingly, the number of cases of asbestos disease has also risen.

The use of asbestos

Asbestos is an extremely versatile material. The ability of asbestos to split into fibres has been one of its more valuable properties, but it is these fibres and their splitting which has provided them with their pathogenic quality. It is comparatively cheap with large resistance to both heat and friction. It is extremely strong and can be mixed with cement and resins and made up to be sprayed like paint. Asbestos cement products, such as roofing sheets, pipes and gutterings, are an example of one major use. Vast quantities have been used in insulation, not only for boilers and pipework but as thermal insulants and fire resistant screens in, for example, ships and railway carriages. Woven into cloth it is used for fireproof clothing, for fireproof curtains, and made into mattresses stuffed with loose asbestos fibre to cover awkward areas requiring insulation. It is used in brake and clutch linings, in battery cases, in the gland packings of bearings, and as filters in distilleries and breweries. A thousand uses is a suggested estimate.

ASBESTOS DISEASE

The first recorded case of asbestosis (fibrosis of lungs due to inhalation of asbestos) was observed by Doctor Montague Murray of Charing Cross Hospital, London, in 1900 (Murray, 1907). His patient was 33 years old and had worked in a carding room making asbestos cloth for a mere 10 years. Murray recorded that his disability was far more incapacitating than the physical signs elicited suggested and that he was the sole survivor of the 10 men who were at work in that carding room when he commenced employment. Post-mortem later showed widespread pulmonary fibrosis and marked pleural adhesions. During the next 30 years, other workers reported series of cases of fibrosis of the lung which were considered to be attributable to asbestos exposure. However, it was the report of Merrewether and Price (1930) that led, in the United Kingdom, to the introduction of the Asbestos Industry Regulations 1931. With hindsight it is regrettable that these regulations only applied to the manufacture of asbestos products and not to the use of these products by other workers. They were, however, the first attempt by any country to control the potential hazards of asbestos. Merrewether (1933) reported on the difficulties inherent in the diagnosis of asbestosis, drew attention to its insidious onset and the latent or maturation period that occurred before frank disease developed. He further suggested that there was a dust datum level below which the disease did not develop. He noted that the average age of death from asbestosis was 40·8 years compared with one of 54·1 years for sufferers from silicosis.

The thesis that there was an association between exposure to asbestos and cancer of the lung was recorded by Wood and Gloyne (1934). During the thirties workers in many countries drew attention to the marked thickening of the pleura that occurred in persons exposed to asbestos dust. Wagner et al. (1960) first annunciated the association between asbestos exposure and mesothelioma.

During the years that have passed since Murray first described what may be termed the 'index case', many papers have appeared on the problems associated with asbestos. Most have contributed something to our knowledge of the asbestos-related diseases, all which develop over a period of years of exposure or afterwards. It is such disabilities and diseases which have always presented a particular challange in the occupational health field. Instant disability from a hazard is always easier to explain and rapidly results in the development of preventive measures. Distant possible morbidity and mortality result in a different viewpoint from both employer and employee, collectively and individually.

Classification

In common with many of the diseases related to occupations it is difficult to differentiate on the appearance of the first signs and symptoms between what may be called 'evidence of exposure' and 'disease'. To take lead, for example, at what stage can we say the individual suffers from lead poisoning as distinct from showing signs from lead absorption? Nevertheless, in the case of asbestos it is convenient to classify both exposure and disease into:

1. Acute pleural reactions
2. Diffuse pleural thickening
3. Pleural plaques
   (a) hyaline
   (b) calcified
4. Asbestosis
5. Carcinoma of the lung
6. Mesothelioma
   (a) pleura
   (b) peritoneum

The possibility that other cancers may be associated with asbestos exposure is not to be overlooked.

Development

Apart from the development of asbestos corns of the skin due to its penetration by asbestos fibres in those handling them, asbestos may enter the body either through the respiratory or the alimentary tract. Both these routes of entry may be of occupational origin, from the general environment, or from the consumption of food and drink contaminated with asbestos fibres. It is with occupational exposure that we are mainly concerned, although the general environmental and public health aspects will be discussed briefly later.

The natural defences of the respiratory tract progressively filter out larger dust particles. Those larger than 5 μm do not reach the lung tissue. Particles in the range of 0·5 to 3 μm are most likely to be retained there and, if not phagocytosed, cause cell damage and the development of asbestos disease. Because asbestos dust is in fibre form its penetrative power is related to the diameter of the individual fibre rather than to its length. Hence quite long fibres, whose diameter is less than 3 μm, can succeed in reaching the alveolae and pleura. The straight amphibole fibres are, by their physical shape, more efficient in passing to the deeper lung tissues than the curly chrysotile ones. Other non-asbestos fibres, with similar dimensional characteristics, can travel as far anatomically; an important point to remember when considering asbestos substitutes.

The development of acute pleural reactions or diffuse pleural fibrosis can occur in asbestos exposure. They may be the sequelae of a pleural effusion which may go undetected, be present or be the harbinger of mesothelioma.

Pleural plaques, both of the hyaline or calcified variety, are associated with exposure to all forms of asbestos, but although asbestos is the most common aetiological factor in pleural plaque formation, it does occur in other circumstances (Jones and Sheers, 1973). The great majority of plaques are found on the parietal pleura. The appearance or prevalence of plaques does not appear to be related to total dust exposure but to an indeterminate minimal exposure. The prevalence of calcification shows wide variation in reported series. The pathology of plaque formation remains obscure. Plaques are rarely found under the age of 30 unless childhood exposure has occurred. Calcification in plaques is unusual with less than 20 years, occupational exposure. It remains to be seen whether these latent intervals in plaque development are increased as a result of the adoption of hygiene standards for asbestos dust. There is no suggestion that either variety of plaque has any deleterious clinical effect or that they are in any way associated with possible later development of mesothelioma.

The development of asbestosis (fibrosis of the lung due to asbestos exposure) is definitely related to total dust exposure, thus confirming

Merrewether's (1933) original thesis of a dust datum level. The time interval between first exposure to asbestos and the development of asbestosis is now in the order of 15–20 years, far longer than that described by Doctor Montague Murray in 1900. The introduction, in the intervening years, of far stricter precautions in the manufacture and use of asbestos products, thus lowering total dust exposure, has undoubtedly been an important factor. As the regulations in most countries become even more stringent it can be expected that this interval will become longer still. Hopefully, asbestosis will then pass into the history of occupational medicine. There is no evidence in the context of asbestosis of differing response to the various forms of asbestos.

Smoking habits effect the development of fibrosis. Weiss (1971) in a study of 100 asbestos textile workers found that the prevalence of pulmonary fibrosis was almost doubled in cigarette smokers when compared with non-smokers.

Carcinoma of the lung can be a sequel to the development of asbestosis. This additional risk is markedly increased in cigarette smokers and the effect is synergistic, not merely additive. Hammond and Selikoff (1973) have suggested that the increased risk of lung carcinoma in non-smoking asbestos workers is small.

Mesothelioma of the pleura is a rare tumour in man but a relationship between it and asbestos exposure has been demonstrated beyond reasonable doubt. However, this is not its sole aetiology. Klima et al. (1976) reported on a series of 13 cases of mesothelioma in which 7 had no proved history of exposure to asbestos. Mesothelioma develops some 30 or more years after first exposure and is not dose related. No connection has been proved between the development of mesothelioma and smoking habits. It is suggested that the risk of mesothelioma developing is asbestos type related in the order of crocidolite, amosite, chrysotile and anthophyllite. The extent of the difference between the various types is not established but crocidolite is probably responsible for the large majority. Similar observations can be made about mesothelioma of the peritoneum.

The incidence of other neoplasma has been investigated in relation to asbestos exposure. Selikoff et al. (1964) and Lumley (1976) have shown that there is a probable increase in gastro-intestinal carcinomas. Possible association with carcinomas of the ovary (Keel, 1960) and the upper respiratory tract have been suggested.

Diagnosis

The diagnosis of asbestos disease rests upon the usual triad of occupational history, the elicitation of symptoms and clinical signs and the results of special investigations.

Before a diagnosis of asbestos disease can be made, a history of exposure is essential. This may only come to light with the taking of the most detailed occupational and even life history, identifying every job which the patient has undertaken and the materials he has used. An exhaustive list of suspect occupations cannot be provided, but this would include those engaged in asbestos mining, asbestos product manufacture, insulators, asbestos sprayers, shipyard workers, engine room personnel in ships, construction and building workers, and others who are known to have used asbestos containing products. The neighbourhood worker must not be forgotten. He suffers occupational exposure although not actually working with the product itself (Harries et al., 1972).

The common symptoms of asbestosis are those of dyspnoea, a productive cough for some months of the year, and possibly pleural pain. The most commonly described clinical signs are those of basal rales or crepitations accompanied by finger clubbing and, in a minority, cyanosis. The extent of the area over which the sounds are heard is indicative of the severity of the lung involvement but early in the disease they are best heard at the lung bases or in the axillae. However, evidence suggests that smoking may be more important in the development of finger clubbing. Cyanosis normally occurs in the later stages of the progression of the disease.

The symptoms and signs to be found in carcinoma of the lung are no different from those when this cancer is of other aetiology. It can be present with symptoms and signs of secondary deposits.

In mesothelioma the presenting symptoms, which are of insidious onset are dull, non-pleuritic pain accompanied by dyspnoea, lassitude and weight loss with signs of either pleural effusion, pleural thickening or abdominal ascites dependent on site (Elmes and Simpson, 1976). Clubbing of the fingers and signs of asbestosis are rare in pleural cases, but more common in peritoneal ones. Although secondary metastases can occur, these are never responsible for the presenting clinical picture.

The measurement of chest expansion is of little value in the diagnosis of asbestos chest disease. The presence of asbestos bodies or fibres in the sputum are of little clinical significance, being merely evidence of exposure to asbestos dust.

Radiographic examination of the chest remains an important diagnostic aid. In addition to the normal postero-anterior view of the chest, it is desirable that additional views are taken, particularly lateral obliques, which enable better visualization of the pleura. The International Labour Office (1972) classification can be used in film reading. The assessment of serial films is of particular value in demonstrating progression (Liddell and Morgan, 1978).

The lung function tests that are of most diagnostic value to the plant occupational physician are those of FVC and FEV_1, as both these can be undertaken with relatively simple equipment. In asbestosis, lung function tests show a picture of a restrictive defect with reduced lung compliance, namely the FVC and FEV_1 are reduced but maintain their normal ratio to one another. However, the picture may be complicated by the presence of a concommitant obstructive defect. In addition, the measurement of the CO transfer factor, which is depressed in asbestosis, is a valuable contributory diagnostic aid that can be offered by a lung function laboratory.

Lung and pleural tissue biopsies can also be performed as confirmatory aids to diagnosis. In mesothelioma the presence of a high hyaluronate level in the pleural fluid is significant.

The diagnosis of asbestos disease must rest on a history of exposure accompanied by clinical or radiological evidence and appropriate lung function results (Society of Occupational Medicine, 1977).

Treatment

No treatment is necessary for those with pleural plaques. If adequate precautions are being taken at the work place removal from asbestos work is not required. Interval medical surveillance should be instituted.

The treatment of asbestosis remains symptomatic with removal from asbestos work and routine surveillance for the possible development of malignant changes.

With proven mesothelioma the drainage of pleural effusion (or ascites) is of value in reducing the burden on the respiratory system. Pleural stripping is theoretically a possible line of treatment although direct operative mortality may be high. Successful operative intervention (in terms of increased life expectancy) have been reported by Klima et al. (1976).

THE PREVENTION OF ASBESTOS DISEASE

The use of asbestos products rather than their mining or manufacture is of most general interest. It is on these aspects that this section will concentrate although the general principles of dealing with the problem are the same.

The protection of the workers against asbestos disease is founded on the basic occupational health principles of:

1. Elimination of a dangerous substance and/or its substitution by a less dangerous one.
2. The partial or total segregation or enclosure of the process.
3. The provision of adequate protective clothing for those exposed to the potential hazard.

Considerable efforts have been made by most countries in the past few years either to eliminate or reduce the amount of asbestos used and to attempt to confine its use to those areas where the risk is small or where no other substitute is available. It is of interest that in European countries the commonest use of asbestos is in cement products for building and pipework. This accounts for over half the European consumption of fibre (Commission of European Communities, 1977). The use of crocidolite is now barred by law in some countries, by which it is hoped to eliminate the majority of the mesothelioma hazard. Others are moving towards this for the same reasons. For insulating pipework and thermal insulation of structures substitute materials such as preformed silicate sections, slag wool, man-made mineral fibre, cork and various foams, are being used. All of these materials do of course produce some dust in the respirable range and concern has been expressed, not only by trade unionists, as to the long-term effects of exposure. The production of tumours in experimental animals exposed to large amounts of such dust (Stanton et al., 1977) has been directly extrapolated to man by those unaware of the difficulties in so doing.

Partial or total enclosure of the process with filtered exhaust ventilation has been practised (or required by law in some countries) for many years in asbestos cloth manufacture. In discrete areas where the dust can be contained, similar measures can be adopted. The workshop machining of asbestos products can be isolated in areas separated from other workers and in which adequate exhaust ventilation can be provided. Special extract systems have been designed to remove the asbestos arising when attending to vehicle brake drums. Local exhaust systems extracting at source can be fitted to power driven tools cutting or abrading asbestos products. As a general rule the more confined the space the greater the potential hazard, a common enough occupational health adage.

Outside the shop situation the objective must be to ensure that the hazard is contained within a clearly defined area and that potential exposure is limited to those required to undertake the task. The surveys by Sheers and Templeton (1968) and Harries et al. (1972) bring home only too clearly the morbidity occurring in neighbourhood workers. In many situations it is possible to classify the potential hazard according to the experience gained from dust measurements of previous tasks. Such a classification can be used to identify those tasks which are extremely dusty (and therefore potentially far more hazardous). These must include the stripping out of old asbestos products, particularly where these are known to contain crocidolite. Needless to say, experience suggests that less dust is made when asbestos products are removed with reasonable care rather than in an orgy of destructive ripping out. Those of a less dusty nature include the installation of new insulation – if asbestos bearing products are used. Minimal dust is produced in the use of cement products, with the caveat that machine cutting, though increasing productivity, makes far more dust than hand cutting of similar materials.

Asbestos containing materials should be separated in stores from other materials and packaging kept intact. Issue of stores to be transported elsewhere may need repacking in polythene.

One of the classic methods of suppressing dust has been by the use of water. It has been found in shipyards that an asbestos mix tends to run off into the more inaccessible places on the deck of an engine room, dries and then has to be chipped off, thus merely transferring the hazard from the pipe overhead to the deck of the ship. However, in other situations, the use of water as a dust suppressant is practical and feasible.

Where old asbestos-containing materials are being stripped out or a new asbestos-containing product used, debris, dusty waste and unusable off-cuts must be separated and placed in impermeable bags for later disposal in a safe manner. When the asbestos work is finished the area should be cleared up by vacuum cleaner, a far more satisfactory method than re-distributing some of the dust with the conventional broom.

Adequate personal protection must be provided for all workers who are potentially exposed to levels of asbestos dust above the threshold limit value. This means the provision of special overalls, normally of nylon, skull caps, gloves, approved dust masks which may be power driven, and 'under-garments' used solely at work. Where crocidolite is handled, PVC overalls with air-fed hoods are the clothing of choice, and replace the overalls, caps and respirators.

Protective clothing needs to be checked periodically and repaired as necessary. It should be sent to the laundry in polythene sacks and damped before handling, thus avoiding contamination of the laundry or its workers. Respirators need to be serviced and filters changed.

Occupational hygiene standards

In the old days the miner used a canary to decide whether a work place was safe. Today we rely on environmental measurements and monitoring. It is this principle that has led to the development of hygiene standards such as those proposed by the British Occupational Hygiene Society (1968, 1973) for use with asbestos.

Asbestos dust can be measured by the gravimetric method using the weight of dust collected in a sample. This method has been found, in practice, to be less satisfactory than that of asbestos fibre counting (Harries, 1971a), and the latter has now become the method of choice.

In fibre counting, measured samples are drawn over a filter of a specific size. The fibres with a length to width ratio of 3 : 1 or greater, a length greater than 5 μm and a width less than 3 μm are then counted by light contact microscopy. The result is expressed in fibres per cm^3. It is extremely important that anyone who engages in dust sampling and analysis is properly trained by an experienced laboratory if the results obtained are to be of any value (National Health and Medical Research Council, 1976; Gibbs et al., 1977).

There appears to be general international agreement, at this point in time, on a hygiene standard based on a threshold limit value (TLV) of 2 fibres per cm^3 with riders concerning the allowable excursions above this level, the length of the sampling period, and with reservations concerning crocidolite. (In the United Kingdom the standard for this substance is 0·2 fibres per ml.) Countries whose current standards are above 2 fibres per

cm^3 are moving towards this standard. In the future it seems that this standard, based on a 99 per cent probability of not developing asbestosis over a working lifetime, will be further reduced.

It is possible to sample asbestos for typing should the actual type be unknown. This is particularly important where crocidolite is suspected as the asbestos type.

To date no reliable direct reading instrument is available to give an instant read out of the environmental status; thus the dust measurement taken refers to the past, albeit none too distant.

The estimation of total exposure of an individual is possible for the asbestos mine worker or asbestos product maker, but for the worker using their products this is, in practice, impossible.

Medical surveillance

Medical surveillance of employees engaged on asbestos work is still a subject for discussion. By what parameters, at what interval or at what gain to the employee and his health are they to be conducted? The physician must take an acurate and detailed occupational history, with particular reference to previous exposure to asbestos or other dusts. He should elicit any symptoms of previous respiratory disease and, in particular, the presence of a productive cough, and undertake a clinical examination of the respiratory and cardiovascular systems. A full plate X-ray of the chest, and estimations by simple spirometry of FVC and FEV_1 complete the tests and enable an assessment of fitness to be made. Subsequent examination should update the occupational history and symptomatology, repeat the clinical examination, X-ray and lung function tests, with the objective of assessing any adverse trends.

For those who work full time dealing with asbestos containing materials the interval of examination should be set at 2 years. For those intermittently working with such materials examination at less frequent intervals appears logical, 4–5 years. (It is assumed that safe working practices are adopted at all times.)

The question is often posed as to what value there is in medically examining asbestos workers. Excluding research, the value lies in

1. The selection process of the initial examination to exclude those with pre-existent respiratory pathology.
2. The removal from the dust of those who, despite precautions or because of lack of precautions, have developed signs of asbestos disease, as although these are normally progressive the dust response relationship suggests that this process will be slowed or halted by removal from exposure (Society of Occupational Medicine, 1977).

Regrettably, however, for those who show signs of asbestos disease (as distinct from exposure), the only advantage of the examination might be their recourse to law for compensation in one form or another.

For those found to be suffering from mesothelioma with its very poor prognosis (the expectation of life from diagnosis to death is in most cases less than 2 years), it could be argued that the medical examination offers nothing.

The role of the medical examination in the case of casual or accidental exposure is of no value except in terms of the employee's morale. A note that such an exposure has occurred would be made in the medical records of the individual.

For the initial screening of large populations to identify cases of asbestos exposure or disease the 100 mm Mass Minature X-ray is the method of choice.

Health education

Success in combating any potential hazard to which the employee may be exposed requires adequate health education of the worker. The axiom of Sir Thomas Legge that 'every worker should be told something of the hazard to which he is exposed' is especially important in this context. The reasons for the need to stick to the approved work methods, the rationale of the environmental control measures and monitoring, the use of the equipment and protective clothing provided for his protection, and the place of the medical examination should be explained. The additional synergistic hazard to the asbestos worker of smoking must be strongly emphasized.

PUBLIC HEALTH ASPECTS

Although not strictly concerned with the occupational health problems of asbestos, the public health aspects are worthy of consideration in that they arise from the occupational use of asbestos. At present there is no established evidence of true environmental exposure in the general public causing an increased incidence of asbestos related disease. On the other hand there is no evidence that there is an exposure threshold below which such diseases, particularly maligancies, will not occur. To prove these points it would be necessary to show an excess of mortality or morbidity due to asbestos in the public at large (Commission of European Communities, 1977).

There is no evidence from the many studies that have been carried out, including those of Auerbach et al. (1977), to show that the ingestion of asbestos fibres in food or drink is a risk to the public health.

Lumley et al. (1971) and others have drawn attention to a possible risk both at work or to the general public, from buildings containing asbestos products. This risk is greatest where it has been used as thermal insulation, if it has become damaged or deteriorated with the passage of time, or has been attacked by the natural fauna of the country concerned.

Baris and Ozesmi (1976) report an increased incidence of asbestos related disease (plaques, fibrosis and mesothelioma) in several villages in

Turkey where naturally occuring asbestos has been used (away from areas in which it is mined or processed) as part of the stucco finishing to dwellings.

Newhouse (1973) has stressed the continuing importance of adequate control of environmental pollution in the neighbourhood of areas where it is mined or processed.

ASBESTOS – THE FUTURE

Use

The association between the use of asbestos and disease has called into question its future as an industrial material. Several countries have placed a total or partial ban on the import and use of crocidolite and it seems probable that more countries will follow suit. This is understandable in the light of non-dose related mesothelioma.

Denmark has, for example, placed a ban on the use of asbestos for insulation work. Harries (1971b) has given a very detailed account of the substitution products used in naval dockyards in the United Kingdom to replace asbestos-bearing ones. Such measures would reduce the amount of asbestos used and therefore the occupational exposure of the worker. Substitution or reduction of asbestos content will remain the future trend.

The replacement of asbestos by non-asbestos products in friction-bearing surfaces or in fire safety measures is not foreseen in the near future (Lewinsohn, 1977).

Its use in the building and construction industry in the form of cement products is economically sound and dust production is containable. Its use in sprayed products or as environmental insulation, already drastically reduced, will cease.

The stripping out of old asbestos, especially where the hazard is not appreciated, either by ignorance or design, will remain a constant source of asbestos disease in future years.

The future of asbestos products cannot be divorced from socio-economic acceptability or from their continuing availability from the earth's mineral resources. Without the mesothelioma risk it could be argued they can be used within certain restrictions and, providing adequate precautions are taken, with safety.

It is difficult to see to what other uses asbestos might be put, although its use in roadmaking has been considered. Whether in the light of the publicity given to asbestos related disease this would be acceptable to the public, is a matter of considerable doubt.

Medical

Many cases of asbestos disease will continue to arise in future years from previous exposures even if the use of all asbestos material were to cease today. With the long latent period in the development of mesothelioma this period may be as long as the next 50 years.

It remains to be seen how the adoption of stricter working practices and the adoption of hygiene standards will affect those workers whose first exposure occured in the last few years. It is to be expected that a dramatic fall in the incidence of asbestos disease will occur in these workers.

Like many diseases the same exposure in different individuals results in a different response, and it is possible that immunological tests capable of predicting the susceptibility of an individual to asbestos dust may be developed.

Lastly there remains the hope that current and future research may offer prospects of definitive treatment to arrest or cure the asbestos related diseases.

REFERENCES

Auerbach O., Cuyler Hammond E, Selikoff I. J. et al. (1977) Asbestos bodies in lung parenchyma in relation to ingestion and inhalation of mineral fibres. *Environ. Res.* **14**, 286–304.

Baris Y. I. and Ozesmi M. (1976) An outbreak of pleural mesothelioma in the village of Karain in Anatolia. *Kanser* **5** (2), 63–76.

British Occupational Hygiene Society (1968) Hygiene standards for chrysolite asbestos dust. *Ann. Occup. Hyg.* **11**, 47–69.

British Occupational Hygiene Society (1973) Hygiene standards for airborne amosite asbestos dust. *Ann. Occup. Hyg.* **16**, 1–5.

Commission of European Communities (1977) *Public Health Risks of Exposure to Asbestos.* Oxford, Pergamon.

Elmes P. C. and Simpson H. J. C. (1976) The clinical aspects of mesothelioma. *Q. J. Med.* **45/179**, 427–449.

Gibbs G. W., Baron P., Beckett S. T. et al. (1977) A summary of asbestos fibre counting experience in seven countries. *Ann. Occup. Hyg.* **20**, 321–332.

Hammond E. C. and Selikoff I. J. (1973) Relation of cigarette smoking to risk of death of asbestos associated disease among insulation workers in the United States. In: *Biological Effects of Asbestos.* Lyons, World Health Organisation, International Agency for Research on Cancer, pp. 312–317.

Harries P. G. (1971a) A comparison of mass and fibre concentrations in shipyard insulation processes. *Ann. Occup. Hyg.* **14**, 235–240.

Harries P. G. (1971b) Asbestos dust concentrations in ship repairing: a practical approach to improving asbestos hygiene in naval dockyards. *Ann. Occup. Hyg.* **14**, 241–254.

Harries P. G., Mackenzie F. A. F., Sheer G. et al. Radiological survey of men exposed to asbestos in Naval Dockyards. *Br. J. Ind. Med.* **29**, 274–279.

International Labour Office (1972) *ILO U/C International Classification of Radiographs of the Pneumoconioses 1971.* Occupational Health and Safety Series, Number 22 (Revised). Geneva, ILO.

Jones J. S. P. and Sheers G. (1973) Pleural plaques. In: *Biological Effects of Asbestos.* Lyons. World Health Organisation, International Agency for Research on Cancer, pp. 243–248.

Keal E. E. (1960) Asbestosis and abdominal neoplasms. *Lancet* **2**, 1211–1216.

Klima M., Spjut J. and Seybold W. D. (1976) Diffuse malignant mesothelioma. *Am. J. Clin. Pathol.* **65**, 583–600.

Lewinsohn H. C. (1977) Asbestosis – a diagnostic enigma. *J. Occup. Med.* **19**, 607–610.

Liddell C. D. K. and Morgan W. K. C. (1978) Methods of assessing serial films of the pneumoconioses. *J. Soc. Occup. Med.* **28**, 6–15.

Lumley K. P. S. (1976) A proportional study of cancer registrations of dockyard workers. *Br. J. Ind. Med.* **33**, 108–114.

Lumley K. P. S., Harries P. G. and O'Kelly F. J. (1971) Buildings insulated with sprayed asbestos: a potential hazard. *Ann. Occup. Hyg.* **14**, 255–258.

Merrewether E. R. A. (1933) A memorandum on asbestosis. *Tubercle* **14**, 109.

Merrewether E. R. A. and Price C. W. (1930) *Report on Effects of Asbestos Dust in the Lungs and Dust Suppression in the Asbestos Industry*. London, HMSO.

Murray M. (1907) *Departmental Commission on Compensation for Industrial Diseases.* Cmd 3495, p. 14, Cmd 3496 p. 127. London, HMSO.

Newhouse M. L. (1973) Asbestos in the work place and the community. *Ann. Occup. Hyg.* **16,** 97–107.

National Health and Medical Research Council (1976) *Membrane Filter Method for Estimating Airborne Asbestos Dust.* Canberra, Australian Department of Health.

Selikoff I. J., Churg J. and Hammond E. C. (1964) Asbestos exposure and neoplasia, *J. Am. Med. Assoc.* **188,** 22–26.

Sheers G. and Templeton A. R. (1968) Effects of asbestos in dockyard workers. *Br. Med. J.* **3,** 574–579.

Society of Occupational Medicine (1977) *Health Screening.* London, SOM, pp. 30–31, 70.

Stanton M. F., Layard M., Tergeris A. et al. (1977) Carcinogenicity of fibrous glass: pleural response in the rat in relation to fiber dimension. *J. Nat. Cancer Inst.* **58,** 587–603.

Wagner J. C., Sleggs C. A. and Marchand P. (1960) Diffuse pleural mesothelioma and asbestos exposure in North Western Cape Province. *Br. J. Ind. Med.* **17,** 260–271.

Weiss W. (1971) Cigarette smoking, asbestos and pulmonary fibrosis. *Am. Rev. Resp. Dis.* **104,** 223.

Wood W. B. and Gloyne S. R. (1934) Pulmonary asbestosis: a review of 100 cases. *Lancet* (Dec 22), 1382–5.

6. MAN-MADE MINERAL FIBRES—AN EVALUATION OF CURRENT KNOWLEDGE

J. W. Hill

Fibre morphology

'Solid state carcinogenesis', described by Oppenheimer (1960) when he observed the formation of tumours following the implantation of celluloid squares into rats, introduced the concept that factors associated with morphology rather than with chemistry might initiate tumour induction. As the rat is prone to develop sarcomas, both spontaneously and in response to stimuli as apparently innocuous as saline injections, the relevance of the observations remained in doubt, especially as there was no obvious parallel in human pathology. The hypothesis was to receive striking support however, from intrapleural implantation and inoculation experiments reported by Pott in Germany (Pott and Friedrichs, 1972) and Stanton in the USA (Stanton and Wrench, 1972) in 1972, where both workers found that mesotheliomas were produced in rats by fibres independent of their chemical nature and as widely different as asbestos, glass, magnesium silicate, aluminium oxide and ceramic fibres. Here there was a direct parallel at hand in the form of the known association between asbestos fibres and mesothelioma in man. The immediate problem was that whilst the parallel held for asbestos, the other fibres implicated in the intrapleural work were not known to be associated with lung pathology in humans. Re-evaluation of the experimental data suggested, and later work confirmed, that the common factor between the samples was the presence of fibres possessing extremely narrow diameter. Carcinogenic potential was correlated with the number of fibres less than 0·25 μm in diameter and greater than 8 μm long in the inoculum. Further intrapleural work by Wagner et al. (1976) showed similar responses, but also revealed that glass fibres of 3 μm in diameter and above exhibited no carcinogenic effect. The results of intrapleural implanation studies indicates a spectrum of carcinogenic potential, greatest around the 0·25 μm range of diameter and diminishing with increasing fibre diameter until it disappears at 3·0 μm.

Aerodynamics of the fibre

The aerodynamic behaviour of fibres is mainly determined by their diameter, length having only a minor influence, and Gross et al. (1971) showed that the diameter distribution of fibres found in human lungs at post-mortem suggested a size selection of 3·5 μm and below. Sedimentation is the main factor in deposition of fibres in the lung. Timbrell and Skidmore (1971) used mathematical modelling to show that fibres of 3 μm and below are likely to gain access to the alveoli. Similar results are found in inhalation studies on rats, whose terminal bronchioles are of similar size to their human counterpart. Thus, all three methods are in accord in suggesting that fibres in the carcinogenic range of diameters are also those most capable of penetrating to the alveoli.

There are, nevertheless, considerable differences in the frequency with which different fibres are found in human lungs and pleura. Even in occupationally exposed asbestos workers, chrysotile is less commonly retained than other fibres, and man-made mineral fibres (MMMF) are very rarely found. Attention is drawn therefore to the possibility of other factors which may interfere with access of fibres to the lungs. The curliness of chrysotile gives it an effectively greater aerodynamic diameter which increases the probability of impaction higher in the bronchial tree, resulting in its removal by the muco-ciliary escalator. The cause of the rarity of MMF in the lungs and pleura is unknown at present, but may involve impaction mechanisms (although this seems unlikely) or may result from their fragmentation and removal as cellular debris by macrophages (for which there is some evidence), or may simply be a function of the low airborne concentrations of respirable fibres observed in practice.

Biological effects of fibres

Although fibre length has little influence upon aerodynamic behaviour it is believed to influence the biological effect. In the intrapleural situation, whilst the diameter effect is predominant in initiating carcinogenesis, there is a strong suggestion that within the significant diameter range increasing length potentiates the effect up to 200 μm. Pott and Friedrichs (1972) considered, nevertheless, that lengths below 5 μm were significant in this respect.

Whilst the intrapleural work establishes a dose-response relationship with the number of biologically significant fibres, it is not possible to extrapolate from the intrapleural response into fibre/years for controlling human exposure by inhalation, because of the many intervening variables introduced by the normal lung defence mechanisms. Two further points should be borne in mind. The usual dose introduced intrapleurally is 10–25 mg in the rat. This is altogether disproportionate to any conceivable human exposure, although it must also be said that no minimum point has been observed at which carcinogenic effects are absent. The most important point is that neither human epidemiology nor animal inhalation experiments currently provide any evidence of the occurrence of mesothelioma in relation to glass or mineral fibres (although the opposite is the case with asbestos), and therefore no response exists for the inhalation route to which dose may be equated.

Other factors

While intrapleural work suggests that all fibres of similar diameter are equal in carcinogenic potential at this site, there is evidence that other intervening factors also determine the effects by inhalation. It is clear, for instance, that chrysotile asbestos is materially less dangerous than crocidolite in human exposures although both are equally carcinogenic in the intrapleural site. Apart fom aerodynamic behaviour, consequent upon the wavy shape of chrysotile, there is another way in which asbestos of all types differs critically from glass and mineral wool fibres. This lies in the differing ways in which they fracture. This influences both the reliability of the measurement of their numbers and the estimation of dose. Glass and mineral wool fibres, because of their vitreous nature, can only break transversely into shorter fragments until ultimately they lose their fibrous shape and become effectively spherical dusts. The number of fibres in air, estimated by optical microscopy, correlates broadly with that estimated by electron microscopy, (the only means of resolving diameters of 0·2 μm) for the common forms of MMMF. However, in the case of asbestos fibres, which break down longitudinally into finer fibres, electron microscopy detects very many more fibres than do optical methods. Optical methods may therefore seriously underestimate the real dose of biologically significant asbestos fibres inhaled. The added tendency of asbestos fibres to split into fibrils, as a result of biological action, makes the estimation of the tissue burden of fibres of carcinogenic significance even more complex. The number of fibres potentially contributing to tumour induction are indicated by the large numbers of asbestos fibres in 0·5 diameter range and averaging 5 μm in length found in the lungs of occupationally exposed asbestos workers.

Animal inhalation experiments, however, indicate that the actual rate of tumour induction may not be directly proportional to the numbers of asbestos fibres recovered from the lungs, as similar rates of tumours have been found in association with different quantities of retained asbestos fibres. It appears that other factors may intervene in the biological action of fibres in the lung, one factor being asbestos type and another factor, which is unknown at present, which influences the retention of biological activity in tissue. This may be connected with leaching, and it is known that chrysotile fibres may retain their morphology in the lung, but their biological potency is diminished because of this process. Equally, the rarity of MMMF in lung tissue may reflect the extremely low concentration of respirable fibres (below 3 μm in diameter) encountered occupationally or the ability of the lung to dispose of them. There is considerable consistency between observers in finding very low airborne concentrations of respirable glass fibres ranging in general from 0·02–0·2 fibres/ml in a wide variety of facilities and locations producing insulation wool (averaging 6 μm nominal diameter), and of lower orders of approximately 0·002 fibres/ml in the case of continuous filament production (yarns and textile fibres of 12 μm diameter and upwards).

Sedimentation of fibres

It appears that whilst heavier fibres tend to sediment out of the air rapidly, MMMF in the respirable range tend to remain airborne longer and generally reach equilibrium at the levels indicated above. These observations are compatible with the absence of any current evidence of mesothelioma associated with glass or other MMMF in humans despite long exposures, insofar as the doses are so low, and subject to the question of what lapse or 'latent period' might be expected at such very low dose levels in relation to the duration of observation required to satisfy scientific criteria. This point will be discussed later.

Mesothelioma in Turkey

The question of the dose of biologically significant fibres offered to the lung in terms of number and diameter distribution may be very important, and may well be the determinant in the case reports of mesothelioma from Turkey. Baris (1975) reported clusters of cases of mesothelioma, pleural fibrosis and pleural plaques having an unusually high incidence (about 1 per cent per anum) in certain villages in Turkey. Although at first attributed to environmental exposure to asbestos, detailed investigation failed to substantiate significant exposure and further examination suggests fibres of the zeolite group of minerals as a causal factor, since it is present in great quantities in the villages at hazard but absent from other villages 2 kilometres away where there was no disease. Zeolites are mineral fibres of volcanic origin. These fibres vary in mechanical strength and trace elements, and are composed of sodium aluminium silicate. Like asbestos they are crystalline in structure and not vitreous, which makes the common description 'volcanic glass' incorrect. The fibre concerned is closest to erionite which is one of the many types of zeolite.

The living conditions in the area are extremely dusty because of the combination of arid conditions and the use of volcanic material for road building, house construction and so on. Dust samples have shown very high proportions of fibres with diameters less than 0·25 μm and lengths of 30–100 μm. The low life-expectancy has become a local legend, as those moving from their village in early life may take the risk with them. Those moving into the villages may develop mesothelioma at a later age. The age distribution of the tumours ranges from 12 to 71 years of age with a mean of approximately 46 years.

Conclusions about fibre morphology

Although awaiting full confirmation, these findings give considerable support to the morphological hypothesis of mesothelioma induction, and we now have two examples of natural fibres, both crystalline, producing the disease in humans. It is clear that safety cannot be assumed merely because a fibre is non-asbestiform. Consideration must also be given to its history, to the association with human pathology, to the results of animal and cell culture experiments and to the characteristics of human occupational or environmental exposure in evaluating potential hazards.

History of MMMF

The history of MMMF started with the introduction of rock wool in the late 1800s and saw the manufacture of glass fibres on a production scale in the mid 1930s. The earliest products were insulation wools. The raw materials, rock or slag and glass, were fiberized together by the application of centrifugal force with a stream of hot gases to thin streams of molten material. This inevitably produces a wide distribution curve of diameter in the products which contain substantial quantities of submicron diameter fibres. So that the material could be handled and in order to provide an appropriate matrix of fibres for thermal insulation, binders were applied both in the form of vegetable oils – which are still used today in many forms of rock wool – and in the form of resin binders in the case of glass wool. These binders exercise an extremely important influence in limiting the dust clouds generated from the products. It is therefore technically difficult to extrapolate from diameter distributions of fibres in given products to probable fibre concentration distributions in air. It can be said, however, from examination of limited samples of products made in the 1920s and 1930s, that although the nominal diameter of these insulation wools tended to be greater than those made today (earlier products averaging 14 μm and contemporary products averaging 6 μm in diameter) that the concentrations of fibres of respirable diameter in the products were substantially similar. Having regard to the similarity of the orders of concentration of airborne respirable fibres found at present in different plants, it is reasonable to suppose that concentrations and diameter distributions of airborne respirable fibres were not materially less in the past than they are today. If this view is accepted, then the human epidemiological evidence which is drawn from plants with this history is relevant. Cognizance must be given to the rates of industrial growth in the sense that the MMMF industry has expanded rapidly and only small numbers of people would have been exposed in the early days. Nevertheless, it has been possible to construct cohorts of considerable size (*circa* 1500) and follow their health experience from the 1940s to date. Such cohorts, like all others, will contain many members with continuous exposure throughout the period studied, and some with the minimum of 5 years' exposure. No case of mesothelioma has been observed in MMMF workers, either in these cohorts, or reported by occupational physicians supervising these plants. Cohort studies of this type cover the contingency of occupationally related diseases arising in persons who have left the industry, and follow-up has been extremely thorough. Studies of pensioners have similarly revealed no incidence of mesothelioma. This, combined with the experience of plant physicians, is providing information about a core of employees with long exposures.

Latent period and mesothelioma

The main criticism of these studies lies in the duration of observation in relation to the so-called 'latent' period of induction. It is well known that the development of mesothelioma may be associated with a lapse of 30 or even 40 years, and that the longer periods are sometimes related to environmental exposure to asbestos. It is presumed that the asbestos exposures represent very low level continuous exposures, although the possibility of brief but high exposures may play a part as in the children playing on crocidolite tips, and in the Turkish experience of villages with presumed high level exposure to fibres taking their risk of malignancy with them when they move elsewhere. Furthermore, the risk of developing occupationally caused mesothelioma, even in the asbestos industry, is statistically low. Whether the numbers of cases of exposure for sufficiently lengthy periods in the MMMF industry are large enough must remain debatable at the present time. Confidence is augmented, however, by other related observations.

Pleural plaques

Pleural plaques, commonly found in asbestos workers, can only be regarded as indicating a lung burden of asbestos fibres. Mesotheliomas occur both in patients displaying plaques and in those without them. The absence of pleural plaques in MMMF workers, confirmed by several studies, is in conformity with the rarity of MMMF in lungs and with Gross's similarly negative findings in a limited series of post-mortem studies of the lungs of glass fibre workers. In a life-time inhalation experiment on rats, using high concentrations of glass fibres below 3 μm in diameter, the majority of which were at or below 1 μm diameter, Gross noted 'bland' pleural thickening in a small number of animals. These limited pleural reactions were not accompanied by malignancy or fibrosis, in contrast to similar inhalation experiments with asbestos. These findings are considered by Gross to represent a response to experimental conditions of a severity so far removed from conceivable human exposure as not to permit analogy. Comparable findings have not appeared in humans.

Models of disease

The concept of mesothelioma which emerges is that of a degree of individual susceptibility upon which is superimposed a factor of accumulation of fibres of significant diameters and length in specific target tissue – in this case, mesothelium. This would generate a model in which the probability of the disease, and thus what is described as the lapse or 'latent' period, was equated both with the rate of accumulation of significant fibres at the target tissue, and with their retention of oncogenic potential at that site. The lack of emergence of a mesothelioma hazard over quite lengthy MMMF exposures makes it possible to hypothesize (1) that MMMF of the right size range may not be present in sufficient numbers to produce a significant probability of carcinogenic effect within a lifetime, (2) that the duration of observation and numbers observed remain insufficient to detect a rare tumour and (3) that mechanisms exist in the lung which permit the destruction of glass fibres or prevent their translocation to the pleura. It has been shown that long glass fibres administered to guinea pigs by intratracheal injection become encapsulated in ferro-protein (similar to the formation of ferrugenous bodies); these later assume a beaded appearance and subsequently break into short fragments at the narrowed parts and are then removed by macrophages. Long glass fibres are dealt with in this way more rapidly than asbestos fibres. Short fibres (below about 10 μm) tend to be phagocytosed and removed as cellular debris.

Lung defences and malignancy

It has been postulated that the lung may be capable of dealing with limited numbers of fibres in the above and possibly other ways unless either the dose is so large as to overwhelm the defence mechanisms or the latter are diminished by co-factors such as smoking, infection or toxic dusts. Cell studies show that glass fibres are not cytotoxic, and that in the range of diameter 0·25–1 μm cell constituents are leaked as would be expected when macrophages attempt to engulf particles larger than themselves. These findings would be compatible with the operation of a cellular defence mechanism.

The fundamental basis of the malignant change induced by fibres in the pleural is unknown, but two factors have been identified:

First, tests on bacteria, have shown neither asbestos nor glass fibres to exhibit mutagenicity. While further tests using mammalian cells are needed, it has been suggested that the mechanism of action in the pleura may be similar to the Oppenheimer effect.

Second, an explanation for the specificity of the diameter range has been offered in terms of the diameter of a rigid fibre needed to transfix, but not kill, a cell. If the cell were destroyed a foreign body reaction would be likely and the detritus removed by the muco-ciliary escalator, whereas it is postulated that a damaged cell might release substances which could continue to act chemically. Enzymes such as lactic dehydrogenase and other substances are indeed released, but as yet there has been no positive demonstration that they are the carcinogenic agents. Nevertheless, the size relation of fibres of 0·5 μm diameter and below needed to transfix cells of approximately 10 μm diameter finds support in both Timbrell's own work aligning asbestos fibres with macrophages, and fits the observations of the intrapleural experiments.

A further suggestion by Maroudas et al. (1973) drew attention to the correlation between the numbers of fibres long enough to sustain cell growth in fibroblast cultures (20–200 μm) and the numbers of similar fibres in Stanton's experiments (Stanton and Wrench, 1972). Whilst this is in conflict with Pott's findings (Pott and Friedrichs, 1972) of carcinogenic potential in fine fibres as short as 5 μm in length, the way is opened to explore both length and diameter characteristics of pleural oncogenesis.

Bronchial carcinoma

In view of its different characteristics and probably different aetiology, bronchial carcinoma requires separate discussion. The possibility of any increased risk associated with MMMF exposure arises from no theoretical considerations beyond an analogy with the fibrous form. Gross found inhalation of asbestos in rats produced carcinomas (as well as mesothelioma and fibrosis) but this was not the case with glass fibres. In a large cohort study in the USA Bayliss et al. (1976) found no excess in overall mortality and no increase in deaths due to malignancies of the respiratory tract. No adverse experience was noted in Enterline's study of glass fibre pensioners (1975). A further cohort study of workers in a plant manufacturing glass fibre yarn, strand and roving was conducted by Enterline (1977). The nominal diameters were 6–13 μm, and 8 μm respectively, and the average fibre count was 0·02 fibres per cm^3 of air – typical of this 'textile' type of manufacture where fibres are manufactured by a high speed drawing process given a narrow distribution of diameters and an extremely low concentration of airborne respirable fibres. No excess mortality was observed from malignant respiratory disease, but there was a significantly raised mortality due to coronary heart disease, and an excess in the rate of pancreatic and urinary tract cancer. The coronary heart disease increase reflected the local rate, which was itself high, and the pancreatic cancer and probably the urinary tract cancer seemed unlikely to relate to the glass fibre exposure.

These details have been given to draw attention to the difficulties of epidemiological technique. Demographic variations, both in disease-specific and overall death rates, are well known (for example, compare local variations in the rate of carcinoma of the bronchus in the UK and Scandinavia). Further difficulties arise because such studies are retrospective and it is difficult to evaluate other significant influences such as smoking habits. Thus, in the cohort investigated by Bayliss et al. (1976) above, in which the primary hypothesis was to test whether glass fibre caused malignant respiratory disease, secondary analysis showed a statistically significant excess of deaths in the category 'non-malignant respiratory disease excluding influenza and pneumonia'. The mortality both from all causes and from respiratory malignancy was slightly less in the glass fibre workers than in the controls. The controls constituted the white male caucasian population of the USA, which contains a considerable proportion of rural dwellers. As the glass fibre plants studied drew their population from towns, a high incidence of bronchitis might be expected, but no local comparison was made available. Selection of workers with occupational histories of mining and pottery-making may also have influenced this observation.

Enterline's study (1975) was directed to cover both malignant and non-malignant respiratory deaths and not surprisingly, failed to confirm Bayliss et al.'s findings (1976). Preliminary reports of a further study in the USA by NIOSH suggest that a cohort of mineral-wool workers, whilst showing no statistical significant increase in any cause of death category, revealed an excess risk in the greater than 30-year latency group, for the categories 'digestive and respiratory cancer' and 'non-malignant respiratory disease'. Full details of this paper are not yet available but it appears that the excesses referred to were of doubtful statistical significance and it has already been criticized in terms of the small size of the initial cohort and the even smaller size of the numbers of cases which could be analysed for 30-year latency. It also appears that smoking and drinking habits were not considered.

Limitations of epidemiological and other studies

It has to be recognized that epidemiological methods cannot prove causal relationship by themselves and that observations of health experience are always likely to display random variation, due to statistical clustering and independent factors, such as smoking, diet and many other things. Dispassionate assessment, therefore, demands the demonstration of a systematic trend of a statistically significant nature, preferably supported by evidence suggesting a causal relationship. No such systematic trend can be found in the epidemiological evidence currently available for MMMF, in spite of the extensive studies which have been conducted.

A scientific discussion should concern itself with establishing facts, but a proper concern for safety makes it necessary to examine attitudes. Two are commonly adopted: *first* that a material is dangerous until proved safe; and *second* that a material is safe until proven dangerous. Discussion along these lines can only result in assertion and counter-assertion, and although giving rein to great philosophical debate has little relation either to the scientific or to the real world. A moment's thought about the risks of car driving or air travel shows that sensible guidance should not be derived from statements of attitude but rather from estimates of probability. The evidence presented should be examined in this light.

MMMF's fibrosis and lung function

In the next area to be considered is where the evidence is sufficient to conclude that MMMFs do not cause fibrosis of the lung and do not adversely affect lung function in humans. Studies in several countries, involving large scale X-ray surveys, detailed lung function tests and the administration of questionnaires about symptoms of bronchitis are all in agreement that no fibrosis or impairment of lung function can be attributed to MMMF.

Further support is gained from Gross et al.'s (1976) series of 20 post-mortem examinations of glass fibre workers' lungs in which he could find no tissue alteration or disease attributable to glass fibres.

Animal inhalation experiments show that the reaction to glass fibre is that of mobilization of macrophages. Following the experiment by Gross, previously referred to, in which he administered glass fibres entirely in the respirable range, he considered the material to be a 'nuisance dust' insofar as (1) the alveolar architecture remained intact, (2) there was minimal stromal proliferation consisting mainly of reticulin and (3) that the tissue reaction was potentially reversible. Glass fibres behaved similarly whether they were coated with starch, or phenol formaldehyde resin binder, or were uncoated.

In the early days of this type of animal experiment some tissue reactions were observed, which are considered to represent endemic bronchitis in rats, or to be artefacts consequent upon the technique of intratracheal injection insofar as they disappeared with time and were not observed in inhalation series.

A point of academic interest may be raised regarding the effects of fibre length by experiments using paired samples of long and short fibres. Long fibres are active and short fibres are inactive in producing fibrosis after intratracheal injection in guinea pigs. Asbestos showed a response parallel to human findings and glass fibres showed a response which was minimal. These findings relate to direct tissue contact response without the intervention of the normal lung defence mechanisms and are found neither in inhalation experiments nor in human lungs.

The absence of fibrosis induction by MMMF may be of additional interest when it is recalled that many of the carcinomas of the lung, found in asbestos workers, occur in the areas of maximum fibrosis.

The negative findings of the cross-sectional type of X-ray and lung function study are also reflected in the extremely small number of human cases in which disease and glass fibres have been associated. Three separate cases of chest illness have been reported with occupational exposures where there was a considerable lag between cessation of exposure and the onset of illness (Bezjack, 1957; Kahlau, 1947; Murphy, 1961). In all three cases, bacterial infection has been the dominant feature and the glass fibre exposure may have been incidental rather than causative. One case reported as 'fibreglass pneumoconiosis' appears to have had bronchiectasis as its basic diagnosis. A small number of workers have been reported as having asthmatic symptoms but other factors were not excluded. In the absence of the emergence of any regular pattern or trend, the insubstantial number of reports, most of which fail to withstand critical evaluation, can be seen against the perspective of the very extensive use of MMMF. It is reasonable to conclude that these fibres act similarly to any other non-specific (nuisance) dusts in exacerbating pre-existing chest disease.

Other possible effects of MMMF

In the upper respiratory tract, MMMF have been reported as producing irritation, mainly in the form of sore throats and occasional minor nose bleeds. These symptoms have been less well documented, as they attract less interest, but would be accepted as occurring in unusually dusty conditions by experienced occupational physicians. No information exists upon which suitable limit values could be estimated. A great deal of variability exists in the concentration of the sizes of fibres likely to contribute to upper respiratory tract irritation, apart from the difficulty of making reliable observations of this type of complaint. Basic principles indicate that the fibres of larger diameter and greater length are those likely to be filtered out and deposited in the upper respiratory tract where they might contribute to irritation. These heavier fibres are just those which sediment out very rapidly from dust clouds and this property accounts for the very rapid fall-off of gravimetric estimations which is usually observed between dust generated at waist level and estimations in the breathing zones. Similarly, gravimetric estimations are likely to fall very rapidly within a distance of a few feet. Representative sampling to take account of these steep gradients often requires notice to be taken of the position and characteristics of the dust source; sawing at bench level as an effectively continuous operation requiring a different technique to intermittent application of insulation material perhaps above the head. In the first instance, a time weighted average might be appropriate whereas in the second the question arises whether peak concentrations might reflect irritant potential better, in which case arbitrary decisions may have to be made as to the duration of each sample. The absence of reliable data on complaints of irritation makes the choice of options difficult. The constitution of the sample must also be remembered. Gravimetric samples tend to contain about 10 per cent of glass in fibrous form. The remaining 90 per cent comprises glass and resin fragments together with other mineral material. Although there is no scientific evidence to identify the fibres as the cause of upper respiratory irritation their presence is probably the main difference between this and other general dusts. Quantification of this problem is clearly beset by serious technical and practical difficulties. If arbitrary levels are chosen at which the wearing of masks is advised, an exchange may be being made between a hypothetical upper respiratory tract irritation and a real problem of skin irritation. The latter may be minimized by the use of cloth masks as opposed to a rubber facepiece. These are usually sufficient to stop pharyngitis and other like problems in highly dusty conditions where masks are indicated. It is sufficient to trap relatively large diameter fibres in order to prevent upper respiratory tract irritation.

Dust counts

Standard techniques are recognized for collecting and counting airborne respirable fibres. These involve sampling at flow rate of 2 litres per minute through membrane filters. The porosity of these filters has to be sufficiently large to permit an air flow adequate to secure capture of fibres, and this makes it difficult to use filters with a porosity below 0·5 μm diameter and 0·8 μm porosity is usually used. While fibres less than this diameter are therefore theoretically capable of passing the filter,. the error introduced is likely to be constant, and the method can be accepted as offering a satisfactory reference point.

The counting convention is to count all fibres in the field by optical or electron microscopy. In plants producing fibres of large nominal diameter there is little difference in the numbers estimated by either method, although, as the nominal diameter falls to 1 μm and below, the numbers determined by electron microscopy increased significantly.

In contrast to asbestos dust clouds it is quite characteristic of MMMF that very high gravimetric estimations are commonly associated with extremely low respirable fibre counts, as would be expected from the aerodynamic behaviour indicated previously. In production areas, gravimetric determinations in excess of 10 mg per m^3 are still found to contain an average of only about 0·2 respirable fibres per ml or less. The highest counts rarely exceed about half a fibre per ml. The diameter distribution varies with distance from the source, 2·5 μm diameter being typical of the median of a production plant, this being found commonly with lengths averaging about 50 μm. With increased sedimentation, the further one goes from the source of dust the thinner and shorter the fibres tend to be. Secondary processes might have a median diameter distribution of about 1·5 μm.

It will be seen that only a fraction of these already extremely low counts are likely to consist of fibres in the 0·2 μm diameter range, and that in the continuous filament part of the industry, where respirable fibre concentrations are of the order of 0·002 fibres per ml, the numbers will be minute by comparison with fibres of known hazard such as asbestos.

In considering the question of the probability of hazard with MMMF the extremely low concentrations of airborne respirable fibres encountered in occupational exposures is of great importance. It must also be recognized that similarly low fibre counts are found in the presence of high gravimetric estimations. The inability of glass fibres to split longitudinally into larger numbers of finer fibrils suggests that these counts represent a valid reflection of dose. The dustiest plants are wool insulation plants and these have been in production since the late 1800s in the case of mineral fibres, and since the mid 1930s in the case of glass fibres, without significant human pathology being reported.

Submicron fibres

A caveat must be made in the case of the introduction in Germany and the the USA, during the last decade, of special purpose fibres entirely in the submicron diameter range. These are made by a flame attenuation process and are usually uncoated. Airborne respirable fibre counts of 30–40 fibres per ml have been observed and in view of the diameter distribution and potentially different mechanical characteristics due to the different method of manufacture, they should be regarded with caution. Their main use is in filters for scientific purposes.

One other application may require special attention and that is the use of glass fibres in paper making where binding is less efficient and high airborne respirable fibre counts are observed but, of course, with wider fibre diameters.

Conclusions

The problems which surround the application of gravimetric limit values have been outlined. The logic of using a fibre count with a view to imposing the wearing of dust masks above some arbitrary level remains debatable in the absence of human responses, particularly since the range of diameters in question are less than the diameter of the pores of most 'approved' respirators, which as with some types of asbestos, may not be completely effective.

In contrast to naturally occurring fibres like asbestos, MMMFs are under engineering control. Technical and economic considerations currently prevent the elimination of submicron fibres, but no doubt work will be directed to this end in the future.

It is essential to find a safe substitute for asbestos because of health reasons, together with the foreseeable exhaustion of natural resources in the next 25 years or so at present rates of usage. The Turkish experience suggests that a policy of prudence would be to utilize only substitutes which have a well-documented history. MMMFs probably represent the most extensively researched material in common industrial use which has presented no hazard. Although negative evidence has special problems in itself, the probability of the safety of MMMF must now be considerable. Fibrosis and impairment of lung function has not occurred in humans. Within the limits of epidemiological evidence carcinoma of the lung does not appear to be a hazard, nor does such an eventuality find any support in animal or cell experiments. Mesothelioma logically requires separate consideration. Subject to the problems of detecting a very rare tumour, and to the long period of induction which might be hypothesized, there has been a total absence of this tumour. The lengthy period of manufacture should also be borne in mind. Chance may well produce such tumours, as in all but one series, some 10–15 per cent of patients in mesothelioma studies have not been found to have occupational exposures to asbestos and must be presumed to occur *per naturam.* The total absence of mesotheliomas in association with MMMF so far is encouraging. Studies are in progress both in animals and in the form of retrospective and prospective epidemiological investigations, which should help to resolve this remaining problem.

Practical decisions have to be made concerning a safe substitute for asbestos and the properties required indicate that substitutes for many applications will need to be fibrous in form. From the above, it will be seen that a thorough knowledge of such potential substitutes is needed, taking account of the airborne concentrations and diameter distribution by which they are characterized, and of indications of possible effects from animal and cell culture experiments, together with validation of the safety of such materials in the light of knowledge of human cases and human epidemiology.

REFERENCES

Baris Y. L. (1975) *Environmental Asbestos Related Diseases in Turkey*. Hacettepe University, School of Medicine, Department of Chest Diseases, Anakara, Turkey.

Bayliss D. L., Dement J., Wagoner J. K. et al. (1976) *Ann. N. Y. Acad. Sci.* **271**, 324–335.

Bezjack B. (1957) *Arh. Hig. Rada* **7**, 338.

Enterline P. E. (1975) *Arch. Environ. Health* **30**, 113–166.

Enterline P. E. (1977) *Mortality among Man-made Mineral Fiber Workers in the United States.* Presented at the 105th Annual Meeting of the American Public Health Association, Washington, D.C.

Gross P., Harley R. A. and Davis J. M. G. (1976) The lungs of fibreglass workers: comparison with the lungs of a control population. *Occupational Exposure to Fibrous Glass. Proceedings of a Symposium, College Park, Maryland, 1974.* HEW Publications No. (NIOSH) 76–151. US Department of Health, Education and Welfare, Washington, pp. 249–263.

Gross P., Cralley L. J., Davis J. M. G. et al. (1971) A quantitative study of fibrous dust in the lungs of city dwellers. *Inhaled Particles III. Proceedings of an International Symposium organised by British Occupational Hygiene Society, London, 1970,* vol. 2. Ed. Walton W. H. Old Woking, Unwin, pp. 671–579.

Hill J. W. (1977) Health aspects of man-made mineral fibres; a review. *Ann. Occup. Hyg.* **20**, 161–173.

Kahlau G. (1974) Tödlische Pneumonie nack Glasstaubinhalation durch Verarbeitung eines Kunststoffes aus Glasswohle. *Frank. Z. Path.* **59**, 143–150.

Maroudas N. G., O'Neill C. H. and Stanton M. F. (1973) Fibroblast anchorage in carcinogenesis by fibres. *Lancet* **1**, 807–809.

Murphy G. B. (1961) Fiber glass pneumoconioses. *Arch. Environ. Health* **3**, 704–710.

Oppenheimer (1960) *Ciba Foundation on Carcinogenesis.*

Pott F. and Friedrichs K. H. (1972) Tumoren der Ratte nach i.p. – Injektion fasergförmiger Staübe. *Naturwissenschaften* **59**, 318.

Stanton M. F. and Wrench C. (1972) *J. Natl. Cancer Inst.* **48**, 797–821.

Timbrell V. (1973) Physical factors as etiological mechanisms. *Biological Effects of Asbestos. Proceedings of a Working Conference, Lyons* 1972. Ed. Bogovski P., Gibson J. C., Timbrell V. et al. IARC Scientific Publications No. 8, International Agency for Research on Cancer, Lyons, pp. 295–303.

Timbrell V. (1976) Aerodynamic considerations and other aspects of glass fiber. *Occupational Exposure to Fibrous Glass. Proceedings of a Symposium, College Park, Maryland, 1974.* HEW Publications No. (NIOSH) 76–151. US Department of Health, Education and Welfare, Washington D. C., pp. 33–50.

Timbrell V. and Skidmore J. W. (1971) The effects of shape on particle penetration and retention in animal lungs. *Inhaled Particles III. Proceedings of an International Symposium organised by the British Occupational Hygiene Society London, 1970*, vol. 1. Ed. Walton W. H. Old Woking, Unwin, pp. 49–57.

Wagner J. C., Berry G. and Skidmore J. W. (1976) Studies of the carcinogenic effects of fiberglass of different diameters following intrapleural inoculation in experimental animals. *Occupational Exposure to Fibrous Glass. Proceedings of a Symposium, College Park, Maryland, 1974.* HEW Publications No. (NIOSH) 76–151. US Department of Health, Education and Welfare, Washington D. C., pp. 193–197.

7. SOME OCCUPATIONAL RESPIRATORY DISORDERS

K. H. Nickol

INHALED PARTICLES

The skin, gut and lungs are more directly and intimately exposed to external agents than any other part of the body. We can cover the skin and select what we swallow but we have to go on breathing. We inhale about 500 litres of air every hour and with it any gaseous or particulate contaminants which it contains. Their biological effects vary from the negligible to the rapidly fatal. Some, like carbon monoxide or lead dust, are rapidly absorbed from the respiratory tract and do their damage elsewhere. Others lodge for a longer or shorter time in the lungs. Their effects depend not only on their biological activity but also on the depth within the respiratory system to which they can penetrate.

Particle deposition

The nose is a major trap for intrusive particles (Proctor et al., 1969). Only about 50 per cent of particles of 5 μm diameter penetrate beyond the nose. Under quiet mouth breathing conditions the fate of inhaled particles depends on their size, shape and density. The larger and heavier particles fall and hit the walls of the air passages (sedimentation) or have too much momentum to be swept round corners with the tide of inhaled air. They strike the bronchial wall on the outside of bends or where the airways divide (impaction).

Most of the smaller and lighter particles are able to maintain their position in the airstream and reach the alveoli. They are, by custom, called 'respirable' although the description is unfortunate since it leaves no suitable term for inhaled particles whose ambition is limited to tracheo-bronchial deposition. There is no sharp dividing line between respirable and non-respirable particles but the critical size is about the diameter of a red blood corpuscle (7 μm). As the bronchi divide the number of air passages increases faster than their reduction in calibre. Their total cross sectional area therefore increases as one proceeds inwards. At least 80 per cent of the total airways resistance is in the larger airways (Editorial, 1973). During inspiration air and particles travel more and more slowly until by the end of the breath all forward momentum has been lost. Alveolar entry of the surviving particles depends on diffusion. This random jostling also causes some particles to hit the bronchial or alveolar walls and indeed prevents the smallest particles from escaping during expiration. This is why the deposition curve (Fig. 7.1) rises for particles smaller than 0·1 μm in diameter. The lowest percentage of deposition is for particles of about 0·5 μm diameter.

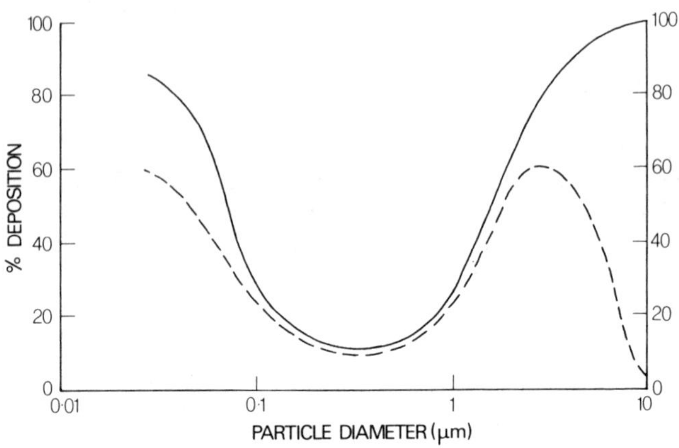

Fig. 7.1. Per cent deposition of inhaled aerosols as a function of particle size. Mouth breathing at rest. Total deposition (——), Alveolar deposition (- - -). Reproduced from *Clinical Aspects of Inhaled Particles,* through the courtesy of Dr D. C. F. Muir and the publishers, William Heinemann Medical Books Ltd.

Particle clearance

Once a particle has landed on a bronchial wall it can progress no further. Caught on the 'ciliary escalator' it is wafted up to the glottis and then swallowed. In rats the cilia beat at about 400 strokes/minute in the terminal bronchioles and about three times as fast in the trachea (Iravani, 1971). This prevents particle congestion as the tributaries merge. Tracheo-bronchial clearance is normally completed within 24 hours (Lippmann et al., 1971).

Alveolar clearance is not quite so efficient. Up to about 40 g of dust may be found in the lungs of deceased coal miners but this represents only some 4 per cent of the total alveolar dust which may have been inhaled throughout a working life. Experimentally the rate of alveolar clearance is usually measured with a scintillation counter after the inhalation of a radio-active aerosol. The half-life clearance rate varies under different conditions from a few days to months (Hatch and Gross, 1964). Most particles which have reached the alveoli are engulfed by macrophages, find their way to the terminal bronchioles and follow the normal pattern of tracheo-bronchial clearance. A few penetrate the alveolar walls and reside in the interstitial tissue, or are taken up by macrophages which carry them to the regional lymph nodes.

The macrophage response is proportional to the alveolar dust burden (Brain, 1971) but not to the biological activity of the material (Hatch and Gross, 1964). Events following initial phagocytosis follow a very different course if the particles are, like quartz, strongly fibrogenic. The macrophages release enzymes which disrupt the phagosomes and free the particles into the cell cytoplasm. Some mechanism as yet not fully understood results in the death and disruption of the cell (Parkes, 1974). This militates against the ciliary clearance of the released particles which are again free to penetrate the alveolar wall and stimulate a tissue reaction. Further waves of macrophages appear and one quartz particle may be ingested repeatedly and kill a succession of them (Morgan and Seaton, 1975). The belief that the fibrogenic activity of quartz is due to its physical sharpness or acidity in solution has given ground to a necessarily more complex hypothesis (Heppleston, 1971).

TREATMENT OF PULMONARY FIBROSIS

The retention of many biologically active dusts causes fibrosis. Attempts have been made to treat both occupational fibrosis and that occuring in conditions such as sarcoidosis, rheumatoid lung and systemic sclerosis. Although aluminium has been shown to reduce quartz-induced fibrosis in experimental animals (Le Bouffant et al., 1977) therapeutic trials in man for periods up to 3 years have proved ineffective (Kennedy, 1956). While experimental evidence has shown that polyvinyl pyridine-*N*-oxide (PVNO) protects pulmonary macrophages from destruction by quartz, therapeutic results in animals (Shlensky, 1970; Weller, 1977) and in man (Antweiler, 1976) have been inconsistent.

Experimentally the lung fibrosis induced by quartz is reduced if iron oxide is also inhaled. In a study of nearly 8000 iron ore miners who also inhaled quartz Reichel et al. (1977) concluded that iron had reduced the degree of fibrosis to be expected from quartz alone.

The treatment of rheumatoid arthritis with steroids, chloroquine and D-penicillamine has provided opportunities to observe their effect on any coincident lung lesions. Davies (1973) has reported improvement in rheumatoid pneumoconiosis treated with chloroquine and steroids. Penicillamine inhibits the cross linking of newly formed collagen (Nimni, 1977) and in 22 patients with systemic sclerosis some improvement in skin and joint changes was observed by Jayson et al. (1977). In the 8 patients with lung involvement no benefit was observed. Immunosuppresive agents are being used by some in progressive sarcoidosis and any success in this field could lead to trials in occupational medicine.

SMOKING

Many aspects of medical research are complicated by the need to take account of the effects of smoking. This is especially important in relation to bronchitis, emphysema and lung cancer. Tracheo-bronchial deposition of inhaled particles is increased by smoking (Lippmann et al., 1971). This might be expected to protect smokers from diseases caused by alveolar deposition but Love and Muir (1976) found that total deposition was increased in smokers and could counterbalance the tendency for deposition to shift centrally. Jacobsen et al. (1977) have found that the attack rate of simple pneumoconiosis in coal miners is not significantly affected by smoking. Tracheo-bronchial clearance is impaired by smoking (Albert et al., 1971; Lippmann et al., 1977) and Sanchis et al. (1971) found that clearance from the larger airways was affected more than that from the smaller, leading to a 'log-jam' accumulation of particles. Airways clearance has been studied in normal and bronchitic rats (Iravani, 1971) and impairment of ciliary activity and mucus transport found in those with bronchitis. Impaired lung clearance has also been found in rats given injections of papaine to induce emphysema (Ferin, 1971).

Delayed tracheo-bronchial clearance could be clinically important in the case of particles which exert a harmful effect while resident in the airways. Increasing the clearance time by 50 per cent may be likened to prolonging an employee's exposure to atmospheric contaminants by several hours' overtime each day. This may be especially important in relation to the carcinogenic effects of radio-active particles and asbestos.

RADIOGRAPHY

Radiography is the most useful aid in the diagnosis and assessment of many respiratory diseases and is often the first indicator of any abnormality. In airways disease without panacinar emphysema or other complications the chest radiograph is usually uninformative (Simon, 1972). Basic interpretation of chest radiographs is described by Turner-Warwick (1973).

If radiographs are being taken for epidemiological purposes in a population at risk from pneumoconiosis guidance about suitable technique should first be sought (Jacobsen et al., 1970; International Labour Office, 1972). Harmony now prevails in the classification of the radiographic appearances of pneumoconiosis (International Labour Office, 1972) in which small rounded and small irregular opacities appear on an equal footing. The Medical Research Council (1942) referred to linear and reticular opacities as representing the early stages of pneumoconiosis. Muir (1974) claimed that improved radiographic technique showed that such reticulation was really nodulation and that the former term had wisely been dropped. Loyalty to the concept of linear and reticular opacities was maintained by McLaughlin (1962). This has received support from Lyons et al. (1974) who in a study of deceased coal miners found a correlation between the extent of small irregular opacities, impairment of Forced Expiratory Volume in one second (FEV_1), and degree of emphysema found at autopsy. No such correlation was found for small rounded opacities.

Amandus et al. (1976) found a significant correlation between irregular opacities and years spent underground mining coal. Interest in irregular opacities has reached the point where combined radiological scores for rounded and irregular opacities have been used (Liddell, 1977). It seems preferable to report them separately until further data have clarified their status.

The techniques for reading serial films for pneumoconiosis are reviewed by Liddell and Morgan (1978) and the balance of advantage concluded to lie with side by side viewing. The technique of xeroradiography with 200 kV exposure is advocated for the study of pleural and linear parenchymal opacities (Glyn-Thomas and Sluis-Cremer, 1977). The possible advantages of using high voltage techniques are discussed by Washington et al. (1973) but no clear advantage emerged.

DIAGNOSIS AND ASSESSMENT OF OCCUPATIONAL RESPIRATORY DISORDERS

Clinical features

The nature of respiratory symptoms and signs is seldom a strong pointer to their occupational cause. Cough, sputum production and dyspnoea are accepted as frequent manifestations of the general burden of disease in many countries. In the past, characterized by small population movements, local differences in the prevalence of respiratory morbidity and mortality were readily accepted and possible occupational factors overlooked. Even close association in time does not ensure that respiratory illness is correctly associated with the relevant cause. It is even more difficult when the symptoms or radiographic changes come about years later, perhaps when the individual has changed his job or retired.

Schilling wrote (1970), 'The occupational cause of a patient's respiratory illness may be detected by a physician in any branch of medicine who takes an occupational history and understands its significance.' He goes on to qualify this statement by pointing out that, 'The epidemiological method... may be the only way of detecting the occupational causes of diseases like lung cancer and non-specific respiratory diseases that commonly occur in the general population.'

Pulmonary function

Pulmonary function tests are a valuable adjunct to clinical inquiry (McKerrow, 1964), though less as a diagnostic aid than as an indicator of the severity of impairment and its change with time as reflected by serial measurements. In all clinical and physiological assessments the possible effects of smoking must be considered, not only because of the obstructive lung disease which it may cause but because of the different behaviour of inhaled particles in smokers and interactions between smoking and a wide variety of substances capable of causing respiratory disease. Some smokers give inconsistent accounts of their habit. On serial questioning they commonly claim to have cut down dramatically but quote the same current consumption as that sworn to on previous occasions (smokers' deception syndrome).

Radiography

A confident diagnosis of occupational lung disease can seldom be made on the basis of radiographic appearances alone. The list of over 70 causes of diffuse nodular or reticular shadowing given by Scadding (1952) could now be considerably extended. Many of the conditions have hallmarks which at least serve to narrow the field of probabilities but his message was that too much reliance must not be placed on radiographic appearances taken in isolation. A group of employees from a flint works was reviewed periodically in a hospital chest department. For some years nothing significant was found but obvious small rounded opacities were then seen in the chest film of a man who had spent some years calcining flint. Some months later the lesions in both upper zones were begining to coalesce. The physician became very excited and visited the works, expecting to find extremely dusty conditions. However, most of the work was enclosed, wet, or done in the open air. At his next attendance the patient had denser upper zone fibrosis and a localized pneumothorax. This is rare, even in pneumoconiosis with progressive massive fibrosis except, curiously, in aluminium workers (Shaver and Riddell, 1947) but diagnostic confidence was unshaken. The patient died some months later and a precise diagnosis eluded the most cunning histologists. One thing was certain; there was no silicosis.

Even if the occupational origin of radiographic changes is correctly assumed, conclusions about their effects on health must be reached with caution. The absence of significant tissue reaction to deposits of tin or barium is securely established and the same is true of the pure iron deposits in welders (Doig and McLaughlin, 1936). But iron is frequently inhaled with silica or other fibrogenic dusts (Stewart and Faulds, 1934; McLaughlin, 1950) and because of its density it may make a disproportionate contribution to the radiographic appearances. It is not easy to make allowance for this even with the help of information from the mineral analysis of lung tissue from deceased workers. Bergman (1970) has shown that the total iron content of pneumoconiotic lungs may exceed that contributed by inhaled particles and the blood content of pulmonary tissue. A technique for measuring the non-haem iron in lungs gives haemosiderin concentrations which are proportional to the pneumoconiosis category in coal miners. Indeed, Bergman and Casswell (1972) suggest that materials like coal mine dust give rise to the appearances of pneumoconiosis mainly through their stimulation of iron deposits in the lungs.

Pulmonary nodules may occur in rheumatoid arthritis but are more common in the presence of pneumoconiosis (Caplan, 1953). Pulmonary rheumatoid nodules may occasionally cavitate (Turner-Warwick, 1969). The occupational physician may see Caplan's syndrome during radiographic surveys and is able occasionally to derive gloomy satisfaction from predicting the later onset of arthritis in a subject with no joint symptoms.

Chest radiography is a mixed blessing. Gone are the days when one can see major radiographic changes but tell the patient only what is 'good for him'. Increasingly the burdens of uncertain diagnosis, unknown prognosis and ineffective treatment have to be shared between physician and patient. The overall benefit of sensibly organized radiographic surveys of employees exposed to relevant occupational hazards is undoubted but the time, money and effort involved must be justified by making the best possible use of the information obtained. Even so, the inexorable chain of events started by certain positive findings means that some are destined to suffer through one's best endeavours. A former asbestos worker known to have minimal lung fibrosis developed a dense oval radiographic opacity unaccompanied by symptoms or change in physical signs. The overwhelming probability that this was a carcinoma dictated its removal but histology showed it to be a mass of asbestotic fibrous tissue. Only consequent on the operation has the patient had any respiratory dysfunction.

Professional relationships

Most doctors know little about the conditions under which their patients work or about the likely interactions between work and health. It is, nevertheless, right that they should take account of medical conditions which they believe, or their patients claim, to be occupational. Where there is no medical colleague at the place of employment their problems of informed assessment are great, but the existence of an occupational medical service enables professional relationships to be established and information shared. Under such conditions doctors writing to the occupational physician serve their patients best by presenting any advice or request in medical rather than in managerial terms. The observation that a patient's asthma is aggravated by dusty work defines the problem and leaves the occupational medical service freedom of action in seeking a solution. The bald request for a patient's transfer to another plant fails to define any environmental problem which is suspected and neglects the possibility of its solution within the working group with which the patient is familiar. In small workplaces where the medical service may be run by a nurse working on her own, doctors should accept that her local knowledge and occupational medical expertise may be more relevant than superior medical learning.

The work environment

The doctor's or nurse's familiarity with the factory may rely solely on personal observation or may enjoy the benefit of an occupational hygiene service. The correlation of environmental with medical data is often the cornerstone of research into the medical effects of working conditions. Due consideration must always be given to the effects of changes with the passage of time. Present symptoms or radiographic abnormalities may relate to environmental conditions years ago. The change from assessing most airborne particles by mass instead of by particle counting has created a rift between observations made with each technique in spite of formulae devised to make data comparison possible. What is not so apparent is the peaceful revolution by which the use of personal samplers has tended to replace static sampling. Threshold limit values (TLVs) based originally on static sampling may not be valid for personal sampling data where sources of dust generation are widely spaced and the contour lines of dust concentration fall away steeply from each process or machine.

Correct diagnosis and assessment of occupational respiratory disease should be as broadly based as possible; resting on clinical, radiographic and environmental data. The possibility of its existence may come to the attention of the occupational physician in many ways. In addition to the classical presentations through symptoms or abnormal investigation findings there is the stimulus of informed scrutiny of the working environment, fresh knowledge from medical publications and epidemiological observations based on mortality or morbidity data. The stimulus may be the receipt of an offensive solicitor's letter; the vituperation of a shop steward or the snide remarks of a plant manager. One should be ready to learn from all sources in order to fulfill one's duty of care to people who come to work trusting that their health will not be harmed because of the way they earn their living.

BRONCHITIS

It is a matter of common experience that breathing some things makes one cough. As children we met the garden bonfire; as students the effects of unstoppering certain laboratory reagents. Visitors and new employees in some factories are upset by a variety of atmospheric contaminants. In some instances those who continue such work lose their initial symptoms, just as the skin newly exposed to a minor irritant may develop a 'hardening rash' and then recover. Because of the immediacy of the response there is seldom any argument about the environmental cause and either the problem is resolved at source or the exposed employees leave, recover or endure. Consideration of occupation and chronic bronchitis is more difficult.

For epidemiological purposes symptoms are generally assessed by using the Medical Research Council questionnaire (Medical Research Council, 1976) or some modification designed to provide the answer to a particular inquiry. The wording of the questions and the way they are posed have been carefully planned and any alterations or additions may be found to bias the results.

Symptoms are often correlated with measurements of ventilatory capacity such as the Forced Expiratory Volume in one second (FEV_1) and Forced Vital Capacity (FVC) or the Peak Expiratory Flow (PEF) rate. In a proportion of chronic bronchitics reduction in all these indices is found giving a physiological picture of mixed restriction and airways obstruction, the latter usually predominating.

Mortality and morbidity data demonstrate relationships between chronic bronchitis and social class, smoking and geographical location. The variation of Standardized Mortality Ratios with occupation is at first sight equally striking but the same differences are seen in the wives as in their husbands working in contrasting environmental conditions (Medical Research Council, 1966).

Surveys of bronchitis and/or ventilatory function have been reported for a wide range of occupational groups. Doll et al. (1965) reported an increased mortality from bronchitis among gas workers, especially those in horizontal retort houses. No further support was found when the survey was extended (Doll et al., 1972), perhaps because of intervening improvements in working conditions. Bronchitis has also been found to be associated with the coke industry (Walker et al., 1971), foundry work (Lloyd Davies et al., 1971; Mikov 1974; Joder, 1976), newspaper workers (Moss et al., 1972) and gold mining (Wiles and Faure, 1977). Joder found no more bronchitis among those foundry workers exposed to irritant fumes but Lloyd Davies et al. found a slightly increased prevalence of the sputum-chest-illness syndrome among iron and steel moulders, iron furnacemen and crane drivers.

An extensive investigation in South Wales steelworks (Lowe et al., 1968; Lowe, 1969; Lowe et al., 1970) showed only a small increase in bronchitis among steelworkers compared with controls. The effect, if any, of occupation was, as in most surveys, overshadowed by the larger effects of smoking. Higgins et al. (1968) found significantly lower FEV_1 values among elderly coal miners and ex-miners, even in those without pneumoconiosis. A significant association was found between increasing dust exposure and the prevalence of bronchitis in British coal miners aged 35–44 but not for those over 45 (Rae et al., 1971). For most of this study dust exposure was estimated by counting particles in the size range 0·5–5·0 μm. The authors note that this technique of dust assessment (whose main purpose was related to pneumoconiosis) may not be the most suitable when considering airways disease, for which particles larger than 5 μm in diameter may be at least as important. Yet two of the most potent causes of bronchitis, cigarette smoking and urban air pollution, are characterized by particularly small particles. The fact of the matter is that in seeking to correlate bronchitis with occupational environments we do not know what is the most relevant material to sample and whether the material collected should be studied by mass, surface area of other parameters. The study of coal miners was extended by Rogan et al. (1973)

who found a progressive reduction in FEV_1 with increasing cumulative exposure to respirable airborne coal mine dust. Given the same dust exposure, however, the FEV_1 was no lower in those with pneumoconiosis than in those without. The significance of bronchitis surveys was admirably reviewed by Gilson (1970).

When one comes to look for specific causes for the small excess of bronchitis in certain occupations the findings are no more dramatic. Doll et al. (1965, 1972) incriminate the products of coal carbonization, and Wiles and Faure (1977) found a dose-response relationship between the degree of bronchitis and amount of dust inhaled, as measured by particle counting in gold mines. Lowe et al. (1970) had concluded that for their steel workers: 'If there is any relation between respiratory disability and atmospheric pollution in the two steelworks it is so slight that none of the three approaches to the problem was sensitive enough to detect it.' The effect of smoking was clearly demonstrated, with heavy smokers being about three times more likely to suffer from chronic bronchitis than non-smokers.

Experimentally the effects of smoking, bronchitis and emphysema can be separated but it is difficult to distinguish the effects of bronchitis from those of emphysema in field surveys. Emphysema is relatively rare in non-smokers and apart from the chronic effects of cadmium poisoning does not appear to have primary occupational associations. Certain occupational causes of bronchitis such as exposure to cotton dust clearly have an immunological component and the finding that deficiency of α_1-antitrypsin is associated with obstructive airways disease in relatively light smokers (Mittman et al., 1973) raises the possibility of genetic factors in relation to occupational bronchitis and perhaps the prospect of protecting the most susceptible individuals from potentially harmful environments.

OCCUPATIONAL LUNG CANCER

It has been suggested that four out of every five cancers may have their origin in the environment (Clayson, 1967; Boyland, 1977) and that the working environment plays a large part. Primary cancers in some sites, such as the nose or scrotum, are rare in the absence of occupational factors but lung cancer is so common that a small increase in its incidence from occupational causes is difficult to demonstrate. If non-occupational causes for a particular type of cancer can be discounted it seems reasonable to expect the employer to do all that is possible to stop the cancers by eliminating the hazard at source. If, on the other hand, the cancer is one occurring frequently in the general population a considerable excess of observed over expected cases must occur before occupational factors are established. The employer's objective in such situations could be the reduction of the particular cancer among his employees to the incidence prevailing in the general population. As cancers may take many years to develop the employer may have a responsibility to past as well as to present employees in order to facilitate early diagnosis. It is not normally possible to tell in the individual if his cancer is occupational or if he would have developed it anyhow, but in epidemiological terms occupational cancers tend to occur at an earlier age. In some situations the incidence of other primary tumours is greater than that expected.

The list of threshold limit values published annually by the American Conference of Industrial Hygienists includes substances recognized or suspected to be carcinogenic in man. To some, but not to all, a TLV is assigned. Hatch (1972) says of exposure to hazardous agents, 'The occurrence of zero response at an exposure level above zero does not identify an absolute no-response bench mark but simply reflects the limit of sensitivity of the particular kind of response being measured. A threshold dose so determined has no certain meaning, therefore, as an index of safety.' He goes on to distinguish between exposure levels which cause impairment and those causing disability. This concept has been recognized by the British Occupational Hygiene Society in promulgating an environmental standard for exposure to chrysotile dust; but they made it clear that the standard did not relate to the carcinogenic potential of asbestos. If the earliest detectable response to an environmental hazard is cancer and no concentration of the carcinogen can be shown to exert a nil effect there remains the burden of proposing an environmental standard below which the incidence of cancer is judged to be 'acceptable'. Hitherto 'acceptable' has meant all right with the medical advisers and managers. In future it will depend increasingly upon acceptance by those exposed to the risk.

As factors other than occupation are shown to affect the incidence of cancers, their possible interaction with occupational factors must be considered. With regard to lung cancer, smoking habits, age and sex are clearly pertinent. Some national laws now limit the freedom of employers to pick and choose who shall work for them. Leaving aside legal restraints it would seem logical to employ a population rich in non-smoking, elderly women in an occupation associated with lung cancer. An even greater refinement might be the exclusion from hazardous work of those with a high level of the enzyme aryl hydrocarbon hydroxylase which is associated with the metabolism of chemical carcinogens (Kellermann et al., 1973).

In some cases where an occupation predisposes to lung cancer the exact carcinogen has not been identified. The various substances met with in industrial practice cannot be treated as independent variables to be manipulated one at a time to see what happens. Studies of occupational cancer must therefore be concerned at times with pure substances, at other times with mixtures whose components have not been tested separately and yet again with industrial populations in whose midst there is an unknown carcinogen at work.

Chromates

Bidstrup and Case (1956) investigated the incidence of lung cancer in three factories producing bichromates from ore. Of 59 deaths which occurred during almost 6 years' observation 12 were from lung cancer. The expected number was 3·3 and the excess, especially in workers under 55, was highly significant. Enterline (1974) also found a respiratory hazard among chromate workers which appeared to be lessening with the introduction of new plant. A cohort study of workers producing chromate pigments (Langard and Norseth, 1975) also revealed an excess of lung cancers. Bidstrup (1978) has found that it is prudent for workers to have chest radiographs every 8 months in order to detect cancers at an operable stage. Fortunately they tend to be peripheral and some may be removed by local resection. In a mortality study of workers at 3 chrome pigment factories Davies (1978) has found an increase in lung cancer associated with zinc chromate but not with lead chromate. An effect was demonstrable after exposure for as little as one year but no further cases have yet been seen following improvements in working conditions in about 1954.

Haematite mining

Faulds and Stewart (1956) examined the post-mortem records of 180 haematite miners and found lung cancer in 9·4 per cent. They considered the possibility that the mines contained radioactive material but found no evidence of this. It was therefore natural to contemplate an association between the cancers and the finding of sidero-silicotic nodules in the miners' lungs. However, Boyd et al. (1970), reporting a continuing excess of lung cancers from the same mining area, some of which apparently arose from sidero-silicotic nodules, also noted the finding of high radon concentrations in the air of three of the mines and this may well be responsible for the cancers.

Nickel workers

The finding of an excess number of cases of lung and nasal cancer in the nickel refiners in South Wales was reported by Doll (1958) and Morgan (1958). Though many have since assumed the carcinogen to be nickel carbonyl the original authors felt that the handling of nickel containing ores was a more likely cause. Changes in the process appear to have eliminated the hazard but investigations to determine the precise cause are continuing (Doll et al., 1977). Konetzke (1974) found lung cancers, including multicentric growths, among workers exposed to both nickel and arsenic. Both have been found to be carcinogenic in animals. Skin and lung cancers had also been reported in workers handling inorganic arsenic compounds by Hill and Faning (1948).

Other causes

An excess of lung cancer has been found among gas workers (Doll et al., 1965, 1972; Kawai et al., 1967). Workers on coke ovens have been found by some to have an increased lung cancer risk (Lloyd, 1971; Redmond et al., 1972; Mazumdar et al., 1975) but Davies (1977) found no excess of deaths from lung cancer, other malignant neoplasms or respiratory disease generally. It is conceivable that the overall figures conceal a smaller group bearing a lung cancer risk, but the data could not validly be divided into groups with differing environmental conditions. In other studies it was the oven topmen who had the greatest cancer risk. Lloyd (1971) found a positive correlation between lung cancer and the temperature of coal carbonization.

Moss et al. (1972) and Greenberg (1972) have demonstrated an excess mortality from lung cancer among newspaper workers and suggest prospective studies to elucidate the cause. The carcinogenic effect of the chloromethyl ethers has been demonstrated by many authors (Figueroa et al., 1973; Weiss and Boucot, 1975). The usual exposure is to chloromethylmethyl ether containing a small amount of (bis)chloromethyl ether. The cancers tend to be undifferentiated and to occur in relatively young men. Weiss and Figueroa (1976) interestingly found an inverse relationship with smoking.

Many other substances and processes have fallen under suspicion of causing lung cancer. There has been a tendency for speculation about the possible effects of oil mist on the lungs to be handed on from publication to publication gathering confidence from repetition. Waterhouse (1971) has reported an excess of subsequent primary cancers in various sites, including the lung, among men already known to have scrotal cancer; but good evidence of an excess of lung cancer is still lacking for the many populations of workers exposed to oil mist.

The knowledge that exposure to wood dust may be associated with cancer of the paranasal sinuses (Acheson et al., 1968) has naturally led to surmise about lung cancer in similar situations. So far, apart from asthma from certain wood dusts, only minor lung changes have been reported (Michaels, 1967). Evidence concerning the possible carcinogenic action of cadmium has recently been reviewed (British Occupational Hygiene Society, 1977) but not yet found to justify any conclusion.

SILICEOUS PNEUMOCONIOSES

The earth's crust is rich in silica and many forms have industrial applications (Parkes, 1974). In the era before mechanization man's exposure to dusty atmospheres was limited and the prevalence of respirable particles generally low. Pneumoconiosis is known to occur in Transkei women who use siliceous stones to grind corn indoors (Editorial, 1968); but it is likely that silicosis became commoner when work such as quarrying, mining and tunnelling was done in confined spaces and when mechanical aids increased the speed of dust generation and reduced more particles to respirable size. Desert dwellers have long been considered free from silicosis in spite of being surrounded by such quantities of sand. Bar-Ziv and Goldberg (1974) describe silica dust particles in the lungs of 54 Bedouins presenting among routine hospital autopsy material. Mild fibrous scarring was found but no classic silicotic nodules. They attribute the relative inertness of the particles to their being 'old', as distinct from the freshly broken down material found in factories. This hypothesis is supported by Browne (1973) who says that recently fragmented siliceous particles have a much more powerful surface activity; that is, they are more potentially dangerous and that polished sand is not particularly dangerous.

The contribution of silica to the chest diseases of miners was not at first apparent because of their exposure to other substances, adverse environmental conditions and the prevalence of tuberculosis and other chest diseases. The capacity of respirable free silica to cause pneumoconiosis is firmly established and, as the material is used so widely, workers in a large number of industries are at risk. In practice exposure is frequently to mixed dust of crystalline silica and other materials such as coal, metals or silicates. It is a laborious business sorting out the contributions to chest disease of these various constituents and the ways in which one may modify the pulmonary reaction to another.

While the development of pure silicosis or mixed dust fibrosis is usually a very slow process, acute silicosis has occurred and parallels the experimental findings in animals overloaded with high doses of silica. An early example was reported by Middleton (1929) in the manufacture of siliceous abrasive soap powders. Dyspnoea, cough and respiratory failure progressed rapidly, and microscopically the alveoli were found to be filled with amorphous material.

Classic chronic silicosis is seen most clearly in those exposed to dusts which have a high proportion of free silica and no other fibrogenic or radio-opaque constituents. There is no doubt that heavy and prolonged exposure can be disabling but, in general, control of dust sources has lessened the prevalence and severity of silicosis. The wider availability of competent radiographic surveys should enable workers to be monitored for dust retention and exposure limited to prevent symptoms, impairment of pulmonary function or shortening of life. In some instances substitution for siliceous materials has lessened the hazards. Examples are the reduced use of siliceous refractories in the ceramics industry (Posner, 1966), the substitution of carborundum and zirconium for sandstone grinding wheels, the use of liquid core washes in place of silica flour used as a foundry parting powder and the displacement of silica by alumina in refractory bricks. The last is especially welcome since some of the silica present in furnace linings is likely to be converted into tridymite and cristoballite at temperatures around 1000 °C and these are more fibrogenic than quartz. The use in foundries of olivine in place of silica sand would eliminate the main source of pneumoconiosis but the substitution is expensive and foundry workers' pneumoconiosis can be controlled by other means.

Foundry workers

Surveys of foundry workers (McLaughlin, 1950; McLaughlin and Harding, 1956; Lloyd Davies et al., 1971; Higgins and Dewell, 1977; Health and Safety Executive, 1977) reveal a picture of lessening prevalence and disability over the years. In most siliceous pneumoconioses, as in coal-workers' pneumoconiosis, the simple radiographic categories are unrelated to respiratory symptoms or to significant impairment of pulmonary function. One must, however, bear in mind that pneumoconiosis has generally been judged only by the appearance of small rounded opacities. The inclusion of irregular opacities in future reporting may alter the apparent position. McLaughlin's cases (1950) included those with progressive massive fibrosis (PMF) but reduction in the disease has enabled Morgan and Seaton (1975) to say that complicated disease appears not to occur in this industry. No case was reported in the Department of Employment survey (Lloyd Davies et al., 1971) but 8 cases of PMF collected in Britain's largest iron foundry include 4 in which foundry work has been the only known source of dust exposure. They had all worked for many years in an earlier and dustier foundry.

Amorphous silica has been regarded as much less fibrogenic than the crystalline forms. Vitums et al. (1977) describe pulmonary changes among 40 workers exposed to fine amorphous silica powder. Eleven had radiographic changes, with nodulation and reticulation mentioned in 3 of them. Lung biopsies in 2 cases revealed a moderate degree of peribronchial and perivascular fibrosis.

Prevalence of pneumoconiosis

Knowledge about the prevalence of pneumoconiosis is patchy. Information on coalworkers' pneumoconiosis is excellent because of the meticulous work of the National Coal Board Medical Service. The prevalence of radiographic changes in South African gold miners is also known because there is a legal requirement for miners to have annual medical examinations while doing dusty work. One survey (Weiss and Figueroa, 1976) of over 2000 workers showed that 6·7 per cent had silicosis. Surveys of foundry workers show a prevalence of small rounded opacities in or above category 1/0 to vary from about 3 to 34 per cent. Unless virtually all the employees have chest radiographs it is idle to draw firm conclusions about prevalence. Published statistics of those receiving pneumoconiosis benefit in Britain are of limited relevance. Not only are the criteria for awarding benefit not made public but workers who have not been X-rayed do not know if they may have reached the category of pneumoconiosis which seems generally to attract benefit.

Hygiene standard for silica

The widely accepted hygiene standard for crystalline silica has remained at 0·1 mg of respirable free silica/m^3 of air for a considerable time. It is not easy to collect epidemiological data with which to support or to challenge this, but ideally one would wish to see threshold limit data for a variety of industries because of the additive or retarding effects on fibrosis of mixed dusts. Utidjian (1975) recommends reducing the TLV to 0·05 mg/m^3 while Higgins and Dewell (1977) calculate that the radiological boundary between categories one and two would be reached on average after fifty years' work exposed to 0·14 mg/m^3 respirable free silica. In considering this higher concentration one should bear in mind the contribution to the radiological score made by iron retained in the lungs and the retarding effect of iron on fibrosis caused by silica in ferrous foundries.

Talc

Chemicially pure talc is hydrous magnesium silicate, with a formula intriguingly like that of chrysotile asbestos, another fibrous silicate. The composition of talc as mined is very variable. Many commercial grades contain crystalline silica, asbestos and other minerals. The physical structure also varies. Cosmetic grades of talc are in the platy form and contain little or no asbestos and few other impurities (Hildick-Smith, 1976; Pooley and Rowlands, 1977). McLaughlin et al. (1949) described a case of pneumoconiosis in a talc worker in whom the pulmonary reaction was probably due to a mixture of talc and asbestos. Subsequent descriptions of lung changes have varied with the composition of the talc. Léophonte (1975) suggested that three forms of talc pneumoconiosis should be recognized: talco-silicosis, talco-asbestosis and pure talcosis. Hildick-Smith (1977) found no radiographic or pulmonary function changes in miners of cosmetic grade talc, but a higher incidence of deaths from respiratory disease in miners of talc containing more that 5 per cent crystalline silica. Fine et al. (1976) studied 80 workers exposed to industrial grade talc and found a reduction in FEV_1 in 27 men with more than ten years' exposure compared with controls. There were, however, no radiographic changes. Kleinfeld et al. (1974) followed up a group of talc workers in whom they found an excess of lung cancer and in some a severe pneumoconiosis leading to cor pulmonale. The talc contained tremolite, anthophyllite, carbonates and a small amount of silica. Hildick-Smith (1976) concluded, however, that pure cosmetic grades of talc present no hazard to health. It does seem that a particularly severe pneumoconiosis may occur in workers with commercial talcs and it may be that the combined effect of talc and other dusts is more than additive.

CADMIUM

Cadmium is a ductile metal which is valuable for its anti-corrosion and anti-sparking properties. Hazards associated with extraction of cadmium from zinc and other ores and the preparation of cadmium containing alloys, brazing components and metal coatings should be recognized and controlled. There is, however, hidden danger when materials not known to contain cadmium are heated.

Acute cadmium poisoning presents initially like metal fume fever but may be much more serious. Pat Wardhan and Finckh (1976) describe a case of fatal cadmium fume pneumonitis in a man who had been welding cadmium-plated drums. Chronic poisoning is characterized by dyspnoea due to panacinar emphysema accompanied by little or no cough or sputum. Chowdhury and Louria (1976) studied the influence of trace metals on human α_1-antitrypsin and found that cadmium alone reduced the concentration. This provides one possible explanation for the mechanism of emphysema production but it is uncertain whether chronic effects occur in cadmium workers who have not also suffered from acute poisoning in the past. Here, as in the case of beryllium and some other metals, features such as the latent interval between exposure and symptoms suggest an immunological mechanism.

Cadmium is rapidly absorbed from the lungs (Editorial, 1969) and can accumulate in the liver and kidneys. Most cadmium workers after many years of exposure excrete a protein of low molecular weight in the urine, detectable by chemical testing but not by boiling, and associated with renal tubular damage. If exposure stops the proteinuria may diminish (Tsuchiya, 1976).

Rats fed with cadmium may develop hypertension and an increase in renal cadmium concentration is found in some patients with hypertension but there is no evidence of hypertension in cadmium workers (Friberg et al., 1974). It has been suggested that cadmium may cause human cancers but evidence is insufficient to draw any conclusions (British Occupational Hygiene Society, 1977).

The hygiene standard for cadmium has recently been reviewed by an Occupational Hygiene Committee (British Occupational Hygiene Society, 1977) which supports the existing TLV at 0·05 mg/m^3 for respirable cadmium dust. A special short exposure limit for not more than 10 minutes is proposed at 2 mg/m^3, but in spite of cadmium's solubility in body fluids no special limit is recommended for larger particles which deposit in the airways. Prolonged exposure to the insoluble compounds of cadmium, however, does not appear to cause proteinuria or pulmonary damage.

BERYLLIUM

Beryllium is a strong, light, non-magnetic metal which in use is generally mixed with other materials, especially in the form of an alloy with copper. Many of the early cases of poisoning arose from its use in making fluorescent lighting elements but this application has now ended. Acute poisoning should no longer occur but Van Ordstrand et al. (1945) described 90 patients with airways involvement and 38 cases of acute pneumonitis of whom 5 died. Most patients surviving an attack of pneumonitis make a complete recovery but a few later develop the picture of chronic poisoning. The chief manifestations are due to a granulomatous reaction in the lungs, histologically identical with that seen in sarcoidosis. Lesions also occur in other tissues and in a case described by Agate (1948) in a research physicist, sarcoid-like granulomata were found on liver biopsy.

Only a proportion of exposed workers may develop beryllium poisoning. There is good evidence that immunological reactions are involved. The role of hypersensitivity had already been suggested by Van Ordstrand et al. (1945) and in 2 cases described by Norris and Peard (1963). This was supported by the finding of sarcoid-like skin lesions on taking biopsies from the areas of positive beryllium patch tests. Evidence now suggests that patch testing can cause beryllium sensitization and that it is inadvisable. Resnick and Morgan (1971) found a constant increase in the levels of immunoglobulin (IgG) in patients with chronic berylliosis; but over 80 per cent of subjects with long exposure to beryllium had raised IgG levels although very few developed disease. Raised IgG levels cannot therefore be regarded as a diagnostic test. The beryllium macrophage migration test (Jones Williams, 1977; Price et al., 1977) similarly demonstrates the presence of beryllium hypersensitivity, but without the risk of sensitizing patients in whom the test is negative.

The differentiation from sarcoidosis may be very difficult. They should both be regarded as systemic disorders but sarcoidosis may involve tissues which beryllium does not, such as the uveal tract. The nodular and irregular radiographic opacities may be identical and both may show increased hilar shadows. The demonstration of greatly enlarged hilar lymph nodes, however, favours sarcoidosis. A positive Kveim test points to sarcoidosis and it is worth looking for abnormalities of cardiac conduction in difficult cases as myocardial involvement in sarcoidosis is more frequent than generally realized (Fleming, 1974).

COBALT

'Hard metal', consisting of tungsten carbide milled with up to 25 per cent cobalt as a binder, is used for the heat and wear resisting tips and edges of drills, dies and cutting tools. Reports from Germany, where the process was developed, indicated an association between hard metal dust inhalation and pneumoconiosis which in some cases led to respiratory failure. Tungsten, but not cobalt, was found in the lungs of fatal cases and it was natural to incriminate the persistent and major component of hard metal. Tungsten carbide, however, proved harmless in animal experiments and to humans exposed to this material alone. Harding (1950) confirmed earlier indications that cobalt metal powder caused severe capillary damage, haemorrhage and oedema in the lungs of experimental animals. In a comprehensive review Bech et al. (1962) described a respiratory syndrome of cough, dyspnoea and wheezing increasing during the working day. In several of the 232 workers surveyed there were radiographic changes suggestive of pulmonary fibrosis. They clearly suspected cobalt as the causative agent. Cotes and Watson (1971) drew the same conclusion from the study of 12 cases of progressive pulmonary fibrosis of whom 8 died. Bech (1974) described a further 12 cases, including histological material from 7, and postulated that cobalt acts like beryllium by protein binding and the development of hypersensitivity.

REFERENCES

Acheson E. D. et al. (1968) Nasal cancer in woodworkers in the furniture industry. *Br. Med. J.* **2,** 587–597.

Agate J. N. (1948) Delayed pneumonitis in a beryllium worker. *Lancet* **2,** 530–533.

Albert R. E. et al. (1971) The effects of cigarette smoking on the kinetics of bronchial clearance in humans and donkeys. *Inhaled Particles III.* ed. Walton W. H. Old Woking, Unwin, pp. 165–180.

Amandus H. E. et al. (1976) Significance of irregular small opacities in radiographs of coalminers in the U.S.A. *Br. J. Ind. Med.* **33,** 13–17.

Antweiler H. (1976) Treatment of silicosis with polyvinyl pyridine-*N*-oxide (PVNO). *Researches on Chronic Respiratory Diseases, Industrial Medicine.* Luxembourg, Commission of the European Communities (ECSC), pp. 36–39.

Bar-Ziv J. and Goldberg G. M. (1974) Simple siliceous pneumoconiosis in Negro Bedouins. *Arch. Environ. Health* **29,** 121–126.

Bech A. O. (1974) Hard metal disease and toolroom grinding. *J. Soc. Occup. Med.* **24,** 11–16.

Bech A. O. et al. (1962) Hard metal disease. *Br. J. Ind. Med.* **19,** 239–252.

Bergman I. (1970) The relation of endogenous non-haem iron in formalin-fixed lungs to radiological grade of pneumoconiosis. *Ann. Occup. Hyg.* **13,** 163–169.

Bergman I. and Casswell C. (1972) Lung dust and lung iron contents of coal workers in different coalfields in Great Britain. *Br. J. Ind. Med.* **29,** 160–168.

Bidstrup P. L. (1978) Personal communication.

Bidstrup P. L. and Case R. A. M. (1956) Carcinoma of the lung in workmen in the bichromates-producing industry in Great Britain. *Br. J. Ind. Med.* **13,** 260–264.

Boyd J. T. et al. (1970) Cancer of the lung in iron ore (haematite) miners. *Br. J. Ind. Med.* **27,** 97–105.

Boyland E. (1977) Biochemistry of occupational cancer. *J. Soc. Occup. Med.* **27,** 97–101.

Brain J. D. (1971) The effects of increased particles on the number of alveolar macrophages. *Inhaled Particles III.* ed. Walton W. H. Old Woking, Unwin, pp. 209–223.

British Occupational Hygiene Society (1977) Committee on Hygiene Standards: sub-committee on cadmium. Hygiene standard for cadmium. *Ann. Occup. Hyg.* **20,** 215–228.

Browne R. C. (1973) Health hazards of siliceous materials. *Practitioner* **210,** 518.

Caplan A. (1953) Certain unusual radiological appearances in the chest of coalminers suffering from rheumatoid arthritis. *Thorax* **8,** 29–37.

Chowdhury P. and Louria D. B. (1976) Influence of cadmium and other trace metals on human α_1-antitrypsin: an *in vitro* study. *Science* **191,** 480–481.

Clayson D. B. (1967) Chemicals and environmental carcinogensis in man. *Europ. J. Cancer* **3,** 405–416.

Cotes E. O. and Watson J. H. L. (1971) Diffuse interstitial lung disease in tungsten carbide workers. *Ann. Intern. Med.* **75,** 709–716.

Davies D. (1973) Treatment of rapidly progressive rheumatoid pneumoconiosis. *Br. J. Ind. Med.* **30,** 396–401.

Davies G. M. (1977) A mortality study of coke oven workers in two South Wales integrated steelworks. *Br. J. Ind. Med.* **34,** 291–297.

Davies J. M. (1978) Lung cancer mortality of workers making chrome pigments. *Lancet* **1,** 384.

Doig A. T. and McLaughlin A. I. G. (1936) X-ray appearances of lungs of electric arc welders. *Lancet* **1,** 771–775.

Doll R. (1958) Cancer of the lung and nose in nickel workers. *Br. J. Ind. Med.* **15,** 217–223.

Doll R. et al. (1965) Mortality of gasworkers with special reference to cancers of the lung and bladder, chronic bronchitis and pneumoconiosis. *Br. J. Ind. Med.* **22,** 1–12.

Doll R. et al. (1972) Mortality of gasworkers – final report of a prospective study. *Br. J. Ind. Med.* **29,** 394–406.

Doll R. et al. (1977) Cancers of the lung and nasal sinuses in nickel workers; a re-assessment of the period of risk. *Br. J. Ind. Med.* **34,** 102–105.

Editorial (1968) Domestic silicosis. *Lancet* **1,** 289.

Editorial (1969) Cadmium. *Lancet* **2,** 1346.

Editorial (1973) Small particles in small airways. *Lancet* **2,** 948–949.

Enterline P. E. (1974) Respiratory cancer among chromate workers. *J. Occup. Med.* **16,** 523–534.

Faulds J. S. and Stewart M. J. (1956) Carcinoma of the lung in haematite miners. *J. Pathol. Bact.* **72,** 353–366.

Ferin J. (1971) Emphysema in rats and clearance of dust particles. *Inhaled Particles III.* ed. Walton W. H. Old Woking, Unwin, pp. 283–291.

Figueroa W. G. et al. (1973) Lung cancer in chloromethyl methyl ether workers. *N. Engl. J. Med.* **288,** 1096–1097.

Fine L. J. et al. (1976) Studies of respiratory morbidity in rubber workers. *Arch. Environ. Health* **31,** 195–200.

Fleming H. A. (1974) Sarcoid heart disease. *Br. Heart J.* **36,** 54–68.

Friberg L. et al. (1974) *Cadmium in the Environment.* Cleveland, Chemical Rubber Co.

Gilson J. C. (1970) Occupational bronchitis? *Proc. R. Soc. Med.* **63,** 857–864.

Glyn-Thomas R. and Sluis-Cremer G. K. (1977) 200kV xeroradiography in occupational exposure to silica and asbestos. *Br. J. Ind. Med.* **34,** 281–290.

Greenberg M. (1972) A proportional mortality study of a group of newspaper workers. *Br. J. Ind. Med.* **29,** 15–20.

Harding H. E. (1950) Notes on the toxicology of cobalt metal. *Br. J. Ind. Med.* **7,** 76–78.

Hatch T. F. (1972) Permissible levels of exposure to hazardous agents in industry. *J. Occup. Med.* **14,** 134–137.

Hatch T. F. and Gross P. (1964) *Pulmonary Deposition and Retention of Inhaled Aerosols.* New York, Academic.

Health and Safety Executive (1977) *Some Aspects of Pneumoconiosis in a Group of Mechanised Iron Foundries.* Joint Standing Committee on Health Safety and Welfare in Foundries. Third Report of the Sub-committee on Dust and Fume. London, HMSO.

Heppleston A. G. (1971) Observations on the mechanism of silicotic fibrogenesis. *Inhaled Particles III.* ed. Walton W. H. Old Woking, Unwin, pp. 357–369.

Higgins I. T. T. and Dewell P. (1977) Medical and environmental studies in an iron foundry – with special reference to pneumoconiosis. *Br. Cast Iron Res. Assoc. J.* Report 1252, 51–54.

Higgins I. T. T. et al. (1968) Chronic respiratory disease in mining communities in Marion County, West Viriginia. *Br. J. Ind. Med.* **25,** 165–175.

Hildick-Smith G. Y. (1976) The biology of talc. *Br. J. Ind. Med.* **33,** 217–229.

Hildick-Smith G. (1977) Talc – recent epidemiological studies. *Inhaled Particles IV.* ed. Walton W. H. Oxford, Pergamon, pp. 655–664.

Hill A. B. and Faning E. L. (1948) Studies in the incidence of cancer in a factory handling inorganic compounds of arsenic. Mortality experience in the factory. *Br. J. Ind. Med.* **5**, 1–6.

International Labour Office (1972) *ILO U/C International Classification of Radiographs of the Pneumoconioses, 1971.* Occupational Safety and Health Series No. 22 (Revised). Geneva.

Iravani J. (1971) Clearance function of the respiratory ciliated epithelium in normal and bronchitic rats. *Inhaled Particles III.* ed. Walton W. H. Old Woking, Unwin, pp. 143–146.

Jacobsen G. et al. (1970) Essentials of chest radiography. *Radiology* **95**, 445–450.

Jacobsen M. et al. (1977) Smoking and coalworkers' simple pneumoconiosis. *Inhaled Particles IV.* ed. Walton W. H. Oxford, Pergamon, pp. 759–771.

Jayson M. I. V. et al. (1977) Penicillamine therapy in systemic sclerosis. *Proc. R. Soc. Med.* **70**, 82–87.

Joder P. (1976) Silikose, Chronische Bronchitis und Rauchgewohnheiten. *Schweiz. Med. Wochenschr.* **106**, 239–244.

Jones Williams W. (1977) Beryllium disease: pathology and diagnosis. *J. Soc. Occup. Med.* **27**, 93–96.

Kawai M. et al. (1967) Epidemiological study of occupational lung cancer. *Arch. Environ. Health* **14**, 859–864.

Kellermann G. et al. (1973) Aryl hydrocarbon hydroxylase inducibility and bronchogenic carcinoma. *N. Engl. J. Med.* **289**, 934–937.

Kennedy M. C. S. (1956) Aluminium powder inhalations in the treatment of silicosis of pottery workers and pneumoconiosis of coal miners. *Br. J. Ind. Med.* **13**, 85–89.

Kleinfeld M. et al. (1974) Mortality experiences among talc workers; a follow up study. *J. Occup. Med.* **16**, 345–349.

Konetzke G. W. (1974) Die Kanzerogene Wirkung von Arsen und Nickel. *Arch. Geschwulstforsch.* **44**, 16–22.

Langard S. and Norseth T. (1975) A cohort study of bronchial carcinomas in workers producing chromate pigments. *Br. J. Ind. Med.* **32**, 62–65.

Le Bouffant L. et al. (1977) The therapeutic action of aluminium compounds on the development of experimental lesions produced by pure quartz or mixed dust. *Inhaled Particles IV* ed. Walton W. H., Oxford, Pergamon, pp. 389–400.

Léophonte P. et al. (1975) Les pneumoconioses par le talc. *Rev. Fr. Malad. Resp.* **3**, 363–384.

Liddell F. D. K. (1977) Radiological assessment of small pneumoconiotic opacities. *Br. J. Ind. Med.* **34**, 85–94.

Liddell F. D. K. and Morgan W. K. C. (1978) Methods of assessing serial films of the pneumoconioses. *J. Soc. Occup. Med.* **28**, 6–15.

Lippmann M. et al. (1971) The regional deposition of inhaled aerosols in man. *Inhaled Particles III.* ed. Walton W. H. Old Woking, Unwin, pp. 105–120.

Lippman M. et al. (1977) Factors affecting tracheo-bronchial mucociliary transport. *Inhaled Particles IV.* ed. Walton W. H. Oxford, Pergamon, pp. 305–318.

Lloyd J. W. (1971) Long term mortality study of steel workers. V, Respiratory cancer in coke plant workers. *J. Occup. Med.* **13**, 53–68.

Lloyd Davies T. A. et al. (1971) *Respiratory Disease in Foundrymen. Report of a Survey.* Department of Employment. London, HMSO.

Love R. G. and Muir D. C. F. (1976) Aerosol deposition and airway obstruction. *Am. Rev. Respir. Dis.* **114**, 891–897.

Lowe C. R. (1969) Industrial bronchitis. *Br. Med. J.* **1**, 463–468.

Lowe C. R. et al. (1968) Bronchitis in two integrated steelworks. I, Ventilatory capacity, age and physique of non-bronchitic men. *Br. J. Prev. Soc. Med.* **22**, 1–11.

Lowe C. R. et al. (1970) Bronchitis in two integrated steelworks. III, Respiratory symptoms and ventilatory capacity related to atmospheric pollution. *Br. J. Ind. Med.* **27**, 121–129.

Lyons J. P. et al. (1974) Significance of irregular opacities in the radiology of coal workers' pneumoconiosis. *Br. J. Ind. Med.* **31**, 185–195.

McKerrow C. B. (1964) A review of methods of measuring respiratory function. *Trans. Assoc. Indust. Med. Offrs.* **14**, 2–6.

McLaughlin A. I. G. (1950) *Industrial Lung Diseases of Iron and Steel Foundry Workers.* London, HMSO.

McLaughlin A. I. G. (1962) Observations on the diagnosis of pneumoconiosis, with special reference to radiography. *Trans. Assoc. Ind. Med. Offrs.* **12**, 74–89.

McLaughlin A. I. G. and Harding H. E. (1956) Pneumoconiosis and other causes of death in iron and steel foundry workers. *Arch. Environ. Hlth* **14**, 350–378.

McLaughlin A. I. G. et al. (1949) Talc pneumoconiosis. *Br. J. Ind. Med.* **6**, 184–194.

Mazumdar S. et al. (1975) An epidemiological study of exposure to coal tar pitch volatiles among coke oven workers. *J. Air Pollut. Control Assoc.* **25**, 382–389.

Medical Research Council (1942) Chronic pulmonary disease in South Wales coal-miners. 1, Medical studies. *Special Report Series No. 243.* London, HMSO.

Medical Research Council (1966) Chronic bronchitis and occupation. *Br. Med. J.* **1**, 101–102.

Medical Research Council (1976) *Short Questionnaire on Respiratory Symptoms.* London, HMSO.

Michaels L. (1967) Lung changes in woodworkers. *Can. Med. Assoc. J.* **96**, 1150–1155.

Middleton E. L. (1929) The present position of silicosis in industry in Britain. *Br. Med. J.* **2**, 485–489.

Mikov M. I. (1974) Chronic bronchitis in foundry workers in Vojvodina. *Arch. Environ. Health* **29**, 261–267.

Mittman C. et al. (1973) Antitrypsin deficiency and abnormal protease inhibitor phenotypes. *Arch. Environ. Health* **27**, 201–206.

Morgan J. G. (1958) Some observations on the incidence of respiratory cancer in nickel workers. *Br. J. Ind. Med.* **15**, 224–234.

Morgan W. K. C. and Seaton A. (1975) *Occupational Lung Diseases.* Philadelphia, Saunders.

Moss E. et al. (1972) Mortality of newspaper workers from lung cancer and bronchitis, 1952–66. *Br. J. Ind. Med.* **29**, 1–14.

Muir D. C. F. (1974) Pneumoconiosis and byssinosis. *Br. J. Ind. Med.* **31**, 322–328.

Nimni M. E. (1977) Mechanisms of inhibition of collagen crosslinking by penicillamine. *Proc. R. Soc. Med.* **70**, 65–72.

Norris G. F. and Peard M. C. (1963) Berylliosis: report of two cases, with special reference to the patch test. *Br. Med. J.* **1**, 378–382.

Parkes W. R. (1974) *Occupational Lung Disorders.* London, Butterworth.

Pat Wardhan J. R. and Finckh E. S. (1976) Fatal cadmium fume pneumonitis. *Med. J. Aust.* **1**, 962–966.

Pooley F. D. and Rowlands N. (1977) Chemical and physical properties of British talc powders. *Inhaled Particles IV.* ed. Walton W. H. Oxford, Pergamon, pp. 639–646.

Posner E. (1966) Diagnosis and management of industrial chest disease. *Br. Med. J.* **1**, 525–529.

Price C. D. et al. (1977) Role of in vitro and in vivo tests of hypersensitivity in beryllium workers. *J. Clin. Pathol.* **30**, 24–28.

Proctor D. F. et al. (1969) The nose and man's atmospheric environment. *Arch. Environ. Health* **18**, 671–680.

Rae S. et al. (1971) Chronic bronchitis and dust exposure in British coalminers. *Inhaled Particles III.* ed. Walton W. H. Old Woking, Unwin, pp. 883–894.

Redmond C. K. et al. (1972) Long-term mortality study of steelworkers. VI, Mortality from malignant neoplasms among coke-oven workers. *J. Occup. Med.* **14**, 621–629.

Reichel G. et al. (1977) The action of quartz in the presence of iron hydroxides in the human lung. *Inhaled Particles IV.* ed. Walton W. H. Oxford, Pergamon, pp. 403–410.

Resnick H. and Morgan W. K. C. (1971) Immunoglobulin levels in berylliosis. *Inhaled Particles III.* ed. Walton W. H. Old Woking, Unwin, pp. 589–597.

Rogan J. M. et al. (1973) Role of dust in the working environment in the development of chronic bronchitis in British coal miners. *Br. J. Ind. Med.* **30**, 217–226.

Sanchis J. et al. (1971) Regional distribution and lung clearance mechanisms in smokers and non-smokers. *Inhaled Particles III.* ed. Walton W. H. Old Woking, Unwin, pp. 183–188.

Scadding J. G. (1952) Chronic lung disease with diffuse nodular or reticular radiographic shadows. *Tubercle* **33**, 352–365.

Schilling R. S. F. (1970) Industrial dust diseases. *Human Environment and the Respiratory System.* London, Health Horizon.

Shaver C. G. and Riddell A. R. (1947) Lung changes associated with the manufacture of aluminium abrasives. *J. Ind. Hyg.* **29**, 145–157.

Shlensky B. (1970) Polyvinylpyridin-*N*-oxid und die Entwicklung der Silikose bei Ratten nach Inhalationen des Quartzstaubes aus einer Stahlgusputzerei. *Int. Arch. Arbeitsmed.* **26**, 179–188.

Simon G. (1972) Radiology in the diagnosis of bronchitis and emphysema. *Trans. Soc. Occup. Med.* **22**, 74–75.

Stewart M. J. and Faulds J. S. (1934) The pulmonary fibrosis of haematite miners. *J. Pathol. Bact.* **39**, 233–253.

Tsuchiya K. (1976) Proteinuria of cadmium workers. *J. Occup. Med.* **18**, 463–466.

Turner-Warwick M. E. H. (1969) Rheumatoid arthritis, rheumatoid factors and lung disease. *Br. J. Hosp. Med.* **2**, 507–513.

Turner-Warwick M. E. H. (1973) Basic interpretation of the chest radiograph in health and disease. *Medicine* **13**, 832–834.

Utidjian H. M. D. (1975) Criteria documents. 1, Recommendations for a crystalline silica standard. *J. Occup. Med.* **17**, 775–781.

Van Ordstrand H. S. et al. (1945) Beryllium poisoning. *J.A.M.A.* **129**, 1084–1090.

Vitums V. C. et al. (1977) Pulmonary fibrosis from amorphous silica dust, a product of silica vapour. *Arch. Environ. Health* **32**, 62–68.

Walker D. D. et al. (1971) Bronchitis in men employed in the coke industry. *Br. J. Ind. Med.* **28**, 358–363.

Washington J. S. et al. (1973) A comparison of conventional and grid techniques for chest radiography in field surveys. *Br. J. Ind. Med.* **30**, 365–374.

Waterhouse J. A. H. (1971) Cutting oils and cancer. *Ann. Occup. Hyg.* **14**, 161–170.

Weiss W. and Boucot K. R. (1975) The respiratory effects of chloromethyl methyl ether. *J.A.M.A.* **234**, 1139–1142.

Weiss W. and Figueroa W. G. (1976) The characteristics of lung cancer due to chloromethyl ethers. *J. Occup. Med.* **18**, 623–627.

Weller W. (1977) Long term test on rhesus monkeys for the PVNO therapy of anthracosilicosis. *Inhaled Particles IV.* ed. Walton W. H. Oxford, Pergamon, pp. 379–386.

Wiles F. J. and Faure M. H. (1977) Chronic obstructive lung disease in gold miners. *Inhaled Particles IV.* ed. Walton W. H. Oxford, Pergamon, pp. 727–734.

8. OCCUPATIONAL DERMATOSES

R. J. G. Rycroft

Occupational dermatoses are skin diseases primarily caused by the working environment. It is now widely accepted that they are the commonest occupational diseases of the industrialized world. Occupational skin diseases do not often stop people working and only very rarely kill. Official statistics compiled from time lost from work and compensation, though disturbing enough in themselves, are therefore only the tip of an iceberg. A survey of skin disease in a large light engineering factory, for example, found three times as many employees had occupational dermatoses than statistics based on time lost and compensation suggested (Squire et al., 1950). These authors were also well aware that even their figures were incomplete since they were derived from patients reporting skin problems to the factory medical department. Many cases of equal severity would probably have gone unreported.

These figures seem to fly in the face of reason. Occupational dermatoses should be among the most preventable of all diseases (Gellin, 1972). It is perhaps this discrepancy which, above all else, makes the study of occupational dermatoses of such potential benefit to industrialized society. This chapter reviews some attitudes of mind, ways of thinking and methods of investigation which are of proven value in this field. It also points out some approaches to occupational skin problems which do not yet seem to have been adequately explored. First, though, let us not forget that all technique is impoverished without the underlying ability to observe accurately and record our observations simply and clearly. It is an ability that the great writers and the very best journalists have in abundance but one that the rest of us must strive after. We have been left few better models than this description of ageing from Shakespeare: 'Have you not a moist eye, a dry hand, a yellow cheek, a white beard, a decreasing leg, an increasing belly?' (*Henry IV* (*2*) I, ii).

DIAGNOSTIC ACCURACY

The acurate diagnosis of individual patients is the cornerstone of all medical enquiry and occupational dermatology is no exception. The process leading to the diagnosis of an occupational dermatosis can be seen as centred around three key questions:

1. Is it eczema (dermatitis) or not?
2. If eczematous (dermatitic), is it primarily caused by external factors in contact with the skin or not?
3. If contact eczema (contact dermatitis), is the contact factor a skin allergen (sensitizer) or a skin irritant? (Or are factors of both types, or the additional factor of sunlight, involved?)

The two terms, eczema and dermatitis, are now used to mean the same thing by most dermatologists; an inflammatory skin condition characterized by redness, swelling, small fluid-filled blisters, oozing of this fluid, scaling, cracking or thickening of the skin.

Is it eczema or not?

Most, but not all, occupational dermatoses are eczematous or dermatitic reactions to external contact factors in the working environment. The importance of the first critical decision therefore is that it separates all skin rashes into two groups; the eczematous, with a high risk of being occupational, and the non-eczematous, with a low risk of being occupational. It is a decision which can usually be made by the trained eye but which can sometimes be extremely difficult. Psoriasis and eczema, for example, can be hard to tell apart when only the hands are involved. Additional techniques such as skin biopsy may be required.

In spite of the importance of this division there are a wide variety of non-eczematous dermatoses which can be occupational. Skin cancer can be caused by mineral oil, white patches of depigmentation by phenolic chemicals, urticarial wheals by contact with tobacco leaves and itchy lumps by the Pyemotes mite that causes grain itch (Hewitt et al., 1976). At least one skin problem consists of what the skin does to the job rather than vice versa: the 'ruster', whose sweat ruins ferrous-metal products (Buckley and Lewis, 1960). The significance of separating eczematous dermatoses from these and many other conditions is that special lines of investigation are required to tell whether or not an eczema is occupational.

Is it contact dermatitis or not?

Many forms of eczema have nothing to do with skin contact with external factors and are therefore unlikely to be occcupational. These eczemas are usually termed endogenous or constitutional and often subdivided into atopic, seborrhoeic, varicose and discoid types, largely on the basis of their distribution over the body surface. The causes of endogenous eczemas are not yet fully known. Other eczemas can be shown to be caused by external factors in contact with the skin and these are referred to as exogenous or contact dermatitis. Contact dermatitis may or may not be occupational but it is essential to distinguish it from endogenous eczema which can never be. Endogenous eczemas may of course occasionally be exacerbated by occupational factors.

Endogenous eczema and contact dermatitis can often be distinguished by a detailed history and a careful examination. The history in suspected occupational cases should concentrate on the duration and timing of the dermatitis in relation to the patient's work. The main feature to establish from an examination of the skin is the distribution of the dermatitis over the body. It is therefore preferable to examine the whole skin surface in a good light. Even in the best hands, however, a full history and examination has been shown to miss at least 10 per cent of occupational dermatoses (Malten et al., 1971). Cement dermatitis, for example, can mimic discoid eczema. It is to a skin testing technique known as patch testing that we must turn for increased accuracy in resolving the second question. Patch testing becomes essential when we arrive at the third diagnostic step.

Is it allergic or irritant?

Irritant and allergic contact dermatitis have too many features in common for clinical evaluation to be reliable. Each has certain characteristic features in the acute stage but these rapidly became blurred as the dermatitis becomes chronic. Irritants are substances which directly damage the skin if they are in contact with it at an adequate concentration for a sufficient length of time. Allergens (sensitizers) on the other hand may produce no direct damage at the time of first contact but after a varying period of time evoke an allergic response in the body (sensitization). It is the allergic reaction that occurs in the skin when the previously sensitized individual next meets the sensitizer that produces dermatitis. Common occupational irritants are strong alkalis, strong acids and solvents while chromates, epoxy resin and rubber-processing chemicals are examples of occupational sensitizers.

Patch testing is a procedure which can only positively answer the third question above in favour of allergy. It is a test for allergens and not for irritants. A diagnosis of irritant contact dermatitis is usually made at present from the history and examination of the patient and the prior knowledge of the medical attendant; a visit to the workplace and usage tests there may be helpful additional aids. There is only one way to learn how to patch test and that is to do it. It is an investigation which sounds deceptively simple. A series of suspected allergens is strapped to the skin for 48 hours. The skin will react to whichever allergen the patient is allergic. The major difficulty is not so much in the technique itself but in the interpretation of its results. If the false positive reaction is the bane of the beginner, the missed allergen is surely the Achilles heel of the more experienced. A false positive reaction is a positive patch test reaction not due to allergic sensitivity (Wilkinson et al., 1970); it may be caused by factors as diverse as irritancy of the test substance and the presence of active eczema elsewhere on the body. Even the experienced can all too easily omit to patch test a patient with the one allergen to which he is sensitive; an allergen will then be missed in spite of negative patch test results. To some extent this can be avoided by the routine use of a series of common allergens in every patient (Fregert, 1974).

It is one thing to demonstrate an allergic sensitivity and quite another to show that the allergen is relevant to an occupation. The relevance of both allergens and irritants is more easily established in occupational cases if the medical attendant can do two things. The first is to visit the workplace and the second is to work with occupational hygienists and toxicologists. Visiting the working environment in the company of an occupational hygienist with an interest in dermatoses is an ideal combination. A single such visit may often be sufficient to make the diagnosis but several may sometimes be necessary and a full scale survey may be indicated if the problem appears to be widespread or new. The skills of the hygienist and toxicologist can be essential first in the identification of potential allergens and irritants in the workplace, second in the detection of allegens to which sensitivity has already been established, and later in the design of a prevention programme.

Diagnosis in practice

As an example of many of the diagnostic points outlined above, as well as others, the recent studies of Emmett and co-workers are difficult to improve on (Emmett, 1977; Emmett et al., 1977a). They were confronted by the fact that 5 out of 26 workers formulating a new kind of printing ink, which is dried by ultraviolet light, had dermatitis. Non-irritating dilutions of the many chemicals used in these inks were established and used for patch testing. Four of the 5 men gave positive patch test reactions. All 4 men reacted not only to chemicals known as polyfunctional acrylic monomers present in the ink but also to a chemically related monomer to which they had never previously been exposed; this is the phenomenon of cross-sensitization (Wilkinson et al., 1970), which can cause confusion if it goes unrecognized. The fifth man was diagnosed as having irritant contact dermatitis since these acrylic monomers were irritants as well as allergens; hence the low concentrations that had to be used for patch testing in order to avoid false positive reactions.

In another plant, 4 men working with similar but not identical inks complained of exaggerated skin reactions to sun exposure. Three of the 4 had developed dermatitis. On patch testing as before only 2 of these 3 gave positive reactions to polyfunctional acrylic monomers. Laboratory toxicological techniques were then employed to identify other chemicals in the inks which were capable of absorbing the wavelengths of sunlight. These chemicals were then tested on the skin of employees both with and without complaints of sun sensitivity. Almost all subjects tested gave positive reactions if their skin was exposed to these chemicals but only if they were then also exposed to sunlight; standard patch tests were negative. The occurrence of sun-related dermatitis in all 3 men, whether sensitized to acrylic monomers or not, was now explicable. Their dermatitis was not dependent upon specific sensitivity, but to particularly heavy occupational exposure to sunlight-absorbing chemicals in the inks. Phototoxic reactions such as this are important variants of irritant dermatitis; the irritant or toxic effect of a phototoxic chemical is dependent upon the additional factor of sunlight.

EPIDEMIOLOGICAL APPROACH

A visit to the workplace as part of the diagnosis of an individual patient often results in the discovery of other employees with skin complaints. Or we may be asked at the outset to evaluate a suspected outbreak of dermatitis in a factory. However we arrive at the investigation of a working population, rather than an individual, an awareness of epidemiology immediately becomes a necessity. The epidemiology of skin disease can be said to mean the study of its distribution in populations and the factors which determine that distribution. Because this study invariably has to be conducted on samples of whole populations, statistics becomes the essential partner of epidemiology. Few epidemiological studies of occupational dermatoses have yet been carried out. But it is to epidemiology and statistics that we must look for help with two of the major problems in occupational dermatology.

The first of these arises because of the high level of skin problems in the general population. Only estimates are available for the background level of dermatoses in most communities but together these run to many percentage units. This leads to particular difficulties in the study of conditions such as occupational skin cancer where there are important non-occupational causes of the identical disease. More generally it makes it hard to assess the significance of, say, a 10 or 15 per cent prevalence of skin complaints in a working population. This could represent the sum total of all non-occupational skin disease in a group. Equally it might indicate the presence of contact dermatitis from a fairly strong allergen or from a weak irritant. Diagnostic methods often resolve the dilemma but, especially if irritant dermatitis is suspected, a comparison of the work group with a control group not exposed to the same occupational factors may be invaluable.

Sometimes highly specialized techniques may be required to resolve this first type of problem; often the application of the simplest principals of epidemiology will suffice. An example of the latter was the work of a dermatologist who was employed to examine employees with skin rashes at a large manufacturer of photographic chemicals. He was well acquainted with a skin disease called lichen planus which he saw from time to time in the rest of his practice. It was when he made the epidemiological observation that rashes looking like lichen planus were more frequent in the factory population than in the population outside that he made a new discovery. The combination of his clinical acumen and his epidemiological awareness resulted in the recognition that certain colour film developing chemicals could cause a lichen planus-like skin eruption (Buckley, 1958).

The second major problem in occupational dermatology which requires epidemiological methods for its solution is the analysis of multiple factors. It is difficult to think of a single occupational dermatosis which is caused by one factor alone. Even an allergic contact dermatitis needs a susceptible host. Many types of irritant contact dermatitis are dependent upon a large number of different factors and are described as having a multifactorial causation. Dermatitis from contact with soluble cutting oils is such an example. The specification of the cutting oil, the susceptibility of the machine operator's skin and the degree of exposure of the skin to the cutting oil are just a few of the variables involved. Epidemiological and statistical methods exist both for the gathering of such data and for its analysis into reliable results. As new questions are asked new techniques may need to be devised. This is an exciting field and one which calls for the close co-operation of clinicians, epidemiologists and statisticians (and computers!).

PREVENTION

The prevention of occupational skin disease is the end to which all endeavour discussed in this chapter is aimed. Recent studies have stressed that it may be even more important to prevent occupational dermatitis than perhaps we realized (Fregert, 1975). A questionnaire was sent to 846 patients diagnosed two to three years previously as having occupational contact dermatitis (irritant and allergic). Sixty-five per cent replied. From their answers it was possible to determine that only one quarter of them were healed, one half had periodic symptoms and a full quarter of them still had permanent symptoms. Furthermore there was no difference in outcome between those who had changed or stopped work and those who had continued in the dermatitis-inducing occupation. Although it is possible that the worst affected patients might have been more likely to reply to the questionnaire, this is a striking reminder of the consequences of failure in the primary prevention of occupational dermatitis.

The breadth of the contribution that preventive medicine can make to our health and safety has been perceptively analysed by Stallones (1977). He identified three overlapping areas of prevention:

1. That carried out by the community as a whole, often via its elected representatives.
2. That carried out by health and safety professionals.
3. That effected by the attitudes of individuals within the community.

All three of these areas would appear to be relevant to occupational skin health. The first of them is likely to play an increasingly important role in the future. The community, through its elected representatives, is responsible for the enactment of legislation on occupational dermatoses. It is also responsible for seeing that enacted legislation is actually adhered to and enforced. The case for properly implemented legislation being the most effective form of preventive medicine historically is difficult to refute. Stallones (1977) cites the example of the relative impacts of child labour laws and of polio vaccination, arguing that the former saved far more lives than the latter. Legislation is also a shaper of individual attitudes just as individual attitudes are vital to its framing in the first place.

The International Contact Dermatitis Research Group (Pirilä et al., 1971) have published a comparison of legislation on occupational dermatoses in 13 European countries and California. The authors stressed that special laws to cover the compensation of occupational skin disease encourage the identification of causal agents. This is itself an important contribution to future prevention. Legislation banning or restricting the use of proven causes of allergic contact dermatitis exists in many countries, such as Denmark (paraphenylenediamine), West Germany (persulphates in flour) and Czechoslovakia (nickel plating). Results have been encouraging. But this type of legislation has highly complex social, economic and political implications which have to be responsibly considered (Calnan, 1970). Milton Friedman, the 1976 Nobel Laureate in economics, has articulated many of the deep suspicions that the commercial and business world can have, at least initially, of government legislation that appears to affect their freedom of action. He has spoken, for example, of 'the internal threat coming from men of good intentions and good will who wish to reform us. Impatient with the slowness of persuasion and example to achieve the great social changes they envisage, they are anxious to use the power of the state to achieve their ends and confident of their ability to do so' (Friedman, 1962). Fortunately on matters of health, the business world is usually more willing to respond to legislative pressure than on most other issues. It may nevertheless be more effective to present proposed advances in occupational skin health as good business (and good trade unionism) than to argue from premises as vague as the common good. In order to do this convincingly however we need studies such as detailed cost-benefit analyses which are at present only available in the crudest terms. This is another area where further research is needed in the future.

REHABILITATION

Rehabilitation of patients with occupational dermatoses has always been an implicit part of their treatment. The clinician wishes to restore the patient to his or her original job or, when indicated, to a suitable alternative. However, it has been found in some other medical specialties that if the rehabilitatory function of medical treatment is made more explicit it can be more successful. One of the first organized centres for the rehabilitation of patients with skin diseases was set up by the British Army at Ragley Hall during the Second World War and much was learnt from the experience. Since 1964 centres for the rehabilitation of patients with chronic skin eruptions have been established at Louisana State University and the University of Maryland School of Medicine in the United States. Robinson and his co-workers (1971) have reported on their progress to date.

Assessment in these centres was undertaken by teams of four professionals; physician, clinical psychologist, social worker and vocational counsellor. Ten factors were identified as being significant in the prediction of success or failure of rehabilitation. These were:

1. Degree of impairment
2. Chronicity
3. Expected response to treatment
4. Intelligence of patient
5. Past work or school performance record
6. Emotional stability
7. Personality
8. Influence of socio-economic factors
9. Influence of other physical defects
10. Motivation.

The point was made that rehabilitation is an expensive and time consuming part of medical care though it is highly important. Since all candidates are unlikely to be successfully rehabilitated the authors proposed these factors as a predictive guide. If a numerical value from 1–10 was assigned to each factor the total score was found to reliably predict success or failure. Successful rehabilitation was defined as attending training for gainful employment or being gainfully employed.

The relevance of factors affecting the rehabilitation of patients with chronic skin conditions to that of patients with occupational dermatoses might perhaps be questioned. First, however, we have already mentioned the disturbing statistics of Fregert (1975) that show at least a quarter of occupational cases still active after two to three years. Second, it is now widely accepted that the more time a patient loses from his job the more difficult it becomes for him to return to work (Robinson, 1965). Hence it seems likely that a large number of patients with occupational dermatoses will benefit from rehabilitation while their skin disease is still active. In large organizations employees can often be transferred to another job either temporarily or permanently. In smaller organizations this can be impossible. Robinson (1965) has suggested that sheltered workshops may therefore fulfil a useful function. Existing industrial rehabilitation units however, are seldom considered for patients with occupational dermatoses. Perhaps a rather different type of unit is required; it certainly seems to be a topic worth re-examination.

MOTIVATIONAL PSYCHOLOGY

Why do some factories have more dermatitis than others with the same work processes? What are the characteristic features of workplaces with consistently low levels of dermatitis as compared with those doing the same job which have consistently high levels of dermatitis? These are the kind of questions to which epidemiology and psychology might be expected to have made contributions, yet published studies on these problems are almost non-existent. Material that is available largely consists of the opinions of professionals with varying degrees of first-hand experience of the workplace. These are of course of great value but studies putting these hypotheses to the test are rare. Fortunately, more work has been carried out on similar questions that confront professionals in the field of occupational safety. I believe we can learn a great deal from their findings which is relevant to occupational dermatoses.

Cohen (1977) has published a lucid review of three different fields of research that have been carried out on companies with excellent safety records. He collected evidence from:

1. Opinion polls of company officials or other personnel knowledgeable in job safety.
2. Analysis of safety practices common to companies with outstanding safety performance.
3. Comparisons of safety programme practices in companies with high work injury experience versus those with low injury rates (matched as far as possible for all other factors).

The overall conclusions of his survey were listed as seven factors which were consistently associated with companies with low work injury rates. These were:

1. Strong management commitment to safety. This commitment, it was stressed, was overt and personal rather than implied and indirect.
2. Close contact and interaction between workers, supervisors and management. Informal contacts were of far more benefit than formal contacts such as safety committees.
3. A stable work force with a large core of married, older workers with long length of service in their jobs.
4. A high level of housekeeping.
5. Well-developed selection, job placement and advancement procedures.
6. Safety training practices involving early indoctrination and follow up.
7. Evidence of added features or variation in conventional safety procedures. An example of this was the design of safety posters with specific local relevance by the employees themselves rather than the use of mass-produced posters.

The importance of this list of features to occupational dermatoses is the strong possibility of its relevance, if appropriately adapted, to occupational health as well as to occupational safety. Moreover it is a list of characteristics which could probably be passed off in a school of business studies as being those that promote productivity without a murmur of disbelief. This research seems to imply that similar factors might promote both profits and occupational skin health.

The first factor was not put at the head of the list by chance. It is a fact that the plant with currently the best safety record in the whole of the United States is run by a manager who personally carries out a safety inspection of the whole of his factory every morning. It takes him 2 hours. It has become customary to blame the attitudes of workers on the shopfloor for high levels of occupational dermatitis in the plant. Should we perhaps spend more time exploring the attitudes of management? This same factory makes more fuss over a 'near-miss' than many others would over an injury itself. This is in some respects analagous to the encouragement of voluntary reporting of minor skin rashes among employees, which can be an excellent practical approach to the prevention of more severe dermatoses. The attitudes of the medical and nursing staff are crucial to the success of such a programme.

MECHANISM AND BIOLOGICAL SUSCEPTIBILITY

Why do some people become sensitized and not others? Why do some people suddenly become sensitized after years of peaceful coexistence with an allergen? These questions and many others involve the mechanism of contact dermatitis and the biological variation in susceptibility to both allergens and irritants throughout the human population. We are still far from knowing the complete answers to most of these questions but many significant advances have been made.

Allergic contact dermatitis from chrome has received a great deal of attention because it is a common occupational sensitizer. Chromium can exist both as a trivalent ion (for example, chromium sulphate) and as a hexavalent ion (for example, sodium chromate). It appears from occupational and patch testing studies that the hexavalent ion is allergenic while the trivalent ion is not. However if trivalent chromium is injected into the skin of patients previously sensitized to hexavalent chromium it provokes an allergic reaction. It has been proposed, therefore, that trivalent chromium is a potential allergen which may be thwarted by its inability, under normal circumstances, to penetrate the outer layers of the skin. This is likely to be connected with the very low solubility of chromium in the trivalent form.

Majeti and Suskind (1977) have demonstrated a phenomenon in guinea pigs which is of great potential relevance to occupational allergic contact dermatitis. Perfumes are complex mixtures of many chemicals, as are many industrial contactants. The perfume component cinnamaldehyde, which is an effective sensitizer on its own, fails to sensitize guinea pigs in the presence of eugenol, another common perfume ingredient. The mechanism of this 'quenching' phenomenon is not yet established.

Sensitizers vary in their sensitizing power and irritants vary in their irritant potential. DNCB (2-chloro-1, 3-dinitrobenzene), for example, is such a potent sensitizer that it sensitizes practically everybody it comes into contact with in sufficient concentration. Other sensitizers are less efficient, as also are mild irritants; some individuals become sensitized or irritated and others do not. Our knowledge at present in this area is almost entirely empirical and is therefore a poor predictive guide in the individual case. Atopic eczema sufferers, for example, are generally regarded as being more susceptible to occupational irritants. But from time to time one sees men with atopic eczema in dirty engineering jobs who claim never to have lost a day's work because of their skin. This susceptibility therefore does not appear to be consistent; nor does it extend to sensitizers (Cronin et al., 1970). There is a great need for further work on reliable tests which will predict how an individual's skin will react to potential sensitizers and irritants.

PLACE WITHIN OCCUPATIONAL HEALTH

Occupational skin diseases do not exist in a vacuum but rather in the context of the rest of occupational medicine. It is only too easy when focusing on an occupational skin problem to miss an associated condition of another system. Rosin (colophony) and epoxy resin systems have only recently been described as causing asthma (Fawcett et al., 1976, 1977), whereas it has been known for some time that they could both cause allergic contact dermatitis. Phototoxic dermatitis from pitch has long been recognized but phototoxic keratoconjunctivitis from the same material has only lately been reported (Emmet et al., 1977b).

The skin is also an important route of absorption for many poisonous chemicals such as organophosphorus pesticides. Its anatomy and physiology are therefore relevent to many internal and systemic disorders as well as to dermatoses. Certain chlorinated aromatic hydrocarbons, including the dioxins, cause a severe skin eruption known as chloracne, but their systemic absorption has also been described as attacking the liver, the kidneys and the nervous system. It is uncertain at present whether the dermal or respiratory route of absorption predominates (Taylor, 1974). Skin lesions resembling those of porphyria cutanea tarda (PCT) have also been seen in severe industrial poisoning incidents. This raises the possibility that the effects of these chemicals on the liver can subsequently be reflected in the skin, because PCT is caused by liver damage.

THE FUTURE

There is nothing more likely to increase the pace of progress in occupational dermatology than a realistic acceptance of our own ignorance. Many observations remain to be made and many that already have been made still await explanation. Why, for example, does hand dermatitis so often continue long after its original cause has apparently been eliminated? A large number of conflicting or alternative hypotheses demand experimental discrimination. Why does repeated contact with some skin irritants appear to evoke increased resistance ('hardening') and other skin irritants, or perhaps other circumstances, produce decreased resistance ('cumulative insult dermatitis')? Several deeply rooted beliefs and generalizations deserve critical evaluation. What really is the role of emotional factors in occupational skin disease?

New chemical products are being developed at an ever increasing rate and our present laboratory test procedures remain screening tests rather than reliably predictive of the possible effects of these chemicals on the human skin. It is sometimes not until a product is marketed that its true dermatitic potential is realized. Further work is needed on the development of better tests.

Doctors, nurses, occupational hygienists and safety advisors are continually being asked questions about occupational skin diseases and potential skin hazards to which no one yet knows the answers. It may be wiser to allow such questions to generate testable hypotheses than to attempt to supply answers before they are reliably known. Something of the spirit of this anonymous eighteenth century writer may also be appropriate to professionals now working in this area. The extract is from a memorial found inside the steeple knob of St. Margaret's Church in Gotha, Germany, dating from 1784, which is quoted in full by Oppenheimer (1954): 'The arts and sciences blossom, and our vision into the workshop of nature goes deep. Artisans approach artists in perfection; useful skills flower at all levels. Here you have a faithful portrait of our time. Look not proudly down upon us, should you stand higher or see farther than we, but rather recognise how with courage and strength we raised and supported your standard. Do the same for those who come after you and rejoice!'

REFERENCES

Buckley W. R. (1958) Lichenoid erruptions following contact dermatitis. *Arch. Dermatol.* **78,** 454–457.

Buckley W. R. and Lewis C. E. (1960) The ruster in industry *J. Occup. Med.* **2,** 23–31.

Calnan C. D, (1970) Skin Disease of occupational origin. *The Glaxo Volume 33,* Greenford, Glaxo Laboratories Ltd, pp. 44–50.

Cohen A. (1977) Factors in successful occupational safety programmes. *J. Saf. Res.* **9,** 168–178.

Cronin E., Bandmann H. - J., Calnan C. D. et al. (1970) Contact dermatitis in the atopic. *Acta. Derm. Venereol. (Stockh.)* **50,** 183–187.

Emmett E. A. (1977) Contact dermatitis from polyfunctional acrylic monomers. *Contact Dermatitis* **3,** 245–248.

Emmett E. A., Taphorn B. R. and Kominsky J. R. (1977a) Phototoxicity occurring during the manufacture of ultraviolet-cured ink. *Arch. Dermatol.* **113,** 770–775.

Emmett E. A., Stetzer L. and Taphorn B. (1977b) Photoxic keratoconjunctivitis from coal-tar pitch volatiles. *Science* **198,** 841–842.

Fawcett I. W., Newman Taylor A. J. and Pepys J. (1976) Asthma due to inhaled chemical agents-fumes from 'Multicore' soldering flux and colophony resin. *Clin. Allergy* **6,** 577–585.

Fawcett I. W., Newman Taylor A. J. and Pepys J. (1977) Asthma due to inhaled chemical agents-epoxy resin systems containing phthalic anhydride, trimellitic acid anhydride and triethylene tetramine. *Clin. Allergy* **7**, 1–14.

Fregert S. (1974) *Manual of Contact Dermatitis.* Copenhagen, Munksgaard, pp. 48–59.

Fregert S. (1975) Occupational dermatitis in a 10-year material. *Contact Dermatitis* **1**, 96–107.

Friedman M. (1962) *Capitalism and Freedom.* Chicago, The University of Chicago, p. 201.

Gellin G. A. (1972) *Occupational Dermatoses.* Chicago, American Medical Association, p. 1.

Hewitt M., Barrow G. I., Miller D. C. et al. (1976) A case of Pyemotes dermatitis. *Br. J. Dermatol.* **94**, 423–430.

Majeti V. A. and Suskind R. R. (1977) Mechanism of cinnamaldehyde sensitization. *Contact Dermatitis* **3**, 16–18.

Malten K. E., Fregert S., Bandmann H. - J. et al. (1971) Occupational dermatitis in five European dermatological departments. *Berufsdermatosen* **19**, 1–14.

Oppenheimer J. R. (1954) *Science and the Common Understanding.* New York, Simon and Schuster. pp. 113–114.

Pirilä V., Fregert S., Bandmann H. J. et al. (1971) Legislation on occupational dermatoses. *Acta Derm. Venereol. (Stockh.)* **51**, 141–145.

Robinson H. M. (1965) Rehabilitation: a problem for the dermatologist. *Arch. Dermatol.* **91**, 198–205.

Robinson H. M., Pass C. and Silverstein E. H. (1971) The rehabilitation index. *Arch. Dermatol.* **103**, 174–179.

Squire J. R., Cruickshank C. N. D. and Topley E. (1950) Occupational skin disease. *Br. Med. Bull.* **7**, 28–41.

Stallones R. A. (1977) Challenges to preventive medicine in the last quarter of the 20th century. *J. Occup. Med.* **19**, 245–248.

Taylor J. S. (1974) Chloracne: a continuing problem. *Cutis* **13**, 585–591.

Wilkinson D. S., Fregert S., Magnusson B. et al. (1970) Terminology of contact dermatitis. *Acta Derm. Venereol. (Stockh.)* **50**, 287–292.

9. TOXICITY TESTING

M. A. Cooke

Ballantyne (1977) has written of the growth of instant, unqualified experts in toxicology and of the 'check-list' type of toxicity testing which has arisen in recent years due to the introduction of legislation such as the Health and Safety at Work Act of 1974 and other legislation. This proliferation of legislation is especially marked in the United States of America and the European Economic Community. It imposes burdens on a society which is ill-equipped with facilities and trained toxicologists to satisfy all the needs specified by the mandatory requirements and advisory documentation. It may not fully allow for the ability of nature to adjust to change and to deal with contamination on a reasonable scale. The cost of controls must also enter into the situation. Cooke (1978) has spoken of the philosophy of safety evaluation and has emphasized the opinion of many authors that there is no such perfection as absolute safety – all activity has its hazards and the cost of safety evaluation and implementation has to be taken into account in relation to the benefit it is likely to bestow. A primitive community in a malaria-ridden swamp may well be prepared to run the risk of high-accumulation of an insecticide such as DDT compared with the almost certain illness and frequent death from inadequately controlled malaria. Toxicity studies are expensive and the cost has to be borne by the community. A full programme of toxicity testing for every chemical, let alone for mixtures and final products, would be impossible in terms of cost and manpower requirements and we have to seek a compromise which will result in an acceptable level of safety and yet not unduly limit production of those chemicals we require if we are to ensure the prosperity of our industry, the employment of our workforce and the feeding, clothing and housing of our population.

The national approach to these problems varies. It has been traditional in the UK in the past to keep mandatory health legislation to a minimum and to work to the principle of 'best practicable means' or what is 'reasonable'. Guidelines have proved popular and voluntary Codes of Practice have achieved great success, a typical example being the UK Pesticide Safety Precaution Scheme. It is to be hoped that the Health and Safety Commission will support and continue this philosophy rather than impose a regulatory approach which is not only expensive but frequently counter-productive, if not unenforceable, on an absolute and equitable basis. A compilation of the chemicals involved is in itself a monumental task, as evidenced by the difficulties encountered in the USA in the registration of chemicals under the Toxic Substances Control Act. Legislation can become so complicated and unworkable as to defeat its purpose and the cost of implementation may become so high as to impose unacceptable economic burdens on less opulent societies. The essential need is to be aware of the possibility of a hazard and to assess its type and magnitude to a degree that the hazards can be controlled to the satisfaction of the worker, consumer or other citizen exposed to its effect.

The toxicity testing programme can then be seen as a dynamic need and not a check list necessity. Careful epidemiological monitoring may suggest the incidence of untoward events which indicate an extension of testing. It is likewise necessary to monitor the reliability of animal testing, for the results of this may not be relevant to man. It is indeed a basic principle that no animal testing or *in vitro* system of laboratory testing can ever guarantee absolute safety for man. At best they indicate potential hazards which must be balanced against degree of risk. The human subject must be the eventual indicator of the validity of the system. Human testing, where applicable, may be the system of choice but the test protocol must be relevant to usage, and one has to ensure a reasonable level of safety for the participants who should be fully aware both of the reasons for the testing and of the potential hazards involved.

The toxicologist has a difficult problem in view of the conflicting views *first* of those who consider that materials should be 'fully' tested, *second* of those who consider we should not use humans for testing, and *third* of those who do not consider animal testing, with its potential for discomfort or pain, is justified. *In vitro* systems such as organ or tissue cultures can only give limited data, due to the modifying influence *in vivo* of the whole organ system. Coupled with these constraints he has to take into account the financial viability of the programme and the value to the community of the development of the specific project.

A commercial or industrial organization may not have an employee who is a toxicologist and may therefore have to seek outside assistance. The final evaluation of the need and design of any test protocol should be a team project in which a human biologist should play the leading rôle – the medical toxicologist and the occupational physician should play an important part and desirably one should lead the team. The evaluation of both the toxic potential and the possible benefit of any chemical must be related to the sick as well as to the fit. A safety evaluation programme which is based on the supposition that only fit personnel are exposed is dangerous, for even the fit may become ill before this is apparent to themselves or to the supervising staff concerned.

Testing programmes will differ for new chemicals or existing chemicals which become suspect for one particular effect. However a consideration of new chemicals will cover the relevant points. The actions to be taken may be listed as follows, it being appreciated that all of the items may not be required for a particular usage.

1. SPECIFICATION OF CHEMICAL

The specification must be accurate and include such physical and chemical data, with analytical methods, as may be required to define and designate the material accurately. Details of impurities should be given.

2. LITERATURE SEARCH

The literature search may conveniently include *Chemical Abstracts*, a Toxline search or use of other computerized systems. A convenient source for a Toxline search is:

Blaise Management,
British Library,
Bibliographic Services Division,
7, Rathbone Street,
London, W1P 2AL.

Computerized searches of established banks such as Toxline will only reveal comparatively recent publications and it is desirable to trace older references which may be found in the bibliographies or references in recent papers or from other sources, such as standard text books, manufacturers' leaflets and from other specialists in the field. An increasing awareness of the need to avoid duplication of effort, to minimize cost and to reduce the number of animal experiments, has stimulated joint studies between companies (producer and consumer, joint producers or trade organizations). Some workers, especially those conducting studies for government agencies or trade organizations, give notice of their current research through such publications as *Tox Tips*.

3. ACUTE TOXICITY STUDIES

While the acute, single dose LD50 test is that most commonly demanded and quoted, it only provides very limited information. It has recently become commonplace for national and international environmental agencies to demand such figures, the LD_{50} being that dose which will result in the deaths of half of the animals under test, and then to draw up ranks of relative toxicity such as 'slightly toxic' or 'highly toxic'. Some also extrapolate the data to estimate the probable fatal dose for man – but such extrapolation may be misleading. LD_{50} tests may vary widely between species and it should be evident that there may be equal or greater variations between animal and man.

Nevertheless, an acute oral study may provide evidence of the order of toxicity of the material and serve as a useful prelude to further studies with smaller doses to assess effects on individual organs, such as liver, kidney, blood or nervous system. Balazs (1970) has stressed the importance of assessment of the 'toxic syndrome' rather than reliance on an LD_{50} figure. More recently Sharratt (1977) has indicated that 'commonly done toxicological investigations should be recognized as pilot studies designed to give information on which definitive studies can be based'. He also points out that such studies may discourage marketing of a product or may indicate that no further work is necessary due to low intrinsic biological activity. However, such low activity may not be a sufficient indicator of safety due to long-term changes which can result from the physical properties of chemically relatively inert materials, for example granulomata, fibrosis and even consequent malignant change.

The acute oral test is conducted by feeding a range of single doses calculated on a geometric scale (e.g. X1, X2, X4, and so on) and observing the animal for a specified period (usually 14 days).

Rodents (rats or mice) are usually chosen as the first species for test but other non-rodent species such as dog or monkey are occasionally used. Apart from the acute oral test, acute dermal or inhalation tests may be required if there is likely to be significant skin contact or inhalation risk. In the dermal test, the material, in a suitable medium if necessary, is applied to the skin, usually of an albino rabbit covered with gauze and suitably wrapped, for a specified period. Observation for subsequent death and organ damage is maintained as for the oral test. Inhalation tests are more difficult due to the technical difficulties of maintaining constant atmospheric levels. It is usual to expose the animals for 4 hours and to observe for 14 days, the result being expressed as an LC_{50} (the concentration which will kill half of the animals in the test group).

4. LONG-TERM STUDIES

The acute tests will give an indication of the maximum dose for long-term studies but some range-finding, medium-term tests are usually desirable to obtain the correct levels for a long-term test. The details of the test need expert and careful consideration if the data are to be of relevance to the practical situation. Route of administration, frequency of dose and the use of recovery periods may all be relevant. A 'no-effect' level determination may be of benefit in the industrial sphere but the greater sophistication and accuracy of modern analytical techniques renders such a concept less valid – the expert judgement to decide whether a change in organ structure or function is significant becomes increasingly important. A long-term inhalation study is one parameter by which a Threshold Limit Value (TLV) may be established.

5. SKIN IRRITATION AND SENSITIZATION STUDIES

These studies are usually conducted on the rabbit (for irritancy) and the guinea pig (for sensitization) but in some cases should be confirmed by human studies. Human studies are often deprecated but if carefully controlled entail little risk. It may not be possible to extrapolate animal or *in vitro* tests to man and then the ultimate choice lies between a controlled human trial (or test) or a large scale more uncontrolled usage, with the possibility that adverse reactions may pass unnoticed. The skin lends itself to immediate detailed observation and such tests can be controlled more satisfactorily than many others. This should not however encourage the unskilled or untrained to attempt such tests. The hazard of sensitization of human subjects is always present in skin testing and the choice both of suitable concentrations and of vehicle, and the evaluation of the results require expert and experienced judgement.

Skin irritation tests

Skin irritation tests involve the application of the material under an occlusive dressing. A commonly used test is the Draize skin test as described in the FDA handbook, *Appraisal of the Safety of Chemicals in Foods, Drugs and Cosmetics* (FDA, 1959), although there are several modifications of this test which are in common use. Six rabbits are restrained in stocks, the backs are shaved and one side of each back is slightly abraded. The test material is applied 0·5 ml to each side, and the areas are then occluded. Readings of the reactions which ensue are taken after removal of the patch at 24 hours and again at 72 hours. The final score based on a numerical scoring system for erythema and oedema gives the primary irritation index: 'Compounds producing combined averages (primary irritation indices) of 2 or less are only mildly irritating; whereas those with indices from 2–5 are moderate irritants, and those with scores above 6 are considered severe irritants'. This is not an entirely satisfactory classification since score 0 is graded as 'mildly irritating' and between 5 and 6 is not defined. The scale may be as misleading as those used for LD_{50} tests – it is wiser to rely upon the interpretation by a toxicologist taking intended usage into account. An alternative test, the Repeated Insult Patch Test (RIPT), employs repeated application.

Sensitization studies

Sensitization studies may be of several types of which those most commonly used are based upon the methods described by Buehler (1965) and Magnusson and Kligman (1969). The Buehler test is perhaps more applicable to industrial usage while the Magnusson and Kligman maximization test is applicable to a consumer product where constant contact is most likely. In the Buehler test the material is applied to groups of guinea pigs in the highest non-irritant concentration and left in place for 6 hours. It may be repeated three times weekly for three weeks and is followed by a challenge application two weeks later. The Magnusson and Kligman maximization test combines topical application with the injection of the material and Freund's adjuvant. This adjuvant is a mixture consisting of a mineral oil and an emulsifying agent enriched with heat-killed acid-fast bacteria and increases the immune response. The skin is likewise challenged two weeks after the application with a non-irritant concentration.

Maximization patch tests on human subjects possibly using sodium lauryl sulphate to increase penetration, and with high doses of the material under test are also used (Kligman, 1966; Kligman and Epstein, 1975). Simple patch testing may not correspond to abnormal usage or frequent usage over a long period. Nevertheless maximization tests may be too vigorous. While they may screen out most sensitizers, they may equally exclude some which would be safe for occasional or transient contact, for example material in wash-off preparations such as a shampoo or an industrial chemical to which there is only occasional exposure.

6. EYE STUDIES

An eye test is desirable for materials which may come into contact with the eye, unless the material has been shown to be a significant skin irritant or corrosive, when there is little or no reason for carrying out eye testing. There are two types of test in general use – the Draize eye test (FDA, 1959) and the Federal Register Test (1964). In the Draize test the material is instilled into one eye and the other used as a control. In three of the six rabbits the eyes are unwashed and in the other three they are washed with lukewarm water four seconds after instillation. The eyes are examined at one, two, three, four and seven days to assess the irritant effects.

In the Federal Register Test the eyes are not washed following instillation of the material and the eyes are examined at 24, 48 and 72 hours after instillation. The examinations need to be meticulous and may with advantage use a slit lamp. Fluorescein facilitates examination of the cornea. Ballantyne and Swanston (1977) have stressed the importance of 'studies on the mechanism of production of eye damage and an assessment of the various factors which modify the nature of chemically-induced damage. Such investigations may assist the development of an *in vitro* test method for screening purposes'. They have also suggested four other areas as being worthy of consideration:

1. Histopathological studies.
2. Measurement of intra-ocular tension.
3. Measurement of corneal permeability
4. Measurement of corneal thickness.

7. CARCINOGENICITY STUDIES

With the control of infectious diseases and the higher standard of living in industrial communities there is an increasing incidence of cancer and it is now one of the common causes of death. Boyland (1977) has discussed the suggestion that over 90 per cent of cases of cancer are due to chemical agents. While some are due to endogenous chemicals such as some hormones or tryptophan metabolites, epidemiological studies indicate 'that about 80 per cent of all cancer is due to environmental factors'. Such figures include smoking and dietary, as well as industrial and urban environmental factors. Epidemiological studies to determine the possible causes of cancer are frequently inadequate because of the influence of smoking on such figures and the unreliability of the data relating to smoking habits. Nevertheless we should consider the carcinogenic potential of all new chemicals. For existing chemicals epidemiological studies with all their deficiences may still prove to be the most satisfactory mode of investigation. The choice of tests for carcinogenicity is difficult for the effects are almost invariably long-term. Some consider that animals should be dosed for a lifetime at the maximum sub-toxic dose, but this may be unrealistic in the industrial situation where exposure may be over a comparatively short period and where it is known that the body can cope with small doses. However, account should also be taken of the 'one molecule theory' which implies that one or perhaps only a few molecules are sufficient to induce cancer. Even if this hypothesis is accepted, the risk of such a sequence of events is likely to be extremely small and the probability of cancer occurring in a detectable number of the population will certainly vary with the dose until the maximum incidence is achieved. Other workers consider that lower test dosages are desirable for it has become increasingly apparent in recent years that immunological mechanisms play a large part in the induction, treatment and occasional spontaneous resolution of cancer. Whatever the approach to the dosage schedule, the test should be both long-term and related to the use of the material. The route of administration should thus be related to use – dermal, oral or inhalation. Occasionally materials are administered by subcutaneous or intramuscular injection or by implants, but misleading results may follow due to physical effects on the tissues. A flat solid implant may produce lesions where a similar perforated implant does not do so.

All such tests for carcinogenicity are extremely expensive and in addition, as tests are often over the animal lifetime, rapid answers cannot be supplied. In lifetime studies of this nature where one has to take account of the natural incidence of tumors in the species under test, the choice both of species and of strain is of paramount importance. Even with the same strain, however, Grasso et al. (1977) have found considerable variation in control mice in different laboratories and discuss the problem of common naturally occurring tumors in cancer studies in mice. Careful use of controls is essential in view of the part occasionally played by viruses and the action of infections on immunological mechanisms. Elimination of such infections in long-term testing in laboratories is desirable, but expensive, and needs extra and more specialized staff.

The time (2 years for a rat experiment) and the cost of these procedures has stimulated an interest in short-term tests as indicators of carcinogenic potential. It has been suggested that a battery of such tests may be at least as good indicators of potential carcinogenicity as are long-term animal studies with both the difficulties involved in such techniques and the problems of extrapolation to man. It is likely that a battery of short-term tests would detect over 90 per cent of potential carcinogenicity, but it would also produce a number of false positives. Purchase et al. (1977) have calculated that in a short-term test of 90 per cent accuracy of 1000 chemicals, of which only a minority, say 1 per cent, are carcinogenic, 108 would be positive. Only 8 per cent of them would be carcinogenic on animal testing. Over 90 materials would be falsely rejected. The position could be worse than that for some of the materials producing carcinogenic effects in animals could be safe in man. Thus well over 10 per cent of new chemicals could be wrongly rejected and we might lose valuable materials by so doing. Grasso (1977) has written '. . . false results may be of small moment to those concerned with the sensational aspects of this type of research, but they could deprive the public of some compounds that make a useful contribution to the quality of life'.

It therefore becomes increasingly important that the chemical structure, activity and metabolic pathways are carefully studied before test programmes for carcinogenicity are undertaken although cost factors may determine the early choice of a short-term test even at the risk of losing some useful new chemicals.

There are a large number of short-term tests for carcinogenicity, some of which will also detect potential mutagenicity for the mechanism of induction may be similar – however, not all mutagens are carcinogenic and not all carcinogens are mutagens. The tests may be considered as falling into three categories detecting:

1. Primary DNA damage.
2. Mutagenic effects.
3. Chromosome damage.

Purchase et al. (1977) consider the cell-transformation test and the reverse mutation test (Ames' test; Ames et al., 1975) to be the most accurate in detecting carcinogens. Other short-term tests include:

1. The sebaceous gland suppresssion test.
2. The degranulation test.
3. The subcutaneous implant test.
4. The tetrazolium reduction test.
5. Changes in rough endoplasmic reticulum.
6. Rate of cell proliferation.
7. Measurement of changes in the size of cell nucleus.
8. Changes in biphenyl hydroxylase activity.

The cell transformation test

The cell transformation test involves the addition of the chemical to a cell culture. Some cells will die but others may survive and proliferate in an abnormal fashion. They are then injected into irradiated animals and if the chemical is carcinogenic, tumours may then develop. Various tissue culture systems, modified to take account of carcinogens which require metabolic activation, have been developed.

8. MUTAGENICITY STUDIES

Mutagenicity is the capacity to change the genetic material of a cell in such a manner that the alteration passes to subsequent generations of cells. It may be detected by various types of test. *In vivo* tests include studies in the fruit fly *Drosophila melanogaster* and in animal species. The micronucleus test involves examination of the bone marrow of an animal treated with the test material. The presence of micronuclei in developing erythrocytes is considered to be due to nuclear debris indicative of chromosomal change. The dominant lethal assay system is designed to detect germ-cell mutations. Male rats or mice dosed with test material are mated with undosed females. The females are examined at mid-term for living or dead implantations, which are correlated with numbers of corpora lutea. However, bacterial *in vivo* tests, especially the Ames test and modifications of this (Ames et al., 1973a,b), are relatively speedy and inexpensive and have recently become popular. They are claimed to have a high degree of accuracy, but as pointed out above this may result in a high rejection rate of new chemicals on an invalid basis. However, *in vivo* animal test results may be equally invalid for man. It is prudent to take cognizance of positive mutagenicity studies unless there are adequate data to the contrary, which in the case of currently used materials may be carefully documented human experience.

The Ames test uses several strains of *Salmonella typhimurium*, each of which contains a mutation through which the bacteria require histidine for their growth. If, therefore, the bacteria grow on a histidine deficient medium, when in contact with the test chemical, further mutation must have occurred. By adding liver homogenates, active metabolites from the test material can be detected. Whether the system will be valid for new chemicals as opposed to the existing materials already tested is still a matter for debate. The relevance to potential human mutagenicity is also questioned. Grasso and Grant (1977) have commented that positive results 'cannot be ignored but the significance of bacterial mutation in general as an indication of potential "mutagenicity" in mammals is a hotly debated issue because of the wide phylogenetic differences between bacteria and mammals'.

9. TERATOGENICITY STUDIES

Teratogenicity has not been proved to occur due to industrial exposure. There is, nevertheless, some evidence to suggest that it may have occurred in the past. An increasing awareness of the possibility has followed the thalidomide incident. Teratogenicity testing is, however, a new procedure and attempts to develop short-term screening methods have so far proved unsuccessful. The low incidence of the effects means that considerable numbers of animals must be used because of the concern with low dose levels rather than with near toxic doses.

Capacity for teratogenicity may be studied by using the embryotoxic potential of the material. Pregnant animals are dosed and any toxic effects and fetal abnormalities are noted. It is also possible to derive data by studying the numbers of corpora lutea, implantation sites, resorption sites and resorptions. There are other more detailed parameters which can give an indication of degree of teratogenicity potential, but the tests are extremely difficult to relate to the industrial usage situation.

In view of different reactions in different species it is wise to use at least two species in such tests. This emphasizes the hazards in extrapolation to man, for if there is inconsistency between species, there could be considerable risk in such extrapolation.

10. OTHER REPRODUCTIVE STUDIES

It is possible to study such effects as fertility, including gonadal function, conception rates and several related parameters by dosing animals and studying the reproductive parameter concerned, but again the extrapolation of these data to man requires expert judgement.

The tests described are examples of those which are in general use but it cannot be over-emphasized that a rigid adherence to standard protocols and classification by stereotyped phrases can be wasteful of limited resources and expert technologists. Each chemical and each problem should be considered individually. Testing should be phased, taking into account published work, reactions of chemically related compounds and anticipated uses of the material.

The published work must be studied critically and may have to be rejected if there are obvious discrepancies or if the test methods prove unacceptable by current standards.

The reaction of chemically related compounds may be useful, but small changes in formulation may produce significantly different toxic effects – this is particularly the case if different atoms are introduced into the molecule or if the sites of active atoms (such as the halogens) are varied. Comparison of members of a chemical series may justify grouping: there is considerable evidence that surfactants with 12 carbons in their alkyl chain are more irritant than those with more or less than 12 (Imokawa et al., 1975).

Barnes and Stoner have discussed the toxicology of organo-tin compounds of the general formula $R_{1-4}SnX_{3-0}$, where R is a simple aryl or alkyl group linked direct to the tin and X is a simple or complex anion. They stated that 'the biological properties of each group are distinct and, within any group, vary with the nature of R and are almost independent of the nature of X'.

Dialkyl and trialkyl tin compounds produce quite different toxic effects. Poisoning by dibutyl tin dichloride (DBTC) lacks any prominent features but while it produced inflammatory lesions of the bile duct leading to pancreatitis, perforation and peritonitis in rats and mice, it does not have this effect on rabbits, guinea pigs or cats. DBTC is excreted in the bile and only causes this lesion in species where the bile and pancreatic ducts run a common course. Some other dialkyl tin compounds have a similar effect.

Trialkyl tin compounds have a specific effect on the nervous system, producing cerebral oedema. The tragedy in France many years ago where a dialkyl tin compound was used for treatment of skin diseases, was probably due to a trialkyl tin compound present as an impurity, producing as it did, cerebral oedema. The importance of accurate specification and the effect of impurities was amply demonstrated by this tragedy.

Predicted use should indicate the extent and type of testing. The manufacturers cannot anticipate all possible uses of his product but he can define the uses for which he is giving his advice and for which he has programmed his advisory and testing services. If new uses develop, then the proponent of these should decide the further information necessary and decide, with his supplier, what further enquiry or testing may be required. The only safe alternative would be 'complete' testing of all materials, for natural products are potentially as dangerous as synthetic chemicals.

The purity of materials is particularly relevant to intended use. Modern, sophisticated analytical techniques can detect very low concentrations of noxious impurities in what is otherwise a harmless product and a judgement has to be made of the level which can be accepted. Batches of product will contain varying amounts of impurity, and it would not be practicable to 'batch test' all products by the standard biological techniques at present in use.

However new techniques of *in vitro* testing are under active study. These could detect varying levels of toxic impurities in batches or in products manufactured by different chemical routes. Analytical methods alone may not always achieve this, due to the presence of unanalyzable residues but techniques involving tissue culture may do so. The value of these has been mentioned under carcinogenicity testing.

In vitro tests may also be used for such diverse purposes as measuring the pharmacological activity of steroids, the relative anti-cholinesterase activity of certain organo-phosphorus compounds, and the rapid assessment of phototoxicity. While such tests may indicate no 'toxic effect', they are frequently too sensitive. Even then, however, they may be valuable for ranking purposes. These tests have other limitations for they may not measure metabolic products produced in the intact animal and conversely, may not allow for inactivation by immune or other responses. Some allowance can be made by the inclusion of tissue extracts or homogenates, as in the various modifications of Ames' test at present in use, and 'whole organ' cultures can now be studied.

Whilst it may not be possible to extrapolate the results of these *in vitro* tests to man, it is pertinent to point out that neither can animal tests be used with complete assurance of their relevance to man. There may be considerable difference in the results using differing species and even strains within a species. For this reason, two or more species (e.g. rodent, rabbit or dog) are frequently used and while primate testing would be more valuable, it presents many practical difficulties and dangers of trauma and infection in handling. Hopefully *in vitro* tests will be more widely developed and facilitate rapid screening and some replacement of current animal testing, which some people find unacceptable. Animal testing in the United Kingdom is closely controlled and rightly so. Beecher (1972) quotes a personal communication from Geoffrey Edsall: 'They (the English) are also distinguished for having the most rigid anti-vivisection laws in the world . . . The British have displayed a tendency to be carried away by their emotional reactions in such affairs time and again.'

Although many experiments do not involve pain, insofar as they are experiments to prove safety at acceptable levels, investigations should nevertheless always evaluate carefully the need for testing to ensure 'reasonable' safety, both in manufacture and in use. Ecological studies and tests on other species (e.g. fish) may be required. Cooke (1978) has suggested that the proper criterion for any test results should be that the material is acceptable for manufacture and use by those who are 'nearest and dearest' to us. In the industrial situation, this requires constant vigilance, for new knowledge of adverse reactions may indicate further investigation and those 'nearest and dearest' may be weak, ill or disabled. This emphasizes the need for complete co-operation between members of the health team, the physician, toxicologist, hygienist, nurse, technical, production and marketing managers. The occupational physician must be aware of this need. He should carefully observe the workforce. Through the scientific literature, the media and marketing managers he should be aware of any evidence of adverse reactions, for the final test of safety for man is in man.

From time to time materials in quite general use are found to produce harmful effects. While 'shopping lists' of tests are popular with government and consumer agencies, they are only useful as guidelines and must not be construed as being either completely adequate or sometimes even necessary. An example would be tests required for a chemically inert, insoluble material where fibrogenicity might be a more significant potential hazard than the acute or chronic toxic hazards covered by standard protocols. The chemical and physical nature of the material, its probable use and its mode of manufacture should all be considered when specifying a testing programme. Many industrial organizations do not have such full health teams and cannot do so in the foreseeable future, for trained personnel are and will remain scarce. Full advantage should therefore be taken of the expertise within academic bodies, trade and government agencies. The commercial testing houses are always willing to submit draft programmes which can be presented to independent experts, perhaps those who require the tests, for further comment and, if necessary, approval.

The mortality and morbidity resulting from industrial poisoning is extremely small compared to that from accidents or such self-imposed hazards as smoking, alcohol and overeating, but this should not deter those who work in the field of occupational health from establishing even safer standards than those which we now enjoy, at a cost which does not preclude the use of materials we need and from which we derive pleasure and increased quality of life.

REFERENCES

Ames B. N., Durston W. E., Yamasaki E. et al. (1973a) Carcinogens are mutagens; a simple test system combining liver homogenates for activation and bacteria for detection. *Proc. Natl. Acad. Sci. USA* **70,** 2281–2285.

Ames B. N., Lee F. D. and Durston W. E. (1973b) An improved bacterial test system for the detection and classification of mutagens and carcinogens. *Proc. Natl. Acad. Sci. USA* **70,** 782–786.

Balazs T. (1970) Measurement of acute toxicity. In: Paget G. E. (ed.), *Methods in Toxicology*. Oxford, Blackwell, pp. 49–81.

Barnes J. M. and Stoner H. B. (1959) The toxicology of tin compounds. *Pharmacol. Rev.* **11,** 211–231.

Ballantyne B. and Swanston D. W. (1977) Scope and limitations of acute eye irritation tests. In: Ballantyne B. (ed.), *Current Approaches in Toxicology*. Bristol, Wright, pp. 139–157.

Beecher H. K. (1972) Scarce resources and medical advancement. In: Freund P. A. (ed.), *Experimentation with Human Subjects*. London, Allen and Unwin, pp. 66–104.

Boyland E. (1977) Biochemistry of occupational cancer. *J. Soc. Occup. Med.* **27,** 97–101.

Buehler E. V. (1965) Delayed contact hypersensitivity in the guinea pig. *Arch. Dermatol.* **91,** 171–177.

Cooke M. A. (1978) *A Philosophy of Cosmetic and Toiletry Safety Evaluation*. In preparation.

FDA (1959) FDA Handbook, *Appraisal of the Safety of Chemicals in Foods, Drugs and Cosmetics*, p. 47.

Federal Register Test (1964) *US Federal Register,* 17 Sept., 1964, **29,** FR 13009.

Grasso P. (1977) Short term carcinogenicity tests: you pays your money. . . *Food Cosmet. Toxicol.* **15,** 74–75.

Grasso P. and Grant D. (1977) Short-term tests for carcinogenicity. In: Ballantyne B. (ed.), *Current Approaches in Toxicology,* Bristol, Wright, pp. 218–234.

Grasso P., Crampton R. F. and Hooson J. (1977) *The Mouse and Carcinogenicity Testing,* Carshalton, The British Industrial Biological Research Association.

Imokawa G., Sumura K. and Katsumi M. (1975) Study on skin roughness caused by surfactants. *J. Am. Oil Chem. Soc.* **52,** 479–489.

Kligman A. M. (1966) The identification of contact allergens by human assay. III, The maximization test. A procedure for screening and rating contact sensitizers. *J. Invest. Dermatol.* **47,** 393–409.

Kligman A. M. and Epstein W. (1975) Updating the maximization test for identifying contact allergens. *Contact Dermatitis* **1,** 231–239.

Magnusson B. and Kligman A. M. (1969) The identification of contact allergens by animal assay: The guinea pig maximization test. *J. Invest. Dermatol.* **52**, 268–276.

Purchase I. F. H., Ashby J., Styles J. A. et al. (1977) Short term tests for carcinogenicity. *Ann. Occup. Hyg.* **20**, 293–295.

Sharratt M. (1977) Evaluation of the safety of chemicals. In: Ballantyne B. (ed.), *Current Approaches in Toxicology*. Bristol, Wright, pp. 1–11.

10. THE ROLE OF EPIDEMIOLOGY IN OCCUPATIONAL HEALTH

Michael Alderson

This chapter discusses the application of epidemiology to a range of issues relevant to occupational health; it is method orientated and does not attempt to provide a comprehensive account of the findings from research on specific topics. In order to bridge the gap between method and findings in a relatively condensed form a Table is included which classifies recent papers in the general field of occupational health by method used, subjects and topics studied, and categories of data collected (*pp*. 168–186).

The main body of the text contains relatively few references; however, a selected list of texts is provided at the end for further reading. These provide much more detailed treatment of the issues touched upon in the contribution and signposts to a voluminous literature.

THE RELEVANCE OF EPIDEMIOLOGY

There are two rather different reasons for considering that an understanding of the role of epidemiology is of value. First is the possibility that the individual may carry out some 'studies' himself; these may involve the general review of the preventive and curative work with which the individual is concerned or the mounting of a specific study (either initiated by the preceding review or for some other reason). Very different is the ability to interpret critically the study design, findings, and conclusions of other published work that should stem from a grasp of the principle discussed in this contribution. If this does no more than stimulate an interest in the topic it has succeeded; one of the pioneers in this field was adamant that one learnt not from instruction, but primarily from pursuit of studies under guidance (Ryle, 1948).

A general scheme for epidemiological studies is now described; this is followed by a note indicating in somewhat greater detail approaches that are particularly suited to exploring problems in occupational health. Though a few individuals label themselves as epidemiologists, for many studies they need the expert assistance of statisticians or laboratory scientists. There is also considerable overlap between the work of epidemiologists and ergonometricians, industrial hygienists, occupational psychologists, safety inspectors, and toxicologists. Many useful studies can be carried out by careful thought, diligence, and the 'application of common sense' – the epidemiologist has no prior claim on these attributes over those working in occupational health!

WHAT IS EPIDEMIOLOGY?

Epidemiology may be defined as the study of the determinants of the incidence and prevalence of disease. Perhaps it is more informative to indicate that it is an approach to: (1) studying the distribution and size of disease problems in human populations, (2) investigating the causative factors in the pathogenesis of disease, and (3) providing data essential for the management, planning and evaluation of services for prevention, control and treatment of disease. Three rather different classes of epidemiological study may be mounted:

1. Descriptive.
2. Analytical – in which hypotheses suggested by descriptive studies are explored.
3. Intervention studies which introduce various changes in the environment and measure their impact upon the health of the study population.

A SCHEME FOR EPIDEMIOLOGICAL STUDIES

Fig. 10.1 sets out a general scheme that can be used in pursuing epidemiological studies from the initial generation of a hunch to the final evaluation of the chosen method of intervention. (It is suggested that this figure is examined in detail after reading the text.) In general, epidemiology can contribute to five rather different aspects of disease control:

1. The generation of hunches.
2. The quantification of specific risk factors and the elucidation of intervening and confounding factors.
3. The identification of mechanisms involved in generation of disease.
4. The planning of intervention.
5. Evaluation of the effect of preventive campaigns.

The following notes describe how this scheme may be put into practice, but it must be emphasized at the onset that this is not a rigid framework that must be followed exactly. The actual path to successful intervention may be direct, or very tortuous, and the types of study used may not conform to the precise categories indicated in the figure.

Another issue that requires emphasis is that the scheme has been set out for the pursuit of aetiological studies, followed by some form of primary or secondary prevention. This is by no means the only sequence of topics upon which epidemiology may focus, but it is thought to be the main interest and application in occupational health. Morris (1975) describes the wider uses of epidemiology as covering: the diagnosis of community health; the working of the health services; the quantification of individual risk of disease; the identification of syndromes; completing the clinical picture (i.e. obtaining bias free descriptions of diseases and their natural history); and the identification of causes of disease.

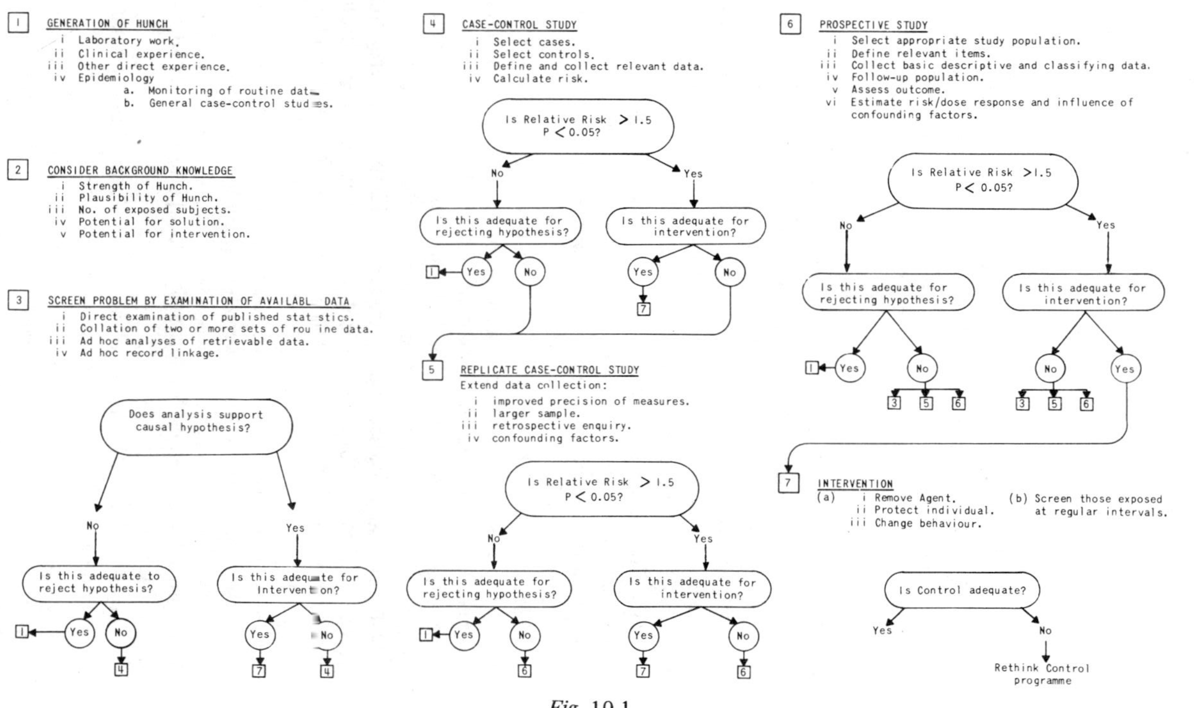
A SCHEME FOR EPIDEMIOLOGICAL STUDIES
Note: This framework is not a Procrustean bed, but indicates the steps that may be taken in aetiological studies from generation of a Hunch to Disease Control. The path can vary, depending on the specific issues involved: progress requires skill and judgement, and collaboration with laboratory and clinical research.
1 GENERATION OF HUNCH
i Laboratory work.
ii Clinical experience.
iii Other direct experience.
iv Epidemiology
a. Monitoring of routine data.
b. General case-control studies.
2 CONSIDER BACKGROUND KNOWLEDGE
i Strength of Hunch.
ii Plausibility of Hunch.
iii No. of exposed subjects.
iv Potential for solution.
v Potential for intervention.
3 SCREEN PROBLEM BY EXAMINATION OF AVAILABLE DATA
i Direct examination of published statistics.
ii Collation of two or more sets of routine data.
iii Ad hoc analyses of retrievable data.
iv Ad hoc record linkage.
Does analysis support causal hypothesis?
No
Yes
Is this adequate to reject hypothesis?
Is this adequate for Intervention?
Yes
No
4 CASE-CONTROL STUDY
i Select cases.
ii Select controls.
iii Define and collect relevant data.
iv Calculate risk.
Is Relative Risk > 1.5 P < 0.05?
Is this adequate for rejecting hypothesis?
Is this adequate for intervention?
5 REPLICATE CASE-CONTROL STUDY
Extend data collection:
i improved precision of measures.
ii larger sample.
iii retrospective enquiry.
iv confounding factors.
6 PROSPECTIVE STUDY
i Select appropriate study population.
ii Define relevant items.
iii Collect basic descriptive and classifying data.
iv Follow-up population.
v Assess outcome.
vi Estimate risk/dose response and influence of confounding factors.
7 INTERVENTION
(a) i Remove Agent.
ii Protect individual.
iii Change behaviour.
(b) Screen those exposed at regular intervals.
Is Control adequate?
Rethink Control programme

Fig. 10.1.

The generation of hunches

It must be borne in mind that there are two rather different issues that need to be considered. *First,* aetiological factors that have been present in the enivronment for many years but have not as yet been identified as harmful need to be investigated. (The expression 'factor' covers a wide range of classes of aetiological agent; these classes are indicated in a later paragraph in this section.) *Second,* there is the very different need to identify the risk to man of new factors released into the environment. Because of the long latent period between the initiation and development of chronic disease, epidemiology will be hard put to quantify the risk thus generated. Henry (1947), when discussing the development of skin epithelioma in men exposed to shale oil, pointed out that there was a median interval of about 45 years between initial exposure and development of the lesion.

Hunches can be derived from clinical experience, from other direct experience, from laboratory investigation, and from epidemiology. A milestone in the identification of carcinogenic factors was the work of Pott (1775), who identified the relationship between scrotal cancer and chimney sweeping, and there are many other examples in the field of malignant disease where clinicians have been the first to suspect a hazard. Epidemiology may contribute to the generation of hunches, particularly through the examination of routine or retrievable statistics. The appropriate techniques are discussed in the following paragraphs. It is important to acknowledge that laboratory investigation has contributed as much to the identification of fresh hazards as epidemiology.

Alderson (1977) has reviewed the value of national mortality statistics, national cancer registration, hospital morbidity returns, and sickness absence data in the identification of fresh hunches. The contribution of these sources of data to fresh leads has been limited, compared with guidance from other fields – a reflection of the very difficult task that is posed when such statistics are expected to identify hitherto unsuspected causes of disease. (Such statistical systems are, however, invaluable for other purposes, and the preceding comment in no way should be taken to imply overall criticism of such statistics.) New developments in the handling of National Vital Statistical systems may increase their power to contribute to this particular issue. These include:

1. Improved techniques for analysing Occupational Mortality data (Fox, 1977).
2. The use of record linkage to provide National Cohort Studies (Office of Population Censuses and Surveys, 1973).
3. The application of grid-codes for the place of residence of patients in the National Cancer Register to facilitate the study of spatial distribution of cancer in relation to a range of demographic and environmental material (Cook, 1977).

Compared with studying general environmental hazards, or risks determined by personal behaviour, there appears to be greater opportunity within industry to obtain retrievable data which contributes to relevant studies. However, personal behaviour and the general environment may be much more important than the industrial hazards. One needs to consider the influence of an individual's genes, sex, age, diet, alcohol consumption, drug taking, smoking habits, presence of other disease, and general environment (chemical, physical and psycho-social). At the present moment, it is inconceivable that monitoring systems to collect this range of data could be established in order to search for variation in the risk of disease in relation to environment and behaviour. This is where the examination of routine statistics can be of value. By probing for variation in the distribution of disease within sub-groups of the population, there is always the hope that pointers to areas warranting more detailed study will arise and, as already acknowledged, clinical observations, individual experiences, and work in the laboratory, can all provide fruitful leads for epidemiological studies.

Does the hunch warrant exploration?

Perhaps the most crucial question faced by a (potential) research worker is which hunch should he pursue; many leads can be thrown up by the activities mentioned above, but only a small proportion will reflect true cause-and-effect relationships. It is suggested that this spotting of hazards is most acute where a relatively small group of individuals have been exposed to an agent that markedly raises the risk of a (relatively) rare form of disease and where those exposed can be readily identified by some particular characteristic of their way of life. Even if a research worker is convinced that there is a lead to a new causal factor, it may not warrant pursuit if:

1. Very few individuals are exposed.
2. The risk to the exposed is a negligible increment on the general patterns of disease.
3. The identification of the aetiological agent is likely to be extremely difficult.
4. Identification of the aetiological agent promises no clear follow-through to intervention.

Screen problem by examination of available data

The first step to be taken in considering a hunch is to review the available or retrievable data in order to see how firm is the proposition. This may be by using directly available published statistics (including commentaries on such statistics) such as the mortality, occupational mortality, and other publications of the Registrar General.

Routine statistics have the great advantage of being on the book shelf and directly available. They are subject to a number of problems:

incompleteness (for example, notifications of infectious disease are notoriously incomplete); inaccuracy (though this is an undoubted fact, judicious interpretation is possible); delay (capture, coding, processing, and publication can take years); retrievability (the system for coding and processing data may result in aggregation, such that desired specificity is lost); inappropriateness (how often is it found that the crucial factor required in a tabulation is not available, and thus the data is useless for exploring the specific issue in question); inflexibility (today's national systems may use yesterday's classification of disease and have difficulty changing to accommodate advances in knowledge); confidentiality (this may prevent release of data for research purposes, when identification of individuals to whom the data relates would occur); acceptance (the potential user may distrust the source or disagree with the findings and thus set up a psychological block to the material).

It may be necessary to manipulate two or more sets of data from different sources in order to probe a particular issue (for example, the Americans have recently been comparing distribution of mortality by county and cause, in relation to known distribution of occupations and industries by county). If the published statistics are not appropriate, or in order to probe the issue more deeply, a special analysis may be carried out of retrievable data; this may be nationally held data that have not been analyzed (for example, the computer-held detailed mortality or incidence material), or data at local level perhaps stored in some information system or merely in written records of industry. The use of such data is discussed in greater detail in the later section on 'Do-It-Yourself Studies'. Another form of special analysis that can be generated from available data is by using linked records; the distinction being that earlier reference has been made to relating two or more sets of data, where the grouped data are contrasted manually; linkage refers to the organization of data relating to individuals that have been acquired on two or more different occasions, even through (two or more) different statistical systems. Some national linkage systems are now being developed; whilst these continue to pose problems of scale and confidentiality there is perhaps scope for *ad hoc* record linkage at local level.

The usual approach is to probe such data for appreciable variation that is compatible with the hypothesis that the associations are causally related. Initially variation may be sought for incidence or mortality by: *person* (age, sex, marital status, occupation, social class, place of birth); *place* (urban/rural, regions of a country, international); *time* (trends within a week or year, or over many years). Great care must be taken to avoid confusing association with causation. Does a common 'unknown' factor cause both the aspects being examined? Could chance or bias lead to the findings? In some circumstances two factors can combine to increase the risk of disease, in others a sequential exposure to first one and then the second factor may be essential or at least greatly increase risk; confounding factors may be present which are associated with risk of disease but neither cause nor increase risk of disease.

Providing this analysis supports the causal hypothesis further studies will then be required, which may either test further the hypothesis, or move straight to initiation of intervention.

Verification that a hazard exists

Where appreciable numbers of employees have been exposed to the suspect factor in the past, a variety of epidemiological studies may be considered. Assuming the appropriate published mortality and incidence statistics do not indicate that the hypothesis is quite untenable, four types of epidemiological study may be mounted:

1. If death certificates exist for an exposed population, it is very simple to carry out a *proportional mortality analysis*;
2. If details of the exposed population can be retrieved and death certificates exist for those that have died, the *person years at risk* can be calculated (tabulated by category of exposure and other relevant variates) and the *observed and expected mortality* examined (such a study is a specific extension of the more general type of cross-sectional study);
3. A *case-control study* may be mounted to collect restrospective data on exposure to the agent and other variates, and the *risk ratio* may be calculated; and
4. For major issues a large scale *prospective study* may be required in an attempt to obtain an unbiased estimate of exposure to the agent and permit examination of a range of confounding factors.

The first two of these are particular examples of studies using 'available' data; they are described in greater detail in the section on 'Do-It-Yourself' studies.

Cross-sectional studies

The simplest type of study that can be launched on people is some form of cross-sectional study; this may be a descriptive study in nature, or it may be testing out the hypothesis that has already been suggested by earlier work. In general a sample of the occupational workers will be identified and contacted; data may be collected through an interview (or self-completion questionnaire), the subjects may be examined, or investigations may be carried out. Before mounting the study careful thought should be given to the study design, which may seek to identify the proportion of individuals with a particular abnormality; a more probing examination occurs when search is made for inter-relationship between other factors and the presence of early or incipient disease. For example, a descriptive study may merely seek to identify the distribution of impaired respiratory function in the workers, while hypothesis testing may explore the relationship between the variation in respiratory function and exposure to particular environmental agents. The study design must be thought out with care. The following points should be considered at the planning phase:

1. Precise definition of the objectives of the study;
2. Link chosen method to these objectives (the type of study and the items collected);
3. Criteria of eligibility for the study population (how will a sample be selected?);
4. Statistical aspects (numbers of subjects required for meaningful results, data recording and processing, method of analysis);
5. Collaboration (obtain permission and agreement of all required to obtain a good response).

The accuracy of the data must be very carefully considered. It is desirable to attempt some internal or external checks on the quality of data, as it is often suprising how random error or bias can occur. There is a comprehensive literature on the problems of validity of 'survey' data, including errors in written or verbal responses, observer error in examination findings, instrument and observer error in investigation results and subject variability. In certain circumstances, a preliminary 'method' study may be required to develop and validate a new technique for obtaining data prior to the launch of a particular study.

Particular attention must be paid to the 'source' of the respondents – are they typical of their general category of workers, or has some overt or hidden bias crept in? In general, it must be considered that all 'populations' are biased. (What are the factors selecting into and out of the group?) Two examples illustrate either aspect of this problem. Ødegard (1956) found an excess of schizophrenia in merchant seamen, due to persons with manifest personality disorder chosing this (isolated) occupation. Schilling (1956) showed that there was under-representation of females with byssinosis in female cotton workers, due to selective exit of affected persons (with no evidence of immunity in the entrants as a whole).

When the study has been launched, the response rate must be monitored; an attempt must be made to obtain some information about non-responders. How biased are they, compared with those co-operating?

In a cross-sectional study information can be collected from the respondents about socio-economic issues, about their present environment at home, at leisure and at work; about their attitudes, knowledge and behaviour. All this information is in response to questions about 'today' and the general plan is to collect data from the representative sample of individuals, some of whom may have identifiable disease (identified by questioning, examination or investigation).

A cross-sectional study can be extended in two rather different ways.

First it can be used as a start point for a case-control study, where individuals with and without the specific abnormality are identified in the screening; more detailed data on associated factors may then be collected from all the cases and a sample of 'controls'. The other way in which the study can be extended is by asking the respondents questions about past history, particularly past history of exposure to potential aetiological agents. One problem about a retrospective study is that the quality of data is in certain circumstances of doubtful validity. Memory may introduce bias due to failure to record long past events, whilst particular recent occurences may differentially influence the recall (Bartlett, 1932). In particular it is often suspect that the patients who have developed disease are more likely to search in their memory for past occurrences compared with the healthy controls.

The appropriate selection of controls is a crucial issue, but one on which it is often difficult to enunciate simple rules. In the industrial environment individuals without the disease being studied but drawn from the same workforce may provide the best general control population; the study could then look at the relative risk of the disease in relation to duration and intensity of exposure to the suspect agent. Matching subgroups can be used; that is, individuals of the same general level of skill or salary can be used as controls. The danger with matching is that it can indirectly match cases and controls to exposure (for example, if age was used as a matching factor and age was directly linked to length of exposure). However, where there is measured variation in exposure to some agent such as dust, it may be useful to match a sample of cases and controls on dust exposure in order that other confounding and intervening variates may be examined more precisely.

Cross-sectional studies, including those involving cases and controls or with extension to retrospective enquiries are relatively economical in use of time and can often be carried out on fairly small samples of individuals. These are two important advantages, particularly if resources are limited and also there is a desire to get a preliminary answer to the questions as soon as possible. The disadvantages of this category of study is that there is a limitation to the issues which they can explore (in the absence of detailed monitoring of environmental exposure in the past it may be impossible to use this technique to relate specific exposures to generation of disease); there is also the problem in the biases already indicated.

Prospective studies

Prospective studies are used to probe in greater detail some specific hypothesis. The general approach is to investigate a sample of individuals and classify their 'exposure' to the suspect agent. The individuals are then followed up and some unbiased valid estimate of outcome is required on all individuals. The concept of the prospective study is thus quite different – it begins with 'healthy' individuals and records in some detail their exposure to various factors, and then follows these individuals up over time (and this may be many years) using accepted techniques to identify the development or death from specific diseases. The advantages of this approach are that it should lead to the collection of unbiased accurate exposure data and permit the examination of a much more comprehensive range of issues. Having decided a particular factor may be relevant as either a causative or confounding variate, it should be possible to include it in a prospective study design – providing a technique exists for measuring it. This is very different in a retrospective study, when crucial data may be unrecorded or irretrievable and the factor thus excluded from the study. The disadvantages are that relatively large numbers of subjects are required; if the subsequent incidence or fatality from the condition being studied is low or very low, very large numbers of individuals will be required. Where the latent interval between exposure and development of the disease is long the study will also be slow to carry out – large numbers will not themselves avoid this need to encompass at least longer than the median latent interval in order to describe adequately the risk of the disease. Because of the need to follow-up large numbers of individuals there is a problem that some may 'drop-out', though in the occupational field this is likely to be restricted to those leaving the industry or retiring and in whom arrangements for special follow-up will be required. A further doubt about the prospective study is the effect that observation can have on behaviour or even generation of disease. This is particularly likely to be a problem where observation may influence exposure to hazard, such as exposure that is closely linked to patterns of behaviour, whilst the incidence or prevalence of certain psychological and psychosomatic diseases may be influenced by the detailed prospective study.

The above comments relate to the traditional prospective study; it is possible to carry out a prospective study 'on the cheap'; this is by the use of recorded data on exposure, and linking this material to other recorded data on outcome in the identifiable individuals. This issue is discussed further in the 'Do-It-Yourself Studies' section at the end of this chapter.

Unravelling mechanisms

The triumph of public health in the middle of the nineteenth century was accompanied by much muddled thinking about the mechanisms of the generation of acute disease. However, by identifying broad 'vehicles' of hazard (such as polluted water, food or air), preventive measures which had a beneficial effect were introduced in the complete absence of scientific knowledge of the mechanisms involved. It is accepted that, in certain circumstances, subsequent detailed research on the vehicle identified the harmful factor (this was sometimes the presence of bacteria or heavy metals). In addition, the specific entry port and also the mode of action for the harmful factor was recognized. Further detailed work on the mechanisms of the generation of the disease resulted in both bacteriological advance and chemical advance. For example, the work on typhoid resulted in the ability to protect against the disease through immunization – without the necessity of completely abolishing the exposure to bacteria. A parallel to this was the development of drugs which have the ability to remove heavy metals from the body and thus reduce the toxic effects long after exposure has occurred. These techniques result in secondary prevention of disease (the following section distinguishes between primary and secondary prevention) and such measures have been effective, even when exclusion of the factor from the human environment has not yet been possible.

What is not clear at the present time is the scope for identifying the mechanisms of generation of chronic disease and the subsequent opportunities to interfere with the disease process in a comparable way. Enhanced knowledge of the generation of the disease is likely to simplify the planning of effective preventive measures. However, it is not clear that the study of the mechanisms will immediately contribute to disease control. (Do we need to know about mechanism at molecule/enzyme/cell/tissue level in order to introduce preventive measures for mental illness, arthritis, chronic bronchitis, or other degenerative diseases?)

Planning prevention

There are three different approaches to prevention. Primary prevention involves removal of the agent from the environment, or removal of the 'vehicle' that transports the specific factor to the susceptible individuals. Secondary prevention aims at diagnosis of precursor abnormalities or the early diagnosis of disease. Tertiary prevention attempts to provide full support and care for those whose disease is beyond curative treatment.

Primary prevention may be tackled by removal of the agent (by closure of the plant or replacement of the agent by some other chemical) or the introduction of measures to reduce the exposure of workers by modifying the plant, modifying the environment, or protecting the worker. Obviously decisions about the appropriate course of action can only be taken where sound information exists. To plan primary prevention one requires information on the relative risk of the disease, and the costs and benefits that stem from interference. When considering prevention, relevant data may not be available to quantify these issues and further discussion will be required in order to clarify the situation with management, union representatives, and workers. Quite different levels of discussion are required when a plant is to be closed, in comparison with the introduction of some protective clothing for individual workers; different people have to make the decision and different people have to alter their way of life. In assisting with planning of prevention, therefore, one needs the best available data, which may have to be collected from *ad hoc* epidemiological studies. Often factual data will not be available on all aspects – and a computer simulation or modelling of the situation may be appropriate in order to spell out the options and the repercussions resulting from different decisions. Primary prevention may require central government action (such as banning artificial colouring or cyclamates) or may depend on individual action (e.g. reducing smoking or alcohol consumption).

Secondary prevention becomes relevant when it is thought that individuals are exposed to particular environmental factors that have put them at risk of chronic disease. It is assumed for the present discussion that early diagnosis is of benefit (the nihilistic view is that early diagnosis merely increases the time for which people are known to have disease but does not influence the actual risk of dying, nor automatically improve their quality of life). There are two rather different aspects to introducing early diagnosis. The first is planned screening of those at high risk of disease, and the second is more general programmes to reduce the delay to diagnosis in those developing the disease. The former can be introduced most appropriately where there is a clear division in the relative risk of different categories of individual to developing a disease.

It is generally accepted that for an appreciable proportion of patients attending for treatment for disease, there has been patient delay and, in certain circumstances, doctor delay. Only with an improved understanding of the factors that influence delay will it be possible to promulgate measures that may reduce this rather distressing aspect of malignant and other chronic disease.

Tertiary prevention can be developed on a pragmatic basis, but it also benefits from epidemiological studies. In particular these should identify the natural history of chronic diseases and quantify the social, psychological, and physical problems faced by patients and their families. It is suggested that the epidemiological approach is highly relevant to all three aspects of prevention since it can quantify the potential for intervention – an essential preliminary phase to planning and initiating action.

Intervention studies

Having selected the appropriate mechanism of prevention it is essential that a planned study is carried out so that the intervention can be assessed. This point has been clearly stressed by Cochrane (1972). In planning such a study, care and thought needs to go into the indentification of the individuals involved in the intervention study, the specific technique to be used to prevent further disease, and the most appropriate arrangements to assess the impact of these measures. The next step is to define the eligibility of the subjects for the study, and in some way randomize their allocation to 'treatment' and control groups (the expression 'treatment' can involve the exclusion of the postulated aetiological factor, the introduction of protective and barrier measures, or the introduction of early diagnosis). The individuals in both treatment and control groups then require careful follow-up with some form of objective assessment. It is desirable to have both subjects and observers unaware of whether the subjects are in the treatment or the control groups; in real life this is often difficult, and care is required to avoid bias. Bias from observation has already been mentioned, and reference is often made to the 'Hawthorne' effect which showed that workers' productivity could be influenced by both advantageous and deleterious changes in their working environment (when each change was associated with increase in productivity). An intervention study in industry will usually involve groups of individuals allocated to treatment and control categories; this requires careful cross-checking to see that both groups are comparable – apart from the planned intervention. It is worth noting that these studies come nearest to the design of 'scientific experiments', compared with observational studies for hypothesis generation and testing that have been discussed in earlier sections.

Where clear evidence of a hazard has been obtained and an agreed method for prevention proposed, it will be ethically objectionable to have a concurrent control group still exposed to the hazard (or using a less sound method of prevention). In such circumstances, data from 'historical controls' will have to be used, though this poses additional problems in interpretation of the results.

'DO-IT-YOURSELF' STUDIES

This section describes two approaches to hypothesis testing that can be relatively easily initiated using retrievable data. They are the kind of studies that individuals in occupational health can carry out with limited resources. They lead to a consideration of how occupational records might be re-organized in order to facilitate the study of hazards or to introduce 'early warning' systems.

Proportional mortality analysis

A relatively simple check of an issue can be carried out where records are available that identify the cause of death in a group of workers. Providing the material identifies each individual's sex, date of death, age at death, and cause of death the analysis can be carried out. The technique tests whether the proportion of deaths from the cause of interest is greater or less than one would expect in relation to deaths from all other causes. The expected figure is calculated by applying the death rates for the country as a whole to the distribution of actual deaths, taking age, sex and calendar period into account (it may also be possible to correct for regional variation or social class effect on mortality). The basic drawback on finding an excess proportion of deaths is that one does not know if the overall mortality from other causes is low, or if the actual death rate for the disease being studied is high. The approach can only be used as a pointer to further work, rather than as a definitive examination of a particular issue.

Prospective study on the cheap

Where there are available records of individuals' work history, with a complete file of data on mortality that has occurred amongst these individuals it should be possible to relate the data on the 'population at risk' to the identifiable outcome presented in the mortality statistics. The occupational records are used to identify each individual in the study, and it is essential to know the individual's date of birth (or age at starting work), date of entry to the occupation, some broad classification of occupational category or exposure, and follow-up status. The latest date known to be alive should be obtained for all individuals, which will include individuals still in the workforce or those retired but known to be drawing a pension. For those individuals who have left the industry it is important that they are traced and for each individual status obtained – either known to be alive or death identified. (These leavers are likely to be different in a number of ways from those staying in the industry; without follow-up information on them the statistics are likely to produce an incomplete or biased result.) For all the deaths that have occurred in the population the date of death and cause of death is required. This material can be manipulated in a standard fashion to generate 'person years at risk' which are tabulated by age and calendar period (they can also be cross-tabulated by level of exposure to the aetiological agent, duration of exposure to the aetiological agent, or latent interval). By applying national age, sex, and calendar period cause-specific mortality rates it is an easy task to calculate the expected numbers of death by cause. A comparison is then made between the number of observed and expected deaths for particular causes. This approach can be used to explore the risk of a specific cause of death, or to examine in more general terms the patterns of mortality of the workers.

Such a study can be carried out providing that the basic occupational records are available, up-to-date status is known for the vast majority of the individuals concerned, and for those that have died cause of death is available. The quality of the results will then depend predominantly on the detail and accuracy of the historical data identifying occupational and other characteristics of the workforce.

INTERROGATION OF A HISTORICAL DATA BASE

The previous section was suggesting the use of retrievable records as a probe of a specific issue. However, many industries are paying increasing attention to the practicality of carrying out such studies, and it is important to bear in mind the fact that the identification of the appropriate exposure in old occupational records can be a somewhat time consuming task. Where such records exist for a large workforce and contain details of chronological job histories, and the industry is relatively complex with exposure to various environmental and other factors, it is appropriate to consider the suitability of making these historical records more readily retrievable than they have been in the past. Conceptually this is in order to carry out the prospective studies on the cheap, but is advocated as a once-off exercise; this would avoid having to go back to the totality of manual records for every specific query raised in the future about the mortality of past employees.

In general, by having such a retrievable historical data base it should be a relatively simple matter to identify all those workers who had been employed in the past on a particular plant or process. Providing follow-up status is available and cause of death for those that have died, the observed and expected mortality should be quickly examined.

A rather different use of this material can be made where there is a need to cross-check on the past exposure of workers dying from a specific and relatively rare disease. If the historical file includes all mortality, it should be a simple matter to identify those individuals dying from the particular disease of interest (e.g. leukaemia), whilst a sample of control subjects can be obtained from the occupational data base. Using this material as a starting-point much more detailed enquiry could be made about the occupational histories of the small sample of subjects dying from leukaemia, and the controls. Such a specific enquiry might identify in considerable depth details of the individual's job history that it was not possible to abstract and include for all workers in the historical data base.

OCCUPATIONAL MONITORING SYSTEMS

An important issue to consider is whether industrial health records can be so organized that they can assist in the establishment of monitoring schemes to detect environmental hazards. There have been two recent reports from the World Health Organisation (1973, 1974) which have suggested that such systems should be established. These reports indicated the need to collect data on environment, the population classified by specific exposure to agents, and follow-up on the health of employees. In order to set up a monitoring system one requires an enlightened management, a labour force which appreciates the value of such an approach, and the availability of a sound industrial hygiene service. These elements are essential prerequisites, but then comes the need to collect, analyse, and interpret relevant data. It does not follow automatically that because more sophisticated data are being fed into a monitoring system that it will automatically provide valuable fresh leads. There are major statistical problems in the analysis and interpretation of such data; the more complex the material fed in (even assuming it is accurate and up-to-date) the greater is the difficulty in interpretation. This is because the number of separate analyses and the range of factors that have to be taken into account increase geometrically; with this increase in complexity of the data base there is always the difficulty of distinguishing between false leads (from random and biased errors in the data) and genuine positive findings of equal statistical significance. The greater the number of separate comparisions that are carried out, the greater the number that will be 'statistically significant' at any chosen level. It may be possible to identify fresh leads and distinguish them from the many false leads by replication and comparision of comparable sub-sets of data, perhaps taking into account the relationship between risk and dose, and time trends.

It is important to remember that relative risk, absolute risk, specificity of risk, number of people exposed, job stability, latent period, and the influence of confounding factors are important in determining whether hazards can be readily identified. In planning such systems consideration needs to be given to the availability of data, the feasibility of data collection, interpretation of the data, processes of decision-making on results from the system, costs and benefits, and confidentiality.

In the section dealing with prevention, reference was made to the need to monitor the impact of any new form of intervention. When a hazard appears to be adequately controlled it is still necessary to establish some surveillance system that continually checks on the number of individuals potentially exposed to the hazard and the generation of the specific disease in question.

REFERENCES

Alderson M. R. (1977) Epidemiological monitoring of indices of chemical hazard. In: Hunter W. J. and Smeets J. G. P. M. (ed.), *The Evaluation of Toxicological Data for the Protection of Public Health.* Oxford, Pergamon, pp. 161–169.

Bartlett F. C. (1932) *Remembering: A Study of Experimental and Social Psychology.* London, Cambridge University Press.

Cochrane A. L. (1972) *Effectiveness and Efficiency: Random Reflections on Health Services.* London, Nuffield Provincial Hospitals Trust.

Cook P. (1977) Personal communication.

Fox J. (1977) Occupational mortality: a new study. *Pop. Trends* **9**, 8–15.

Henry S. A. (1947) Occupational cutaneous cancer attributable to certain chemicals in industry. *Br. Med. Bull.* **4**, 389–401.

Morris J. N. (1975) *Uses of Epidemiology,* 3rd ed. Edinburgh, Churchill Livingstone.

Ødegard Ø. (1956) The incidence of psychoses in various occupations. *Int. J. Soc. Psychiatr.* **2**, 85–104.

Office of Population Censuses and Surveys (1973) *Cohort Studies: New Developments.* London, HMSO.

Pott P. (1775) *Chirurgical Observations.* London, Hawes Clarke and Collings.

Ryle J. A. (1948) *Changing Disciplines: Lectures on the History, Methods and Motives of Social Pathology.* London, Oxford University Press.

Schilling R. (1956) Byssinosis in cotton and other textile workers. *Lancet* **2**, 261–265.

World Health Organisation (1973) *Environmental and Health Monitoring in Occupational Health. WHO Tech. Rep. Ser.* No. 535.

World Health Organisation (1974) *WHO Environmental Health Monitoring Programme.* Report of a WHO Meeting, EHE/75. 1. Geneva, WHO.

RECOMMENDED FURTHER READING

Alderson M. R. (1974) *Central Government Routine Health Statistics.* London, Heinemann.

Alderson M. R. (1977) *An Introduction to Epidemiology.* London, Macmillan. (Note: this revised reprint contains an appendix with definitions.)

Alderson M. R. and Dowie R. (1978) *Health Statistics from Surveys and Special Inquiries.* Oxford, Pergamon.

Together these three texts discuss in greater detail many of the issues raised in this chapter; they provide a critical review of about 2 000 references covering national statistics, chronic disease epidemiology, and medical care studies.

Armitage P. (1971) *Statistical Methods in Medical Research.* Oxford, Blackwell.
A clearly written text that goes further than most non-mathematicians would wish; if it doesn't cover the point of concern to the reader it is long past time to call in the statistician.

Bourke G. J. and McGilvray J. (1975) *Interpretation and Uses of Medical Statistics,* 2nd ed. Oxford, Blackwell.
Deals with application of statistical method, with emphasis upon a basic approach; minimal use of algebra.

Cochrane A. L. (1972) *see* references above.
Clearly demonstrates the extension of randomized controlled trials to a wide range of topics in the medical care field.

Fisher Sir R. (1966) *The Design of Experiments,* 8th ed. Edinburgh, Oliver and Boyd.
Warrants a quick read to grasp some of the fundamentals of the study design.

Hill A. B. (1962) *Statistical Methods in Clinical and Preventive Medicine.* Edinburgh, Livingstone.
Collected papers which clearly unfold a major development in the application of clear thinking to the study design of clinical trials. Also includes some milestones in chronic disease epidemiology.

Morris J. N. (1975) *See* references above.
Stimulating – not a 'textbook', but to be read quickly at the week-end to pick up some fresh ideas.

Moser C. A. and Kalton G. (1971) *Survey Methods in Social Investigation.* London, Heinemann
A useful guide to surveys that can be adapted to issues relevant to occupational health.

QUICK REFERENCE LIST

This is a classification of epidemiological articles that have appeared in the past five years in the *Archives of Environmental Health, The British Journal of Industrial Medicine, The Journal of Occupational Medicine* and *The Journal of the Society of Occupational Medicine.* The aim of this is to indicate the different types of study that have been mounted, the industries or issues that have been explored, and the broad categories of data required. The selection of these articles is somewhat eclectic; reviews and position papers are not included, whilst the emphasis is on studies presenting fresh findings.

The Chapter describes the types of study and needs to be read in conjunction with the very brief notes in the Quick Reference List (QRL). In particular a distinction is drawn between studies using recorded data (even if they link information on population at risk to outcome, such as death, and are thus technically prospective) and *ad hoc* studies where data are specifically collected to illuminate a particular issue.

The entries in the QRL are numbered and have a cross reference number to the QRL key which provides an abbreviated reference for each article.

No.	Type of Study	Industry	Country	Categories of Data	Ref.
A1	Method	Cotton textile plant	US	Persons diagnosed as having byssinosis and controls: exposed to various aerosol extracts; respiratory function measured (to identify agent causing disease)	4
A2	Method	Hospital staff exposed to X-ray	US	Rubidium chloride (^{86}Rb) uptake (to develop test for exposure to X-rays)	2
A3	Method	Viscose factory	Yugoslavia	Administration of disulfiram and subsequent measurement of urinary diethyldithio-carbamates (to develop test for susceptibility to CS_2)	6
B1	Retrievable data: proportional registration/mortality analysis	Dockyards	England	Cancer registrations (expected registrations based on males in locality)	108
B2	Retrievable data: proportional registration/mortality analysis	Pesticide production – arsenic exposure	US	Cause of death of exposed/non-exposed	24

B3	Retrievable data: proportional registration/mortality analysis	Printing presses	US	Cause of death in union members (expected based on US white males)	176
B4	Retrievable data: proportional registration/mortality analysis	Stationary engineers and firemen	US	Cause of death in union members (expected based on US)	181
B5	Retrievable data: proportional registration/mortality analysis	Talc mining and milling	US	Cause of death. Occupational records of environmental measurement (expected proportions from US male mortality)	142
C1	Retrievable data: cross-sectional	Agriculture	E & W	Analysis official records of pesticide poisoning	66
C2	Retrievable data: cross-sectional	Coal mining countries	US	Compared mortality for stomach cancer in coal mining and control counties	19
C3	Retrievable data: cross-sectional	Dynamite factory	US	Identified deaths in local registers for cardio-cerebrovascular deaths and controls. Checked factory records for occupations of decedents	180
C4	Retrievable data: cross-sectional	Hairdressers – apprentices	UK	Reported prevalence of shampoo dermatitis, from all dermatologists	189
C5	Retrievable data: cross-sectional	Manual workers	England	Cause of sickness absence. Occupational records of length service	55
C6	Retrievable data: cross-sectional	Plastics factory	England	Morbidity statistics of dermatitis. Occupational records of products	197
C7	Retrievable data: cross-sectional	Post Office workers	UK	Sickness absence statistics	112
C8	Retrievable data: cross-sectional	Poultry industry	US	Routine records of skin injuries and lesions, and individuals jobs	138
C9	Retrievable data: cross-sectional	Rubber workers	US	Cause of death. Occupational records of decedents and controls	158
C10	Retrievable data: cross-sectional	Steelworkers	England	History; examination; audiometry	193
C11	Retrievable data: cross-sectional	Textile workers	E & W	Detailed analysis of occupational mortality statistics	86
C12	Retrievable data: cross-sectional	Welding in heavy engineering	England	Reported sickness by diagnosis and occupation	192

No.	Type of Study	Industry	Country	Categories of Data	Ref.
C13	Retrievable data: cross-sectional	All employed	Ireland	National statistics sickness absence: claims by cause, sex, calendar period	187
C14	Retrievable data: cross-sectional	Dermatology patients	England	Patients attending dermatologist: diagnosis; work history	198
C15	Retrievable data: cross-sectional	Mesothelioma patients	UK	National Register of patients with mesothelioma, from multiple sources; work history	79
D1	Retrievable data: prospective	Asbestos manfr.	England	History; X-ray; respiratory function; assessed disability; recorded work environment	188
D2	Retrievable data: prospective	Asbestos manfr.	US	Person years at risk; cause of death; recorded measurements of environment	58
D3	Retrievable data: prospective	Asbestos industry	US	Person years at risk; cause of death; work history and measurement of environment	16
D4	Retrievable data: prospective	Asbestos mines and mills	Canada	Person years at risk; cause of death; X-ray; recorded measurement of environment	20
D5	Retrievable data: prospective	Asbestos textile factory	England	Person years at risk; cause of death (expected deaths based on national mortality)	123
D6	Retrievable data: prospective	Asbestos plant	US	Person years at risk; cause of death; work history	183
D7	Retrievable data: prospective	Atomic bomb survivors	Japan	Occupational records of sickness and other absences in exposed and controls	98
D8	Retrievable data: prospective	Chemical plant – chloromethyl methyl ether exposure	US	Person years at risk; cause of death	40

I

D9	Retrievable data: prospective	Chemical plant; dichlorobenzidine exposure	US	Person years at risk; cause of death; records of plant environment	141
D10	Retrievable data: prospective	Chloromethyl ether production	US	Person years at risk; cause of death; occupational records of exposure	184
D11	Retrievable data: prospective	Chrome pigment manfr.	Norway	Person years at risk; cancer registration; recorded measurement of environment (chrome)	94
D12	Retrievable data: prospective	Coal mines	E & W	Cause of sickness absence; regular X-ray; recorded work environment	50
D13	Retrievable data: prospective	Coal mines	E & W	Cause of death; recorded work environment	51
D14	Retrievable data: prospective	Coal mines	US	Person years at risk; cause of death (expected deaths based on white male mortality rates for State)	15
D15	Retrievable data: prospective	Coke-ovens	Wales	Person years at risk; cause of death (expected based on national mortality)	130
D16	Retrievable data: prospective	Compressed air workers	US	X-ray. Recorded work history and measurement of environment	152
D17	Retrievable data: prospective	Construction industry – whole body vibration	US	Sickness absence records by cause; recorded work history	42
D18	Retrievable data: prospective	Cotton mills	US	Person years at risk; cause of death	136
D19	Retrievable data: prospective	Dye industry	Japan	Register of industrial bladder cancers; recorded work history	99
D20	Retrievable data: prospective	Fertilizer factory	Poland	History; cause of sickness absence	114
D21	Retrievable data: prospective	Fibrous glass insulation manfr.	US	Person years at risk; cause of medical retirement; cause of death	30
D22	Retrievable data: prospective	Lead workers	E & W	Cause of sickness absence; blood lead levels; recorded environmental exposure	113
D23	Retrievable data: prospective	Manual workers (recruits)	England	Initial medical records; cause of sickness absence	54
D24	Retrievable data: prospective	Nickel refinery	Wales	Person years at risk; cause of death; recorded work history	119

No.	Type of Study	Industry	Country	Categories of Data	Ref.
D25	Retrievable data: prospective	Pesticide production – arsenic exposure	US	Person years at risk; cause of death	25
D26	Retrievable data: prospective	Petro chemicals	Europe	Estimated person years at risk; recorded deaths from leukaemia; recorded benzene exposure	143
D27	Retrievable data: prospective	Petro chemicals and refinery	England	Recorded sickness absence before and after alteration in shift system	122
D28	Retrievable data: prospective	Plant, laboratory and office staff	US	Screening medical; population at risk; cause of death (expected deaths based on US white male mortality)	154
D29	Retrievable data: prospective	Potash miners and millers	US	Person years at risk; cause of death; recorded work history	134
D30	Retrievable data: prospective	Rubber manfr. – ethylene thiourea exposure	England	All employees: linked to cancer register to check thyroid cancers	201
D31	Retrievable data: prospective	Rubber manfr. – ethylene thiourea exposure	England	Women leavers: identification linked to local birth registers to identify congenital abnormalities	202
D32	Retrievable data: prospective	Rubber tyre manfr.	US	Person years at risk; cause of death; recorded work history	146
D33	Retrievable data: prospective	Rubber and cable manfr.	UK	Person years at risk; cause of death; recorded work history	115
D34	Retrievable data: prospective	Rubber and cable manfr.	UK	Person years at risk; cause of death	82
D35	Retrievable data: prospective	Ship's crews	GB	Recorded sickness absence	104
D36	Retrievable data: prospective	Steel works	US	Person years at risk; cause of death; recorded work history (expected based on other workers not in specific sub-group)	155
D37	Retrievable data: prospective	Steelworks masons	US	Person years at risk; cause of death (expected based on other steelworkers)	161

D38	Retrievable data: prospective	Steelworks pensioners	US	Person years at risk; cause of death (expected other steelworkers; US male)	162
D39	Retrievable data: prospective	Talc miners and millers	Italy	Cause of death; occupational records of decedents and environmental monitoring	159
D40	Retrievable data: prospective	Telegraphists	Australia	Recorded sickness absence	60
D41	Retrievable data: prospective	Tetraethyl lead workers	US	Person years at risk; examination at intervals; cause of sickness absence; recorded work history and measurement of environment	157
D42	Retrievable data: prospective	Vinyl chloride plants	US	Person years at risk; cause of death; recorded work history and subjective exposure	148
D43	Retrievable data: prospective	Vinyl chloride plants	US	Person years at risk; cause of death; recorded measurement of environment	34
D44	Retrievable data: prospective	Vinyl chloride plants	GB	Person years at risk; cause of death; recorded work history and estimated exposure (expected deaths based on E & W mortality)	116
D45	Retrievable data: prospective	Vinylidene plant	US	Annual medical examination; cause of death; environmental monitoring	168
D46	Retrievable data: prospective	Psychiatric patients – rehabilitation	England	Pts. discharged from psychiatric hospitals; subsequent work history from occupational records	46
E1	Cross-sectional	Aluminium pot room	US	History; examination; respiratory function; subjective assessment of work environment	160
E2	Cross-sectional	Asbestos plant	Singapore	History, examination, X-ray, respiratory function	7
E3	Cross-sectional	Battery plant	US	History; examination; hormone excretion; semen analysis; lead in blood and urine to identify 'exposure'	35

No.	Type of Study	Industry	Country	Categories of Data	Ref.
E4	Cross-sectional	Cement and/or asbestos exposure	Italy	History, examination; X-ray; respiratory function	33
E5	Cross-sectional	Cement workers	Yugoslavia	History; examination; X-ray; respiratory function	3
E6	Cross-sectional	Cement workers	Yugoslavia	History; respiratory function	23
E7	Cross-sectional	Chemical workers, farmers, firemen, physicians	Canada	History; examination; respiratory function	22
E8	Cross-sectional	Coal miners	US	History; X-ray chest; respiratory function	139
E9	Cross-sectional	Coir processing factory	Sri Lanka	History; examination; X-ray	95
E10	Cross-sectional	Cotton textile mills	US	History; respiratory function	5
E11	Cross-sectional	Cotton textile mills	US	History; respiratory function; environmental dust measurements	133
E12	Cross-sectional	Electroplating	Egypt	History; examination; haematology; measurement of environment (cyanide)	100
E13	Cross-sectional	Farmers	England	History; serology	67
E14	Cross-sectional	Farmers	E & W	History; respiratory function; serology	101
E15	Cross-sectional	Farmers	Scotland	Serology; microbiology of air samples from byres	126
E16	Cross-sectional	Ferro-alloy production – manganese exposure	Yugoslavia	History; neurological examination; measured environment	120
E17	Cross-sectional	Firefighters	US	History; carboxyhaemoglobin	149
E18	Cross-sectional	Firefighters	US	History; blood gases	164
E19	Cross-sectional	Flax processing	Egypt	History; respiratory function; measurement of environment (dust)	97
E20	Cross-sectional	Grain elevators	US	History; examination; skin testing and serology; respiratory function	11
E21	Cross-sectional	Hardrock miners	Canada	X-rays – repeat readings	118

E22	Cross-sectional	Highway workers	US	History; examination; blood CO and lead; respiratory function; measurement of environment	13
E23	Cross-sectional	'Industrial concern'	US	Patients referred for assessment: psychiatric problem and its effect on functioning; physical health; source of referral	179
E24	Cross-sectional	Kapoc ginning	Sri Lanka	History; examination; respiratory function; allergy testing	125
E25	Cross-sectional	Laboratory technicians: mercury exposure	Belgium	History; clinical chemistry; measurement of environment	10
E26	Cross-sectional	Lumberjacks	Finland	History; examination; X-ray	56
E27	Cross-sectional	Lumberjacks	Finland	History; X-ray hands	150
E28	Cross-sectional	Lumberjacks	Finland	Examination; thenar muscle blood flow; bone mineral content	92
E29	Cross-sectional	Maltings	Scotland	Questionnaire; serology; mycological survey in environment	76
E30	Cross-sectional	Meat packers	US	History; respiratory function	32
E31	Cross-sectional	Mercury exposure (various)	England	History; urinary excretion analysis	70
E32	Cross-sectional	Offices	US	History; perceived stress; examination	172
E33	Cross-sectional	Polyurethane manufacture – toluene diisocyanate exposure	US	History; respiratory function; measurement of environment	140
E34	Cross-sectional	Potash mine	Canada	Examination	144
E35	Cross-sectional	Rock drillers	US	History; examination; serum immunoglobulins	153
E36	Cross-sectional	Rubber factory – dust exposure	US	History; examination; X-ray; respiratory function; measurement of environment	41
E37	Cross-sectional	Rubber factory – talc exposure	US	History; examination; X-ray; respiratory function; measurement of environment	44

No.	Type of Study	Industry	Country	Categories of Data	Ref.
E38	Cross-sectional	Rubber/plastic industry styrene exposure	Netherlands	Urinary mandelic acid; measurement plant environment	74
E39	Cross-sectional	Scientific glassware manufacture	US	History; examination; clinical chemistry; environmental assay mercury	132
E40	Cross-sectional	Sea divers	North Sea	History; examination; respiratory function; recorded work history	117
E41	Cross-sectional	Shipbreakers yard	Sweden	History; renal function; renal biopsy; clinical chemistry	81
E42	Cross-sectional	Shipyard welders	US	History; respiratory function; X-ray; measurement of environment	1
E43	Cross-sectional	Steel bronzing – arsenic exposure	England	Arsenic assayed in hair and nails of workers; environmental measurement of arsenic	205
E44	Cross-sectional	Telegraphists	Australia	History; examination; recorded sickness absence	61
E45	Cross-sectional	Textile mills	Yugoslavia	History; respiratory function	102
E46	Cross-sectional	Vets	N. Ireland	History of brucellosis symptoms	73
E47	Cross-sectional	Vinyl chloride plant	E & W	History; examination; liver function; liver biopsy	121
E48	Cross-sectional	Weavers	Iran	History; examination; BP; noise level at work	167
F1	Cross-sectional + retrospective work history	Biology laboratory	US	History; tests with allergens; work history; measurement of environment	147
F2	Cross-sectional + retrospective work history	Cadmium workers	Belgium	Serum cadmium and lead analysis; work history	71
F3	Cross-sectional + retrospective work history	Coal mines	US	History; examination; X-ray; respiratory function; work history	105
F4	Cross-sectional + retrospective work history	Coal mines	US	History; X-ray; respiratory function; work history	47
F5	Cross-sectional + retrospective work history	DDT production	US	History; liver function tests; serum DDT levels; work history	17

F6	Cross-sectional + retrospective work history	Drop forge – hammermen and helpers	US	History; examination; audiometry; length of work history	174
F7	Cross-sectional + retrospective work history	Electrical industry – exposure to a poly-chlorinated biphenyl	Australia	History; examination; clinical chemistry; work history	43
F8	Cross-sectional + retrospective work history	Filter manfr. – phenolic resin exposure	US	History; respiratory function; work history; measurement of environment	36
F9	Cross-sectional + retrospective work history	Foundry workers	Yugoslavia	History; examination; respiratory function; work history	26
F10	Cross-sectional + retrospective work history	Furniture factory – exposure to western red cedar dust	Japan	History; examination; resp. function; skin test with allergens; work history	135
F11	Cross-sectional + retrospective work history	Garage workers	Denmark	History; examination; clinical chemistry; measurement of environment	129
F12	Cross-sectional + retrospective work history	Granite sheds	US	History; respiratory function; work history; measurement of environment	18
F13	Cross-sectional + retrospective work history	Lead additives in lubricants	Belgium	Blood and urine lead assays; work histories	87
F14	Cross-sectional + retrospective work history	Lead smelter	US	History; examination (esp. for lead effects); biochemistry or blood haematology; nerve conductivity; Zn/P6 levels	48
F15	Cross-sectional + retrospective work history	Monumental masons	Scotland	X-ray; work history; measurement of environment	64
F16	Cross-sectional + retrospective work history	Perlite miners and processors	US	History; examination; X-ray; respiratory function; work history	166
F17	Cross-sectional + retrospective work history	Pesticide handlers – organophosphate exposure	US	History; psychological testing; cholinesterase measurement; work history	29
F18	Cross-sectional + retrospective work history	Policemen	US	History; respiratory function; immunological assessment; lead in hair; work history	8
F19	Cross-sectional + retrospective work history	Rubber factory – tyre curing	US	History; examination; work history; measurement of environment	38

No.	Type of Study	Industry	Country	Categories of Data	Ref.
F20	Cross-sectional + retrospective work history	Rubber industry	US	History; respiratory function; work history	163
F21	Cross-sectional + retrospective work history	Shoe-makers	Italy	History; examination; motor conductivity; work history	107
F22	Cross-sectional + retrospective work history	Smelter	US	History; examination; blood lead; nerve conductivity; work history	177
F23	Cross-sectional + retrospective work history	Steelworks	Wales	History ear disease; audiometry; history noise exposure	200
F24	Cross-sectional + retrospective work history	Vinyl chloride and other chemical works	US	History; examination; respiratory function; work history	165
F25	Cross-sectional + retrospective work history	Viscose factory – carbon disulphide exposure	Italy	History; examination; ophthalmoscopy and electromyography; clinical chemistry; work history	27
F26	Cross-sectional + retrospective work history	Wall-board production	US	History; examination; respiratory function; work history	12
F27	Cross-sectional + retrospective work history	Autopsy series	England	Prevalence of asbestos bodies at autopsy; recorded job history and address in clinical notes	93
G1	Cross-sectional with retrievable data	Activated-carbon production	US	History; X-ray; respiratory function; occupational records used for subjective assessment of exposure	37
G2	Cross-sectional with retrievable data	Rayon plants – CS_2 exposure	US	History; examination; ECG; cholesterol; occupational records of plant environment	145
H1	Retrospective	Asbestos exposure	Australia	Work history for deaths from mesothelioma	109
H2	Retrospective	Bladder cancer patients + case-control	England	Work history	191
H3	Retrospective	Bladder cancer deaths	England	Work history from next-of-kin	78
H4	Retrospective	Cancer patients	US	Routine occupational histories contrasted	169

H5	Retrospective	Cancer patients	US	Occupational histories; expected from census data	170
H6	Retrospective	Dermatitis patients	England	Diagnosis made by patch testing; retrospective enquiry for occupation involved and source of epoxy resin	196
H7	Retrospective	Flax workers	Egypt	History; examination	103
H8	Retrospective	Nasal cancer patients	Denmark	Occupational history	128
H9	Retrospective	Psychiatric patients	England	Psychological questionnaire to cases and controls	199
H10	Retrospective	Medical officers in industry	UK	Questionnaire; personal details; medical career; present post	194
I1	Prospective	Aluminium smelter	US	History; urine chemistry twice yearly; plant history and environmental monitoring	156
I2	Prospective	Asbestos mines	Finland	History; cause of death; work history	80
I3	Prospective	Asbestos cement manfr.	US	History; X-ray; respiratory function; occupational records of dust exposure	28
I4	Prospective	Battery manfr.	England	History; examination; blood and urine estimates of lead levels repeated frequently	185
I5	Prospective	Battery manfr.	Finland	History; examination; blood and urinary lead etc.; measurement of environment	57
I6	Prospective	Battery manfr. – lead exposure	Finland	History; periodic lead and other urine measurements, nerve conduction velocity	31
I7	Prospective	Battery manfr. and lead foundry	Italy	History; examination; blood and urine lead levels; chromosome analyses; measurement of environment	39
I8	Prospective	Benzidine production	US	History; cytoscopy and cytology; cause of death; measurement of environment	9

No.	Type of Study	Industry	Country	Categories of Data	Ref.
I9	Prospective	Cement works	Yugoslavia	History; respiratory function	106
I10	Prospective	Chemical industry	Japan	Urinary metabolite analyses; measurement of environment	69
I11	Prospective	Chloromethyl ether chemical plant	US	History including smoking; examination; respiratory function; description of plant history	178
I12	Prospective	Coal mines	US	History; X-ray; respiratory function; measurement of environment	14
I13	Prospective	Coal mines	GB	History; examination; X-ray; respiratory function; measurement of environment	63
I14	Prospective	Coal miners with pneumoconiosis	Wales	History; X-ray; respiratory function; morbid anatomy at autopsy	77
I15	Prospective	Coal mines	UK	X-ray at regular intervals; recorded work history	83
I16	Prospective	Coal mines	Wales	History; examination; X-ray; cause of death	84
I17	Prospective	Cotton mills	England	History; respiratory function; measurement of environment	52
I18	Prospective	Cotton mills	England	History; respiratory function; measurement of environment	53
I19	Prospective	Cotton mills	England	History; questionnaire on respiratory symptoms; work history; measurement of environment	75
I20	Prospective	Cotton ginnery workers	Sudan	History; respiratory function; measurement of environment	111
I21	Prospective	Detergent manfr.	Australia	History; examination; respiratory function; allergen tests; work history	110
I22	Prospective	Detergent manfr.	England	History; examination; respiratory function; allergen testing; measurement of environment	203

I23	Prospective	Epoxy resin exposure	US	History; respiratory function; measurement of environment	45
I24	Prospective	Farmers	Canada	History; cardiorespiratory function; work history	137
I25	Prospective	Fibre glass manfr.	England	History; X-ray; respiratory function; measurement of environment	59
I26	Prospective	Insecticide manfr.	Netherlands	History; examination; clinical chemistry; recorded plant history	62
I27	Prospective	Insecticide manfr.	Switzerland	History; examination; clinical chemistry; measurement of environment	21
I28	Prospective	Insulation workers	N. Ireland	History; examination at regular intervals; person years at risk; cause of death; (expected deaths based on national mortality)	41
I29	Prospective	Metallurgical Plant	US	History; X-ray; respiratory function; lung biopsy	46
I30	Prospective	Microwave and laser operators	US	History; opthalmic examination at regular intervals; work history	182
I31	Prospective	Polyurethane manfr.	US	History; respiratory function; measurement of environment	127
I32	Prospective	Rayon industry	Egypt	History; clinical chemistry; records of plant environment	68
I33	Prospective	Rubber plant	US	History of smoking; reason for medical retirement; work history	173
I34	Prospective	Telephone co.	US	Pre-employment medicals; subsequent work attendance and job performance	171
I35	Prospective	Textile mills using synthetic fibre	US	History; respiratory function; work history (esp. no prev. exp./exp. cotton/exp. hemp)	49
I36	Prospective	Toluene diisocyanate manfr.	England	History; examination; respiratory function; measurement of environment	96

No.	Type of Study	Industry	Country	Categories of Data	Ref.
I37	Prospective	Uranium mill	US	Screening medical; cause of death	131
I38	Prospective	Viscose rayon/manfr.	Finland	History; examination; ECG; incidence of fatality from IHD; measurement of environment (CS_2)	91
I39	Prospective	Patients having herniorrhaphy	England	History; hernia operation details; subsequent sickness absence; work history	186
J1	Experiment	Orange pickers	US	Clinical chemistry on blood and urine; application of different levels of parathion, with monitored exposure	175
K1	Intervention	Cotton mills	US	History; respiratory function	65
K2	Intervention	Cotton spinning plant	US	History; examination; respiratory function; measurement of plant dust	85
K3	Intervention	Cotton mill	US	History; respiratory function	88
K4	Intervention	Engineering plant – noise exposure	US	History; examination; audiometry at intervals; measurement of environment	151
K5	Intervention	Flax mills	Yugoslavia	History; respiratory function	72
K6	Intervention	Toluene exposure	Switzerland	Respiratory excretion toluene before and after	90
K7	Intervention	Steelworks – manual staff	Enland	Sickness absence before and after vaccination	190
K8	Intervention	Flu vaccine – in volunteers	England	Sickness absence before and after vaccine in volunteers	89
K9	Intervention	Industrial workers – cold prevention	England	Compliance; subsequent colds assessed	195

QUICK REFERENCE LIST KEY

No.	Reference				First author	List No.
1	*Arch. Environ. Health*	(1973)	**26,**	28 – 31	Peters J. M. et al.	E42
2	*Arch. Environ. Health*	(1973)	**26,**	64 – 66	Scott K. G. et al.	A2
3	*Arch. Environ. Health*	(1973)	**26,**	78 – 85	Kalacic I.	E5
4	*Arch. Environ. Health*	(1973)	**26,**	120 – 124	Hamilton J. D. et al.	A1
5	*Arch. Environ. Health*	(1973)	**26,**	183 – 191	Imbus H. R. et al.	E10
6	*Arch. Environ. Health*	(1973)	**26,**	287 – 289	Djuric D. et al.	A3
7	*Arch. Environ. Health*	(1973)	**26,**	290 – 293	Chew P. K. et al.	E2
8	*Arch. Environ. Health*	(1973)	**26,**	313 – 324	Speizer F. E. et al.	F18
9	*Arch. Environ. Health*	(1973)	**27,**	1 – 7	Zavon M. R.	I8
10	*Arch. Environ. Health*	(1973)	**27,**	65 – 68	Lauwerys R. R. et al.	E25
11	*Arch. Environ. Health*	(1973)	**27,**	74 – 77	Tse K. S. et al.	E20
12	*Arch. Environ. Health*	(1973)	**27,**	105 – 109	Wegman D. H. et al.	F26
13	*Arch. Environ. Health*	(1973)	**27,**	168 – 178	Ayres S. M. et al.	E22
14	*Arch. Environ. Health*	(1973)	**27,**	221 – 226	Morgan W. K. C. et al.	I12
15	*Arch. Environ. Health*	(1973)	**27,**	227 – 230	Ortmeyer C. E. et al.	D14
16	*Arch. Environ. Health*	(1973)	**27,**	312 – 317	Enterline P. E. et al.	D3
17	*Arch. Environ. Health*	(1973)	**27,**	318 – 321	Laws E. R. et al.	F5
18	*Arch. Environ. Health*	(1974)	**28,**	18 – 27	Theriault G. P. et al.	F12
19	*Arch. Environ. Health*	(1974)	**28,**	28 – 30	Creagan E. T. et al.	C2
20	*Arch. Environ. Health*	(1974)	**28,**	61 – 68	McDonald J. C. et al.	D4
21	*Arch. Environ. Health*	(1974)	**28,**	72 – 76	Menz M. et al.	I27
22	*Arch. Environ. Health*	(1974)	**29,**	143 – 146	Lefcoe N. M. et al.	E7
23	*Arch. Environ. Health*	(1974)	**29,**	147 – 149	Kalacic I.	E6
24	*Arch. Environ. Health*	(1974)	**29,**	250 – 255	Ott M. G. et al.	B2
25	*Arch. Environ. Health*	(1974)	**29,**	250 – 255	Ott M. G. et al.	D25
26	*Arch. Environ. Health*	(1974)	**29,**	261 – 267	Mikov M. I.	F9
27	*Arch. Environ. Health*	(1975)	**30,**	85 – 87	Cavalleri A.	F25
28	*Arch. Environ. Health*	(1975)	**30,**	88 – 97	Weill H. et al.	I3
29	*Arch. Environ. Health*	(1975)	**30,**	98 – 103	Rodnitzky R. L. et al.	F17
30	*Arch. Environ. Health*	(1975)	**30,**	113 – 116	Enterline P. E. et al.	D21
31	*Arch. Environ. Health*	(1975)	**30,**	180 – 183	Seppalainen A. M. et al.	I6
32	*Arch. Environ. Health*	(1975)	**30,**	269 – 271	Polakoff P. L. et al.	E30
33	*Arch. Environ. Health*	(1975)	**30,**	272 – 275	Scansetti G. et al.	E4
34	*Arch. Environ. Health*	(1975)	**30,**	333 – 339	Ott M. G. et al.	D43
35	*Arch. Environ. Health*	(1975)	**30,**	396 – 401	Lancranjan I. et al.	E3
36	*Arch. Environ. Health*	(1975)	**30,**	574 – 577	Schoenberg J. B. et al.	F8
37	*Arch. Environ. Health*	(1975)	**30,**	578 – 582	Wehr K. L. et al.	G1
38	*Arch. Environ. Health*	(1976)	**31,**	1 – 5	Fine L. J. et al.	F19
39	*Arch. Environ. Health*	(1976)	**31,**	73 – 78	Forni A. et al.	I7
40	*Arch. Environ. Health*	(1976)	**31,**	125 – 130	De Fonso L. R. et al.	D8
41	*Arch. Environ. Health*	(1976)	**31,**	136 – 140	Fine L. J. et al.	E36
42	*Arch. Environ. Health*	(1976)	**31,**	141 – 145	Spear R. C. et al.	D17
43	*Arch. Environ. Health*	(1976)	**31,**	189 – 194	Ouw H. K. et al.	F7
44	*Arch. Environ. Health*	(1976)	**31,**	195 – 200	Fine L. J. et al.	E37
45	*Arch. Environ. Health*	(1976)	**31,**	236 – 240	Sargent E. V. et al.	I23
46	*Arch. Environ. Health*	(1977)	**32,**	62 – 68	Vitums V. C. et al.	I29
47	*Arch. Environ. Health*	(1977)	**32,**	211 – 215	Fairman R. P. et al.	F4
48	*Arch. Environ. Health*	(1977)	**32,**	256 – 266	Lilis R. et al.	F14
49	*Arch. Environ. Health*	(1977)	**32,**	283 – 287	Valic F. et al.	I35

No.	Reference				First author	List No.
50	*Br. J. Ind. Med.*	(1973)	**30,**	1 – 14	Liddell F. D. K.	D12
51	*Br. J. Ind. Med.*	(1973)	**30,**	15 – 24	Liddell F. D. K.	D13
52	*Br. J. Ind. Med.*	(1973)	**30,**	25 – 36	Berry G. et al.	I17
53	*Br. J. Ind. Med.*	(1973)	**30,**	42 – 53	Fox A. J. et al.	I18
54	*Br. J. Ind. Med.*	(1973)	**30,**	64 – 70	Pocock S. J.	D23
55	*Br. J. Ind. Med.*	(1973)	**30,**	64 – 70	Pocock S. J.	C5
56	*Br. J. Ind. Med.*	(1973)	**30,**	71 – 73	Kumlin T. et al.	E26
57	*Br. J. Ind. Med.*	(1973)	**30,**	134 – 141	Tola S. et al.	I5
58	*Br. J. Ind. Med.*	(1973)	**30,**	162 – 166	Enterline P. et al.	D2
59	*Br. J. Ind. Med.*	(1973)	**30,**	174 – 179	Hill J. W. et al.	I25
60	*Br. J. Ind. Med.*	(1973)	**30,**	187 – 198	Ferguson D.	D40
61	*Br. J. Ind. Med.*	(1973)	**30,**	187 – 198	Ferguson D.	E44
62	*Br. J. Ind. Med.*	(1973)	**30,**	201 – 202	Versteeg J. P. T. et al.	I26
63	*Br. J. Ind. Med.*	(1973)	**30,**	217 – 226	Rogan J. M. et al.	I13
64	*Br. J. Ind. Med.*	(1973)	**30,**	227 – 231	Lloyd Davies T. A. et al.	F15
65	*Br. J. Ind. Med.*	(1973)	**30,**	237 – 247	Merchant J. A. et al.	K1
66	*Br. J. Ind. Med.*	(1973)	**30,**	253 – 258	Hearn C. E. D.	C1
67	*Br. J. Ind. Med.*	(1973)	**30,**	259 – 265	Morgan D. C. et al.	E13
68	*Br. J. Ind. Med.*	(1973)	**30,**	284 – 288	El Gazzar R. et al.	I32
69	*Br. J. Ind. Med.*	(1973)	**30,**	289 – 292	Imamura T. et al.	I10
70	*Br. J. Ind. Med.*	(1973)	**30,**	293 – 296	Taylor A. et al.	E31
71	*Br. J. Ind. Med.*	(1973)	**30,**	359 – 364	Lauwerys R. R. et al.	F2
72	*Br. J. Ind. Med.*	(1973)	**30,**	381 – 384	Valic F. et al.	K5
73	*Br. J. Ind. Med.*	(1973)	**30,**	385 – 389	McDevitt D. G.	E46
74	*Br. J. Ind. Med.*	(1973)	**30,**	390 – 393	Slob A.	E38
75	*Br. J. Ind. Med.*	(1974)	**31,**	18 – 27	Berry G. et al.	I19
76	*Br. J. Ind. Med.*	(1974)	**31,**	31 – 35	Riddle H. F. V.	E29
77	*Br. J. Ind. Med.*	(1974)	**31,**	36 – 44	Lyons J. P. et al.	I14
78	*Br. J. Ind. Med.*	(1974)	**31,**	65 – 71	Veys C. A.	H3
79	*Br. J. Ind. Med.*	(1974)	**31,**	91 – 104	Greenberg M. et al.	C15
80	*Br. J. Ind. Med.*	(1974)	**31,**	105 – 112	Meurman L. O. et al.	I2
81	*Br. J. Ind. Med.*	(1974)	**31,**	113 – 127	Cramer K. et al.	E41
82	*Br. J. Ind. Med.*	(1974)	**31,**	140 – 151	Fox A. J. et al.	D34
83	*Br. J. Ind. Med.*	(1974)	**31,**	185 – 195	Liddell F. D. K.	I15
84	*Br. J. Ind. Med.*	(1974)	**31,**	196 – 200	Waters W. E. et al.	I16
85	*Br. J. Ind. Med.*	(1974)	**31,**	209 – 219	Imbus H. R. et al.	K2
86	*Br. J. Ind. Med.*	(1974)	**31,**	224 – 232	Moss E. et al.	C11
87	*Br. J. Ind. Med.*	(1974)	**31,**	233 – 238	Van Peteghem J. et al.	F13
88	*Br. J. Ind. Med.*	(1974)	**31,**	261 – 274	Merchant J. A. et al.	K3
89	*Br. J. Ind. Med.*	(1974)	**31,**	292 – 297	Smith J. W. G. et al.	K8
90	*Br. J. Ind. Med.*	(1974)	**31,**	310 – 316	Guillemin M. et al.	K6
91	*Br. J. Ind. Med.*	(1975)	**32,**	1 – 10	Talonen M. et al.	I38
92	*Br. J. Ind. Med.*	(1975)	**32,**	11 – 15	Karjalainen P. et al.	E28
93	*Br. J. Ind. Med.*	(1975)	**32,**	16 – 30	Doniach I. et al.	F27
94	*Br. J. Ind. Med.*	(1975)	**32,**	62 – 65	Langard S. et al.	D11
95	*Br. J. Ind. Med.*	(1975)	**32,**	66 – 71	Uragoda C. G	E9
96	*Br. J. Ind. Med.*	(1975)	**32,**	72 – 78	Adams W. G. F.	I36
97	*Br. J. Ind. Med.*	(1975)	**32,**	147 – 154	Noweir M. H.	E19
98	*Br. J. Ind. Med.*	(1975)	**32,**	193 – 202	Meigs J. W.	D7
99	*Br. J. Ind. Med.*	(1975)	**32,**	203 – 209	Tsuchiya K. et al.	D19
100	*Br. J. Ind. Med.*	(1975)	**32,**	215 – 219	El Ghawabi S. H.	E12
101	*Br. J. Ind. Med.*	(1975)	**32,**	228 – 234	Morgan D. C. et al.	E14

No.	Reference				First author	List No.
102	*Br. J. Ind. Med.*	(1975)	**32,**	283 – 288	Zuskin E. et al.	E45
103	*Br. J. Ind. Med.*	(1975)	**32,**	297 – 301	Noweir M. H. et al.	H7
104	*Br. J. Ind. Med.*	(1976)	**33,**	9 – 12	Carter J. T.	D35
105	*Br. J. Ind. Med.*	(1976)	**33,**	13 – 17	Amandus H. E. et al.	F3
106	*Br. J. Ind. Med.*	(1976)	**33,**	18 – 24	Saric M. et al.	I9
107	*Br. J. Ind. Med.*	(1976)	**33,**	92 – 99	Abbritti G. et al.	F21
108	*Br. J. Ind. Med.*	(1976)	**33,**	108 – 114	Lumley K. P. S.	B1
109	*Br. J. Ind. Med.*	(1976)	**33,**	115 – 122	Milne J. E. H.	H1
110	*Br. J. Ind. Med.*	(1976)	**33,**	158 – 165	Musk A. W. et al.	I21
111	*Br. J. Ind. Med.*	(1976)	**33,**	166 – 174	Khogali M.	I20
112	*Br. J. Ind. Med.*	(1976)	**33,**	230 – 235	Taylor P. J.	C7
113	*Br. J. Ind. Med.*	(1976)	**33,**	236 – 242	Shannon H. S. et al.	D22
114	*Br. J. Ind. Med.*	(1976)	**33,**	243 – 248	Jedrychowski W.	D20
115	*Br. J. Ind. Med.*	(1976)	**33,**	249 – 264	Fox A. J. et al.	D33
116	*Br. J. Ind. Med.*	(1977)	**34,**	1 – 10	Fox A. J. et al.	D44
117	*Br. J. Ind. Med.*	(1977)	**34,**	19 – 25	Crosbie W. A. et al.	E40
118	*Br. J. Ind. Med.*	(1977)	**34,**	85 – 94	Liddell F. D. K.	E21
119	*Br. J. Ind. Med.*	(1977)	**34,**	102 – 105	Doll R. et al.	D24
120	*Br. J. Ind. Med.*	(1977)	**34,**	114 – 118	Saric M. et al.	E16
121	*Br. J. Ind. Med.*	(1977)	**34,**	142 – 147	Lee F. I. et al.	E47
122	*Br. J. Ind. Med.*	(1977)	**34,**	148 – 150	Gardner A. W. et al.	D27
123	*Br. J. Ind. Med.*	(1977)	**34,**	169 – 173	Peto J. et al.	D5
124	*Br. J. Ind. Med.*	(1977)	**34,**	174 – 180	Elmes P. C. et al.	I28
125	*Br. J. Ind. Med.*	(1977)	**34,**	181 – 185	Uragoda C. G.	E24
126	*Br. J. Ind. Med.*	(1977)	**34,**	186 – 195	Wardrop V. E. et al.	E15
127	*Br. J. Ind. Med.*	(1977)	**34,**	196 – 200	Wegman D. H. et al.	I31
128	*Br. J. Ind. Med.*	(1977)	**34,**	201 – 207	Andersen H. C.	H8
129	*Br. J. Ind. Med.*	(1977)	**34,**	208 – 220	Clausen J. et al.	F11
130	*Br. J. Ind. Med.*	(1977)	**34,**	291 – 297	Davies G. M.	D15
131	*J. Occup. Med.*	(1973)	**15,**	11 – 14	Archer V. E. et al.	I37
132	*J. Occup. Med.*	(1973)	**15,**	15 – 20	Danzigger S. I.	E39
133	*J. Occup. Med.*	(1973)	**15,**	409 – 413	Tuma J. et al.	E11
134	*J. Occup. Med.*	(1973)	**15,**	486 – 489	Waxweiler R. J.	D29
135	*J. Occup. Med.*	(1973)	**15,**	580 – 585	Ishizaki T. et al.	F10
136	*J. Occup. Med.*	(1973)	**15,**	717 – 723	Henderson V. et al.	D18
137	*J. Occup. Med.*	(1974)	**16,**	91 – 93	Gumming G. R. et al.	I24
138	*J. Occup. Med.*	(1974)	**16,**	94 – 97	Cohen J. R.	C8
139	*J. Occup. Med.*	(1974)	**16,**	245 – 247	Amandus H. E. et al.	E8
140	*J. Occup. Med.*	(1974)	**16,**	258 – 260	Wegman D. H. et al.	E33
141	*J. Occup. Med.*	(1974)	**16,**	322 – 344	Gerarde H. W. et al.	D9
142	*J. Occup. Med.*	(1974)	**16,**	345 – 349	Kleinfeld M. et al.	B5
143	*J. Occup. Med.*	(1974)	**16,**	375 – 382	Thorpe J. J.	D26
144	*J. Occup. Med.*	(1974)	**16,**	383 – 387	Williams N.	E34
145	*J. Occup. Med.*	(1974)	**16,**	449 – 453	Lieben J. et al.	G2
146	*J. Occup. Med.*	(1974)	**16,**	458 – 464	McMichael A. J. et al.	D32
147	*J. Occup. Med.*	(1974)	**16,**	465 – 469	Lincoln T. A. et al.	F1
148	*J. Occup. Med.*	(1974)	**16,**	509 – 518	Tabershaw I. R. et al.	D42
149	*J. Occup. Med.*	(1974)	**16,**	543 – 546	Sammons J. H. et al.	E17
150	*J. Occup. Med.*	(1974)	**16,**	552 – 556	Lahinen J. et al.	E27
151	*J. Occup. Med.*	(1975)	**17,**	569 – 580	Gosztonyi R. E.	K4
152	*J. Occup. Med.*	(1975)	**17,**	666 – 667	Sealey J. L.	D16
153	*J. Occup. Med.*	(1975)	**17,**	706 – 707	Knuttson A.	E35

No.	Reference				First author	List No.
154	*J. Occup. Med.*	(1975)	**17,**	708 – 715	Miller J. M. et al.	D28
155	*J. Occup. Med.*	(1975)	**17,**	751 – 755	Mazumdar S. et al.	D36
156	*J. Occup. Med.*	(1976)	**18,**	17 – 20	Dinman B. D. et al.	I1
157	*J. Occup. Med.*	(1976)	**18,**	31 – 40	Robinson T. R.	D41
158	*J. Occup. Med.*	(1976)	**18,**	178 – 185	McMichael A. J. et al.	C9
159	*J. Occup. Med.*	(1976)	**18,**	186 – 193	Rubino G. F. et al.	D39
160	*J. Occup. Med.*	(1976)	**18,**	379 – 386	Discher D. P. et al.	E1
161	*J. Occup. Med.*	(1976)	**18,**	541 – 545	Rochette H. E. et al.	D37
162	*J. Occup. Med.*	(1976)	**18,**	595 – 602	Collins J. F. et al.	D38
163	*J. Occup. Med.*	(1976)	**18,**	611 – 617	McMichael A. J. et al.	F20
164	*J. Occup. Med.*	(1976)	**18,**	628 – 632	Radford E. P. et al.	E18
165	*J. Occup. Med.*	(1976)	**18,**	659 – 670	Gamble J. et al.	F24
166	*J. Occup. Med.*	(1976)	**18,**	723 – 729	Cooper W. C.	F16
167	*J. Occup. Med.*	(1976)	**18,**	730 – 731	Parrizpoor D.	E48
168	*J. Occup. Med.*	(1976)	**18,**	735 – 738	Ott M. G. et al.	D45
169	*J. Occup. Med.*	(1976)	**18,**	787 – 792	Viadana E. et al.	H4
170	*J. Occup. Med.*	(1976)	**18,**	797 – 801	Menck H. R.	H5
171	*J. Occup. Med.*	(1977)	**19,**	107 – 112	Alexander R. W. et al.	I34
172	*J. Occup. Med.*	(1977)	**19,**	119 – 122	Weiman C. G.	E32
173	*J. Occup. Med.*	(1977)	**19,**	263 – 268	Lednar W. M. et al.	I33
174	*J. Occup. Med.*	(1977)	**19,**	333 – 336	Grabowski R. R. et al.	F6
175	*J. Occup. Med.*	(1977)	**19,**	406 – 410	Spear R. C. et al.	J1
176	*J. Occup. Med.*	(1977)	**19,**	543 – 550	Lloyd J. W. et al.	B3
177	*J. Occup. Med.*	(1977)	**19,**	603 – 606	Winegar D. A. et al.	F22
178	*J. Occup. Med.*	(1977)	**19,**	611 – 614	Weiss W.	I11
179	*J. Occup. Med.*	(1977)	**19,**	659 – 663	Rappaport M. et al.	E23
180	*J. Occup. Med.*	(1977)	**19,**	675 – 679	Hogstedt C. et al.	C3
181	*J. Occup. Med.*	(1977)	**19,**	679 – 682	Decoufle P. et al.	B4
182	*J. Occup. Med.*	(1977)	**19,**	683 – 689	Hathaway J. A. et al.	I30
183	*J. Occup. Med.*	(1977)	**19,**	737 – 740	Weiss W.	D6
184	*J. Occup. Med.*	(1977)	**19,**	741 – 746	Pasternak B. S. et al.	D10
185	*J. Soc. Occup. Med.*	(1973)	**23,**	3 – 18	McRoberts W.	I4
186	*J. Soc. Occup. Med.*	(1973)	**23,**	36 – 48	Semmence A.	I39
187	*J. Soc. Occup. Med.*	(1973)	**23,**	53 – 60	O'Quigley S.	C13
188	*J. Soc. Occup. Med.*	(1973)	**23,**	61 – 65	Beverley W. H. A.	D1
189	*J. Soc. Occup. Med.*	(1973)	**23,**	120 – 124	Black M. M. et al.	C4
190	*J. Soc. Occup. Med.*	(1973)	**23,**	125 – 127	Haigh W. et al.	K7
191	*J. Soc. Occup. Med.*	(1974)	**24,**	110 – 116	Anthony H. M.	H2
192	*J. Soc. Occup. Med.*	(1974)	**24,**	125 – 129	Ross D. S.	C12
193	*J. Soc. Occup. Med.*	(1975)	**25,**	28 – 32	Howell R. W.	C10
194	*J. Soc. Occup. Med.*	(1975)	**25,**	38 – 49	Sawtell I. J.	H10
195	*J. Soc. Occup. Med.*	(1975)	**25,**	99 – 102	Carson M. et al.	K9
196	*J. Soc. Occup. Med.*	(1975)	**25,**	123 – 126	Calnan C. D.	H6
197	*J. Soc. Occup. Med.*	(1975)	**25,**	127 – 132	Craigen A. A.	C6
198	*J. Soc. Occup. Med.*	(1976)	**26,**	3 – 8	Wilkinson D. S.	C14
199	*J. Soc. Occup. Med.*	(1976)	**26,**	13 – 20	Ardis M.	H9
200	*J. Soc. Occup. Med.*	(1976)	**26,**	57 – 58	Taylor C. F.	F23
201	*J. Soc. Occup. Med.*	(1976)	**26,**	92 – 94	Smith D.	D30
202	*J. Soc. Occup. Med.*	(1976)	**26,**	92 – 94	Smith D.	D31
203	*J. Soc. Occup. Med.*	(1977)	**27,**	3 – 12	Juniper C. P. et al.	I22
204	*J. Soc. Occup. Med.*	(1977)	**27,**	50 – 57	Wansbrough S. N. et al.	D46
205	*J. Soc. Occup. Med.*	(1977)	**27,**	102 – 104	Clay J. E. et al.	E43

11. POLLUTION ASSESSMENT AND CONTROL

Peter Sutton

Pollution may be defined as any discharge of material, or the outcome of any other human activity, which causes appreciable change in the environment. Thus pollution is what affects the natural ecosystem, the countryside or people, and pollution is itself a consequence of people.

There can be no such thing as a non-polluting human activity. We cannot heat our homes without some form of discharge, direct or indirect. We cannot build our homes without causing pollution (as anyone who lives near a brick works or cement works knows). Even by merely living in the simplest possible manner we breathe, sweat, excrete and so on, thus inevitably having some impact on the environment.

As the number of people in the world increases so the problems of supporting, feeding and housing them and disposing of their waste increase. Indeed, since pollution is a consequence of people it is arguable that population is the first problem to be tackled. In fact, it seems that no international organization and no country (except India) has seriously set out to control population growth. The consequence of lack of control is shown in Fig. 11.1.

This fundamental problem is merely academic to industry and commerce. We have to accept social demands largely as they are if we are to stay in business. The best we can do is to control the impact of our operations as far as is practicable and perhaps to influence government and the public where appropriate.

THE ENVIRONMENTAL TECHNOLOGIST

An industrial works or commercial undertaking has a responsibility – social and statutory – to control the impact of its operations on the neighbourhood. A large organization should have some central co-ordinating group to oversee the environmental control policy and practice of the organization as a whole. Each major processing works should have at least one environmental specialist at a senior technical level: the smaller works or establishment which cannot support a full-time specialist should nominate an appropriate person as part-time environmental specialist and contact. This nominee is likely to be either the works chemist or alternatively the hygienist, medical officer, industrial nurse or safety officer.

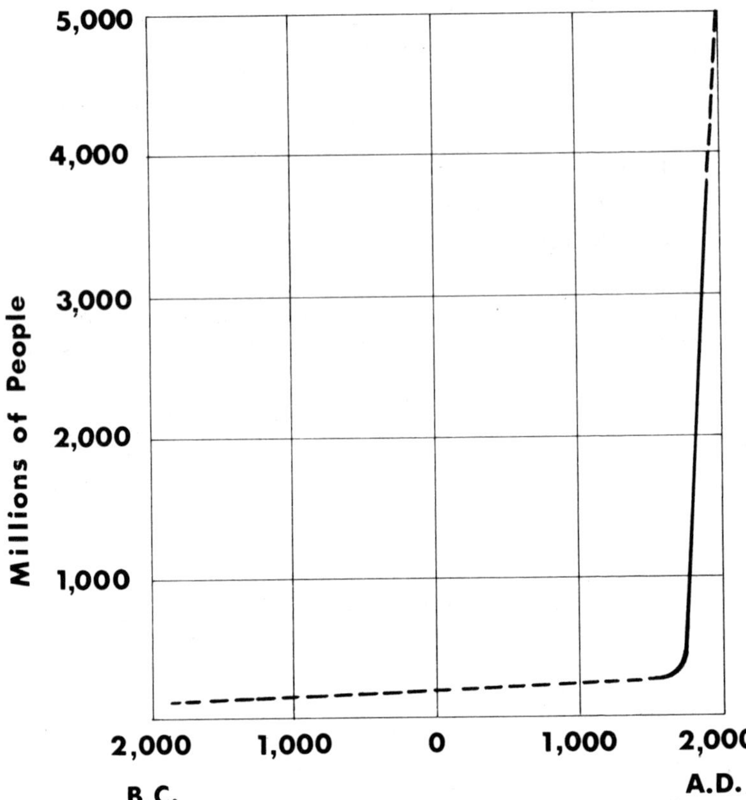

Fig. 11.1. The 'people plague'. The growth of world population. The rapid increase in growth rate in the late 17th and 18th centuries was a result of developments in agriculture and in public health engineering. Population continues to increase at an alarming rate with food production and effluent control scarcely keeping up.

If pollution is seen merely as a matter of chemicals in the air or the water then the works chemist is an obvious choice. However, pollution is really far more than this; it is associated with health effects and with annoyance. The health aspects involve not only people but also plants and animals, both natural and commercial. Thus a health specialist is an appropriate person to deal with it.

In Lymington, a small English south coast town, there was recently much concern over an industrial health problem connected with the boat-building industry. The wives of workers in the boat yards were reported to be complaining that their husbands were losing their sexual potency and they blamed the fumes from the synthetic resins used. At about the same time, a learned paper was published by an ecological research institute reporting a study of pollution of the river Medway, in which one of the parameters of pollution used was the effect on fecundity of female limpets. There is clearly something in common between occupational hygiene and environmental pollution.

ACCEPTABLE POLLUTION

Since any human activity involves some impact on the environment, the criteria of acceptability must be set in terms of the damage or modification which can be accepted. Pollution limits are determined largely by the price that society is prepared to pay for life support, convenience or pleasure.

It is generally accepted now that pollution which might cause death or serious health risk to people must be reduced at least to the threshold risk level – as far as this can be established. Similarly, widespread damage to crops, the countryside and the sea is not acceptable and discharges must be reduced to at least somewhere near the threshold level in this respect or further if practicable.

The natural ecosystem of the Earth has great resilience. The total quantity of water in the world was established long ago and although living organisms have been ingesting and excreting it ever since it is still fit to drink. We are very dependent on the natural regeneration of the ecosystem so it will be helpful first to consider the capacity of this system to absorb and digest our wastes.

NATURAL SYSTEMS OF REGENERATION

Organic material consists of carbon and hydrogen combined with some amount of oxygen, nitrogen, or sulphur and often traces of other elements. Under the action of living organisms and of sunlight, organic

Table 11.1 Simple natural reactions. Degradation of organic material.

Constituent		*Product*
(a) In presence of oxygen (aerobic conditions)		
carbon	$C \rightarrow CO_2$	carbon dioxide
hydrogen	$H \rightarrow H_2O$	water
nitrogen	$N \rightarrow NO_2$	nitrogen dioxide
	or $(NO_3)^-$	nitrate
sulphur	$S \rightarrow SO_2$	sulphur dioxide
	or $(SO_4)^=$	sulphate
(b) In absence of oxygen (anaerobic conditions)		
	$C \ \& \ H \rightarrow CH_4$	methane
	$N \ \& \ H \rightarrow NH_3$	ammonia
	$S \ \& \ H \rightarrow H_2S$	hydrogen sulphide

materials will eventually break down into a series of simpler compounds. This applies to substances made by man, such as detergents or industrial prussic acid, as well as to natural materials, such as dead leaves or human excreta, through some degrade very much more slowly than others.

In some cases, particularly in anaerobic conditions, other more complex compounds such as amines may be formed. Anaerobic products tend to be unpleasant and they account for the malodorous character of stagnant ponds or sweaty socks. Fortunately, they are susceptible to subsequent natural oxidation.

Atmospheric reactions

Plants take in carbon dioxide and give out oxygen; this provides carbon for cell growth. Animals inhale oxygen, which is used for reaction with food substances to release energy, and exhale carbon dioxide. These two processes maintain the oxygen and carbon dioxide levels in the atmosphere virtually constant.

Dead vegetation and animal material rots (degrades) on or in the ground. This is partly an anaerobic process so methane, ammonia, hydrogen sulphide and associated compounds are evolved (Fig. 11.2).

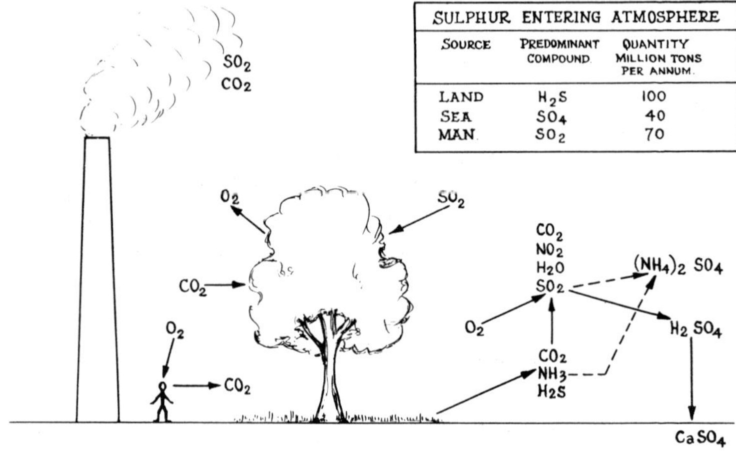

Fig. 11.2.

Further reactions may take place such as the formation of ammonium sulphate $(NH_4)_2SO_4$ from reaction between ammonia, sulphur dioxide and atmospheric oxygen. Sulphur dioxide tends to oxidize to trioxide. It is washed out of the atmosphere either as sulphite or sulphate or possibly as sulphurous or sulphuric acid. This then reacts with alkaline substances such as limestone in the ground. Sulphur is necessary for plant growth and is absorbed by plants out of the air and the ground.

Oxides of nitrogen are also washed out of the atmosphere. They are reactive and eventually form nitrates which are nutrients and provide nitrogen for plant growth.

Sulphates and nitrates are, up to a point, a good thing since they are necessary for plant growth. However, it may be possible to have too much of a good thing, as will be discussed later.

Fossil fuels (coal, oil and natural gas) consist primarily of carbon, hydrogen and some sulphur. Their combustion produces carbon dioxide, sulphur dioxide and water vapour. Coal and oil also contain some inert minerals which produce ash.

The carbon dioxide goes back into the air. The carbon was taken from the air in the first place by plants and the fossil fuel was formed from the remains of plants or of animals which, in turn, had fed on plants. Since man is returning to the atmosphere, in the space of a few centuries, the carbon dioxide which was originally extracted over a period of millions of years, some change in the atmosphere is to be expected. There is some evidence that the carbon dioxide level in the atmosphere is increasing but opinion is divided as to whether this is having or will have any significant effect on the biosphere.

Table 11.2 shows the estimated rate of discharge of sulphur into the atmosphere from natural sources and from human activities.

Table 11.2 Sulphur to atmosphere.

Source	Predominant compound	Estimated quantity sulphur (million tons per year)	
Land-natural	H_2S	100	140 total
Sea-natural	(SO_4)	40	
Human activity	SO_2		70

From the land sulphur appears principally as hydrogen sulphide produced by anaerobic biodegradation. From the sea it is also a biodegradation product and appears partly as hydrogen sulphide but mainly as sulphate since the seas are generally well oxygenated, at least near the surface. Some comes from natural volcanic activity. From human activities it appears mainly as sulphur dioxide from burning of fossil fuels. The sulphur compounds continuously leave the atmosphere by deposition and wash-out and the greater part would eventually reach the sea.

Fossil fuel combustion also produces oxides of nitrogen and, in some cases, hydrocarbon compounds. Hydrocarbons, as well as nitrogen oxides, enter the atmosphere naturally but intensive use of fuels by man tends to produce unnaturally high concentrations.

Aquatic reactions

Similar processes of oxidation and recycling take place in the water (Fig. 11.3).

Again there is a carbon dioxide/oxygen exchange between plants and animal life and oxygen can enter water by diffusion from the air. The oxygen balance is, however, very sensitive. Whereas air consists of 20 per cent oxygen, water can contain in solution only about 10 mg/l (10 parts per million).

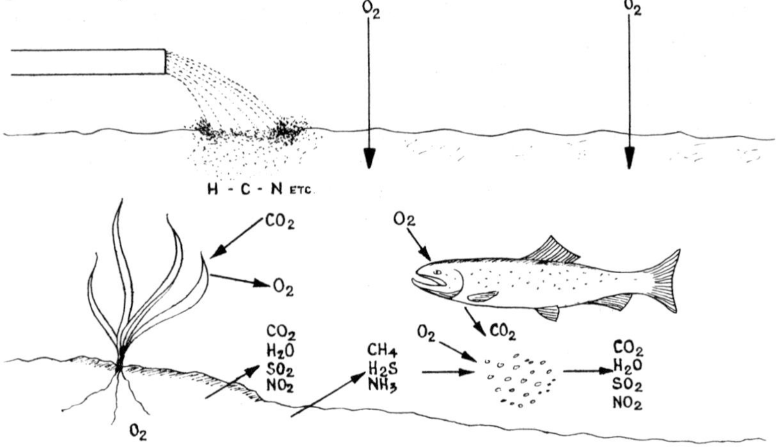

Fig. 11.3.

The mud in a river bed is likely to be at least partly anaerobic in which case degradation of organic materials produces methane, hydrogen sulphide and ammonia. This is often the case in stagnant ponds (which is why methane was first called marsh gas) or in lakes or rivers which receive large amounts of sewage or industrial effluents. Such anaerobic degradation products are malodorous and toxic. In small quantities they are oxidized chemically or by bacterial action in the water but in large quantities they will reduce or even eliminate natural life in the waters. This is why dissolved oxygen in the receiving water and the oxygen demand of effluents are so important as indicators of pollution.

The dissolved oxygen content of water has an effect on the toxicity of dissolved chemicals to fish. A fish requires oxygen at a certain rate so the lower the oxygen content of the water the more water it has to pump through its gills and the more dissolved chemicals it will tend to absorb. Thus the toxicity of ammonia, phenols and metals, for example, increases with decreasing dissolved oxygen.

Domestic sewage consists mainly of organic material dissolved or suspended in water and industrial effluents generally contain organic material. This is digested by the natural water system in the same way as organic matter of natural origin. The natural regeneration system can however easily be overloaded.

Some materials are less susceptible to biodegradation than others. Tar and wax are persistent because they do not disperse easily and so are not readily available for ingestion by organisms. Polythene bags and plastic cups are very persistent.

Some useful synthetic organic materials, such as chlorinated hydrocarbons (which include many pesticides) and some wastes, such as polychlorinated biphenyls (PCB), are very resistant to biodegradation and can accumulate in animal tissues.

Compounds containing metals may change or break down but the metal content remains and some metals (notably mercury and lead) accumulate in animal tissue. The dramatic episode of mercury poisoning in Minamata in Japan was a consequence of mercury in industrial effluents accumulating in fish and then in turn in the bodies of the people who lived largely off locally caught fish.

Table 11.3 Steps in pollution control.

1. *Arrestment*

Removal of pollutants from gaseous or liquid waste stream before discharge; for re-use or for disposal by other less harmful means.

- metal plating works effluent – precipitate metal salts
  re-use or dispose of
- flue gas from coal-fired furnaces – knock out fly ash
  use as aggregate or landfill
- sewage works effluent – settle out sludge
  use as fertilizer or dump at sea or incinerate
- wash water from mineral workings – settle out solids
  re-use water: use solids as landfill

2. *Neutralization*

Treatment of aggressive substance before discharge.

- caustic scrubbing of tail gas from acid manufacture
- pH correction of waste water
- biological oxidation of organic matter in waste water

3. *Dispersal*

Discharge so as to achieve rapid dilution to safe level.

- flue gases to atmosphere by high chimneys
- liquid effluents into tidal waters offshore

Treatment or dispersal?

The environment can accept any discharge without significant damage provided that the discharge is rapidly and adequately diluted and that the rate of discharge does not exceed the rate of removal by natural processes. Most, if not all, substances appear to have a threshold level below which there is no detectable effect. Thus it has been suggested that there are no harmful *substances* but only harmful *concentrations*.

It is quite defensible, up to a point, to dispose of an effluent by kicking it around till you lose it – though it is over-optimistic to assume that 'dilution is the solution to pollution'. A note of warning is sounded by the fact that over the years, as ever more careful studies are made, the observed thresholds of damaging effect are found to be lower than was previously thought. Thus dispersal can be accepted only as the last step in pollution control, following the best practicable pre-treatment as indicated in Table 11.3.

ATMOSPHERIC DISCHARGES

The dichotomy that exists in public attitudes to pollution generally is illustrated by the acceptance of smoking – chimneys must not smoke but people may. This is a facet of the comfortable assumption that pollution is what *they* do, not what *I* do. Even if one regards self-administration of poison in repeated sub-lethal doses to be an inalienable right of the individual in a free society, subjecting others to gratuitous pollution by one's waste tobacco smoke represents an unjustifiable infringement of the rights of others. Administratively the solution is simple – prohibit smoking in public places (smoking should be permitted only in private among consenting adults). Politically and socially, however, society does not appear to be ready for this.

Limits

Pollution does not matter till it reaches something which it will affect, so it is logical to set limits for air pollutants in the form of ground level concentration (bearing in mind that in some cases 'ground level' may be the upper floors of buildings).

Some pollutants are synergistic, that is, the presence of one modifies the effects of another. For example, fine particulate matter and sulphur dioxide are both irritants so the threshold level at which SO_2 affects respiration is reduced in the presence of smoke. This is important in both epidemiological studies and pollution control administration. In typical urban atmospheres the SO_2 and smoke levels at any moment tend to be related partly because they are often discharged together and partly because both tend to accumulate in stagnant air conditions. This has led incautious investigators to ascribe to SO_2 (which is ubiquitous and easy to measure and is therefore popular with research students) health effects which more properly relate to smoke. Experience in many cities during the last twenty years, particularly in Britain, has shown how respiratory effects have decreased as smoke levels have decreased even though SO_2 levels have changed very little.

Although ground level concentration (GLC) is the logical control parameter, it is rather elusive and inconvenient. It is possible to measure the total GLC of, say, SO_2 at a location but often impossible to tell how much comes from any particular local emitter. In addition, the GLC varies with time as wind and weather change. Pollution level is a statistical concept and when quoting GLC figures it is essential to define whether one is referring to, for example, a 3 minute maximum, 1 hour maximum highest day-average in a year, year-round average, or whatever.

The threshold limit values for factory atmospheres are commonly used as a basis for setting neighbourhood limits to air pollutants. The TLV* is based on 8 hour per day exposure of moderately healthy adults to a specific substance. However, neighbourhood limits apply for 24 hour per day exposure to a variety of substances simultaneously for the whole population including infants, the aged and the infirm. Thus a safety factor has to be applied and a short-term (less than 1 hour) calculated maximum GLC of 1/30 or 1/50 TLV for a single emission is commonly used.

The use of best practicable means of emission control can be ensured by setting limits on the actual emissions from the process. Thus specific limits may be applied to emission of dust from cement kilns or sulphate mist from sulphuric acid works based on experience of what can practicably be achieved. Limits of this type are generally expressed in the form of grammes of pollutant per standard cubic metre of flue gas but sometimes as grams of pollutant per tonne of material processed.

Methods of control

Smoke is controlled primarily by efficient combustion, and great improvements have been achieved over recent years. The increased availability of alternatives to coal for domestic heating and industrial processes where flexibility is required (such as pottery kilns and railway locomotives) has facilitated smoke control. The history of smog caused by coal smoke shows how a pollution problem increased with increasing population and use of readily available natural resources but was eventually brought under control by the use of more advanced technology (Table 11.4).

Grit and dust emission is controlled by the use of cyclones, bag filters, electrostatic precipitators, or wet scrubbers. Sulphur dioxide emission is controlled primarily by burning low sulphur fuels. The sulphur content of fuel oils can be reduced in the refining process. There are processes for the flue gas desulphurization but these are still very expensive and not very reliable and the disposal of the sulphurous products is a problem.

Reactive gases generally can be controlled by treatment in wet scrubbers. This, of course, produces a liquid effluent which requires treatment. The GLC of the final effluent gases is controlled by dispersal from high chimneys. Hot flue gas rises in the atmosphere as a consequence of its thermal buoyancy and its efflux velocity. The plume is bent over by

*The precise definition of TLV–TWA (Threshold Limit Value – Time Weighted Average) is the time weighted average concentration for a normal 8-hour workday or 40-hour workweek, to which nearly all workers may be repeatedly exposed, day after day, without adverse effect.

Table 11.4 Smoke and smog. Some notable events.

Year	Event
1273	Use of coal prohibited in London as being prejudicial to health
1306	Renewed prohibition. Execution of one offender
1595	Welsh anthracite (smokeless coal) first brought to London
1801	Manchester Corporation sets up Nuisance Committee on Smoke
1850	Manchester Smoke Inspectorate served over 300 smoke notices
1909	Glasgow smog for 5 weeks; incremental deaths approx. 600
1920	Public Health (Smoke Abatement) Act
1930	Meuse Valley (Belgium) – smog incident death rate 10 times normal. Many cattle affected and slaughtered
1948	Donora (USA) – smog incident. 40% population reported ill
1952	London – 4-day smog; 4000 incremental deaths
1956	Clean Air Act
1962	London – 5-day smog; 750 incremental deaths (last recorded smog incident in London)

the wind and the gas cools as it disperses outwards and is diluted. The effectiveness of a chimney for atmospheric dispersal depends on its height and the total heat content of the flue gas. It is essential that a chimney be high enough to avoid downwash around adjacent buildings (a point commonly overlooked by architects). The degree of dispersal actually achieved is greatly influenced by meteorological conditions.

Some special cases

Smog originally meant merely smoky fog. The word was coined in England in 1905 by the first president of the National Smoke Abatement Society. Photochemical smog, however, is relatively new and is formed principally by reaction of complex hydrocarbons, oxides of nitrogen, possibly oxides of sulphur and ozone or oxygen under ultraviolet light. It can occur only where there is an adequate discharge rate of these pollutants, still air to allow accumulation, and intense sunshine. Thus it is characteristic of densely populated areas particularly where large inefficient petrol-engined cars are used in Mediterranean-type-climate areas in summer. Los Angeles is badly affected and Milan to a lesser degree. It is unlikely that photochemical smog would occur at latitudes above about 45° because insolation is not sufficiently intense (though instances may have occurred further north in Europe in the exceptional summer of 1976).

Pollution knows no frontiers and long-range drift of atmospheric pollution is a matter for concern. Acidity of the rain and rivers in Scandinavia has been blamed on the drift of oxides of sulphur from other western European countries. A major international study was set up to investigate this. The report shows that oxides of sulphur and of nitrogen from other countries do contribute significantly to the acidity of rain and surface waters in southern Norway and Sweden but it is not yet possible to determine these effects numerically because of the many variables involved. It is interesting that the pH of rainfall in east Scotland is similar to that in southwest Scandinavia but this does not appear to affect Scottish forests or fish significantly.

LIQUID EFFLUENTS

It is ironic that historically the principal concern in controlling river pollution has been to allow fish to thrive so that people can catch them for fun. As interest in ecology increases, perhaps society will mature sufficiently to reject angling together with other blood sports.

Limits

The receiving water feels the impact of an effluent at the end of the discharge pipe; there is no equivalent of the virtually uninhabited atmosphere in which initial dispersal and dilution can take place. Thus limits are most commonly set on the concentration of pollutants in the effluent. In setting sensible limits one must consider the rate of dilution in the receiving water and its initial condition. In any case, the best practicable means of effluent quality control should be employed.

The most important single factor is biological oxygen demand (BOD). This is a measure of the total loading on the natural aerobic regenerative system of the receiving water. The standard BOD test involves diluting a sample of the effluent with oxygenated water, seeding with active bacteria, storing for five days and then measuring the oxygen consumed. This is useful for monitoring purposes but in a changing situation the results come rather late for corrective action to be taken. In addition, a very low BOD may mean only that the effluent was toxic to the bacteria and they died. An alternative test is the chemical oxygen demand (COD) where an oxidizing agent (potassium dichromate) is used. This is a relatively quick, easy and reproducible test but the correlation with BOD – that is to say with the natural world – is variable.

Suspended solids have to be controlled since even inert solids can harm the ecology by smothering natural life and by reducing the penetration of sunlight. Limits commonly imposed on effluents into clean rivers with high flow rate or into estuaries are 30 mg/l suspended solids and 20 mg/l BOD (referred to as 30/20 standard). In more sensitive situations, a 10/10 standard may be imposed. In open tidal waters higher concentrations may be accepted. Toxic chemicals, pH and temperature also require control.

Methods of control

The BOD of an effluent is reduced by the logical method of subjecting it to an accelerated biological oxidation process before discharge. This involves passing the effluent through a culture of micro-organisms kept active by intensive aeration. The two common methods are the familiar trickle-beds, still widely used for municipal effluents, and the activated-sludge process which is generally more suitable for industrial effluents. The dead organisms have to be settled out before the effluent is discharged. The resulting sludge is incinerated or possibly dumped at sea.

Solids can be arrested by screening or gravity settling. It is often necessary to add flocculants or demulsifiers to assist the process and sand-filtration is used where high quality effluents are required.

Pollutants which cannot be removed by biological oxidation may be neutralized or precipitated out by chemical treatment.

Some special cases

A problem which commonly arises with rivers is that discharges from one town or factory render the water unfit for use by the next one down stream. It has been suggested that each town should be required to take its domestic water supply from a point downstream of its own sewage discharge – thus creating an incentive to adequate treatment! This is technically feasible but not really necessary provided all discharges and abstractions are controlled by a single authority for the whole length of the river. This system of control has evolved in some countries but international rivers, such as the Rhine, still present administrative problems.

On a larger scale the need for international co-operation in the preservation of the Mediterranean has now been recognized. Large though the sea is, its capacity to digest effluents is finite and it is clear that the discharges from growing population and industry are now approaching the limits of that capacity.

WASTE DISPOSAL

Materials discharged into the air or into rivers are rapidly spread around for all to see. Solid wastes tend to stay where they are put so the practice of dumping rubbish in remote holes in the ground seemed to be a satisfactory means of waste disposal. In the long run, however, the hazards of uncontrolled dumping are immense. Locally, cattle or children stray onto dumps and can be poisoned. More extensively and insidiously, chemicals may be leached out by rain and contaminate natural waters. Percolation through the ground is almost impossible to monitor.

Limits

There are two basic criteria for acceptability of dumping. The first is avoidance of consequential pollution of the ground, of water, or of the air (by gaseous emissions). The second is avoidance of destruction of the countryside by huge quantities of inert waste. China clay waste on Bodmin Moor and colliery waste in the Welsh valleys are examples of this and may have economic implications or may be objectionable for purely aesthetic reasons.

Since measurable pollution is consequential it is not practicable to put numerical limits on waste dumping; each case must be considered individually. Dumping is regarded as acceptable where the geology is appropriate, for example continuous clay basins and mineshafts in impervious strata. Unfortunately it is impossible to be *certain* that the impervious envelope is continuous.

Methods of control

The only thorough method is to process the waste so as to render it inert and inoffensive. In some cases special chemical treatment is appropriate, as with liquid effluents. In many cases, particularly with organic material, incineration is the simplest and most thorough method of disposal. The flue gases, of course, require scrubbing to arrest ash and to neutralize or wash out toxic gases. Domestic refuse can be incinerated to produce inert ash but the flue gas contains such things as hydrochloric acid produced from the PVC inevitably included in modern garbage.

Some special cases

The practice of depositing drums of cyanide waste in open rubbish tips brought the hazards of uncontrolled dumping to the attention of the public in Britain some years ago. The first move by the Government was to require notification of dumping and to make it an offence to deposit waste in such a manner that it might cause a health hazard or pollution in the future. The next step is to control waste dumping by means of licensing but it will be some time before resources of manpower, expertise and adequate disposal facilities are available. (By granting a licence for specific disposal the control authority of course accepts responsibility for any consequences as long as the conditions of the licence are observed). Britain is not alone in having neglected to control the disposal of solid wastes adequately in the past.

Where dumping is permitted, there is risk of reaction between different chemicals which would be relatively harmless individually but which give off harmful vapours when mixed. There has been at least one case of death of a dump operator from this cause and several cases of toxic or noxious gases blowing over nearby housing.

NOISE

Noise may be regarded as a form of pollution but it is more ephemeral than the other forms since it leaves no lasting effect on the environment. Although noise can be a serious cause of annoyance or discomfort in residential areas, numerous social surveys have shown that factory noise is generally far less important than road traffic or aircraft noise and often less important than noise from children, dogs or neighbours.

Limits

Factory noise is most unlikely to reach the hearing damage risk threshold outside the works. In the absence of direct health effects the relevant criterion is annoyance, including disturbance of sleep. An 'acceptable' level is that which will satisfy most people for most of the time.

Industrial noise is more noticeable at night than in the day because the background level of traffic and social noise is less at night. This background noise level is higher in urban areas than in rural areas and people expect, and therefore generally accept, more noise in established industrial localities than in otherwise rural locations where industrial works are newly established. Variation in noise level or character can increase annoyance by drawing attention to the noise and a whine or whistle is particularly annoying.

Typical limits for uniform, characterless industrial noise which would be generally accepted range from about 40 dB(A) at night in a semi-rural locality to about 70 dB(A) in the day in a busy urban area.

Methods of control

Neighbourhood noise can be reduced by enclosure of the noisy machines, either within a single factory building or within separate individual enclosures. (The effect of such enclosure on the noise within in the workshop must, of course, be considered.) Doors, windows or ventilators in a building act as acoustic windows and can let out a considerable amount of noise energy.

Sometimes it is possible to select alternative, quieter machines. For example, there is no excuse now for buying or hiring mobile compressors which are not silenced within an integral acoustic casing. With installed machines it is often necessary to silence only a part of the whole installation; a detailed noise survey is required to identify such cases.

A special case

Air traffic constitutes probably the most objectionable source of noise in terms of intensity and number of people affected. For this very reason commercial aircraft operators are protected against action for noise nuisance by local authorities or members of the public. It is accepted that aircraft cannot operate commercially without creating widespread noise nuisance so people who live near airports must suffer in the interests of commerce. Some progress is being made, slowly, in making commercial aircraft less noisy, but for technical reasons it is unlikely that any great reduction in noise will ever be achieved.

SO WHAT SHOULD *I* DO ABOUT IT?

The primary objective of almost any organization is to remain in business. For a commercial undertaking this necessitates making profits, but for business security it is necessary also to behave in a legally and socially acceptable manner.

Contribution to management decision-taking

The basis for most commercial decisions is return on investment. Pollution control measures, however, are not profitable; at best some small return on material recovered, for example, may offset a part of the cost. Decisions in this area must be made in terms of legal need or social desirability; the financial consideration being that the lowest cost route is chosen to achieve the desired objective. The environmental technologist must be able to express the objective in measurable terms and to see that the action proposed is appropriate and economic. For example, if noise is a cause of complaint, he must be able to identify the source. Is it from the factory, from traffic serving the factory or from elsewhere? If from the factory, is it general plant noise or a single source such as a ventilating fan? In the latter case, noise reduction applied to the whole works would be ineffective as well as costly but silencing the fan would cost relatively little and would achieve the objective of reducing noise annoyance.

The environmental audit

The first thing to do is to evaluate the present environmental performance of the works. This can be done by means of a thorough and formal environmental audit. The areas of concern are:

1. Air pollution.
2. Water pollution.
3. Waste disposal.
4. Neighbourhood noise.
5. Appearance.
6. Consequential effects.

These should be considered in terms of:

1. Legal requirements.
2. Emissions.
3. Impact.

Under legal requirements, identify any consent conditions and any laws, regulations, guidelines or standards relating to emissions. Identify the control authorities and their powers to enter, inspect, test or demand information (and find out whether they have been exerting these powers).

Make a catalogue of all emissions. This involves checking through flow-plans *and* going round the works looking for vents, eductors, drains and dumps. Collect available data on emissions, question its accuracy, make tests where doubt exists. Listen to noises. Look out for intermittent operations and materials handling activity. Talk to the workpeople. Then step back from the works. Look, listen and smell from the outside. Would *you* like to live there? Look at the neighbouring gardens and trees. Paddle out on the river in a small boat. Walk along the shore in gumboots. Come back at night and wander round again inside and outside the works with ears, eyes and nose alert. Then go back through the plant and identify the emissions you missed first time. Include works traffic in your survey.

Find out whether the authorities do any monitoring of pollution or noise levels in the neighbourhood. Read the local paper and take an interest in local council and local pressure group activities to get an idea of local opinion of the works.

From your emission data and from what you see and hear and from evidence of complaints or other comments, decide whether any surveys of pollution levels or noise are required.

All this must be done before the environmental technologist can expect to be taken seriously, can identify what needs to be done and can make a useful and reliable contribution to management decision-taking.

LEGISLATION AND LIMITS

Pollution can be controlled by means of legislation, provided that the legislation is realistic and is enforced. Pollution control is costly and gives no product benefit – it is money poured down the drain to prevent poison going down the drain. Thus controls should be relevant and sufficiently, but not unnecessarily, stringent. The effects on the environment (including people) must be related back to the limits on discharges.

The bureaucrat loves sets of tidy numerical limits, like mg/l in the effluent or kg emitted per 100 t processed. But these numbers can so easily become just harmonized irrelevances. The size or nature of the factory discharging the dirty water is totally irrelevant to pollution; what matters is the size and nature of the lake into which it is discharged.

Trends in legislation

There is much table-thumping now between Britain and other members of the EEC in which Britain advocates a flexible approach, considering the effects on the environment and using the best practicable means of control, while the others advocate the universal numerical limit approach. In practice, the difference is not so great as it appears. The 'British' approach leads naturally to a fair degree of standardization and the 'Euro' approach is inevitably constrained by what is practicable anyway.

A recent development in legislation is adoption of the concept that the polluter should pay. In this, an effluent is taxed on the basis of its polluting effect. A levy is imposed in the form of so many francs, marks or guilders per kg of oxygen demand of an effluent. The justification for the system is twofold. The levy provides a direct economic incentive to a works to improve its effluent and it provides money for the authorities to spend on improving the environment. There are, however, several objections. The ethics of allowing a commercial organization to buy the right to pollute are questionable. Also it is uneconomic for a public authority to try to clean up a river after it has been polluted and of course much of the pollution comes from municipal sewage.

In any case, a pollution tax must be set high enough to encourage a works to employ appropriate pollution control measures but not so high as to demand a degree of effluent treatment which would make the whole enterprise uneconomic. In other words, the pollution tax is merely an oblique and cumbersome way of requiring that best practicable means of control be employed.

It is an inescapable though unpalatable fact that in the long run the public must pay for pollution control. Municipal sewage treatment is paid for by taxes. The cost of factory effluent treatment or the incremental cost of lead-free petrol is part of the manufacturing cost and must be paid by the customer. This cost is paid both as an increase in money price and also as a reduction in the resources available for other purposes.

As standards become more stringent, unexpected constraints may be discovered. There is a general demand for further reduction in sulphur dioxide emissions, and desulphurization of fuel oil or flue gases are practicable methods of achieving this – expensive and difficult, but technically feasible. But removal of pollution in one area may sometimes create problems in another.

Consider the situation in Britain. Sulphur is used in the chemical industry and imports amount to nearly 1 mt/year. But a total of over 3 mt/year is discharged to the atmosphere in flue gases. Thus if about 30 per cent of sulphur in the nation's fuel is recovered we are in balance. If the discharge were cut by more than that we would have a problem – should we then pour sulphur down old mine shafts or ship sulphuric acid out to the North Sea?

In the days when pollution control consisted of treating a few shocking local discharges a piecemeal approach was adequate, but now we are reaching the point where a broader based national and international approach is required.

REFERENCES AND FURTHER READING

CEC (1975) *Damage and Annoyance Caused by Noise*, EUR 5398e. Luxemburg, Commission of the European Communities.

CEC (1977) *State of the Environment, First Report.* Luxemburg, Commission of the European Communities.

Gilpin A. (1976) *Dictionary of Environmental Terms.* London, Routledge and Kegan Paul.

Jones J. R. and Erichsen (1964) *Fish and River Pollution.* London, Butterworth.

Mellanby K. (1972) *The Biology of Pollution.* Institute of Biology Study No. 38. London, Arnold.
Nonhebel G. (1972) *Gas Purification Processes for Air Pollution Control.* London, Newnes-Butterworth.
OECD (1977) *The OECD Programme on Long Range Transport of Air Pollutants.* Paris, OECD.
Sharland I. (1972) *Woods Practical Guide to Noise Control.* Colchester, Woods.
Stern A. C. (1972) *Air Pollution* (3 Vols). London, Academic.
Sutton P. (1971) Noise and the community. *Ann. Occup. Hyg.* **14,** 109–117.
Sutton P. (1975) *The Protection Handbook of Pollution Control**. Alan Osborne & Associates (Books) Ltd. Unit 5 Seager Buildings, Brookmill Rd., London SE8.†
Sutton P. (1977) *The Protection Handbook of Industrial Noise Control,* 3rd ed. Alan Osborne & Associates (Books) Ltd. Unit 5 Seager Buildings, Brookmill Rd. London SE8†.

*With addendum bringing UK legislation up to 1977.
†These books must be obtained direct from the publisher.

12. THE DEVELOPMENT OF OCCUPATIONAL HYGIENE

Derek Turner

INTRODUCTION

Before embarking upon a discussion of the prospects for occupational hygiene it would be profitable to consider its origins and the fundamentals of its practice. The very term occupational hygiene itself is often misunderstood; hygiene is the study of the promotion of health; occupational hygiene, therefore, is this study within the ambit of people's work. The American Industrial Hygiene Association found it necessary in 1959 to publish a formal definition of the subject, even though it had its origins in America. Originally, when it became accepted that many diseases and disabilities associated with various occupations resulted from excessive contamination of the atmosphere in the workplace, engineers were involved with physicians in the design and provision of ventilation systems to improve in some measure the atmospheric purity. They became known as Industrial Hygiene Engineers. The activities associated with atmospheric control increased, however, to the point where industrial hygiene was defined as 'that science and art devoted to the recognition, evaluation and control of the environmental factors or stresses arising in or from the workplace which may cause sickness, impaired health and well-being or significant discomfort and inefficiency among workers or among citizens of the community'. In other words it is concerned with ensuring that work-day activity does not impair the quality of the environment. It has been suggested that a more descriptive title would be Occupational Health Technology; it is felt however that any attempt to change the name now would only compound confusion.

Hygiene covers much more than measuring environmental conditions with reasonable accuracy. It involves consideration of where and when to measure and for how long; the interpretation of the results of measurement in terms of human response; the initiation of appropriate control – appropriate within the confines of the process as it exists. It involves a contribution from many disciplines and is essentially a team job with the hygienist as the co-ordinating agency. It requires a knowledge of human biology, chemistry and engineering, which must be applied within the sphere of practical operation of industry.

Other terms often confused, yet essential to a proper understanding of the aims and activities of the hygienist, are toxicity and hazard. Toxicity is the more absolute term; it is the capacity of a material, once absorbed into the body, to cause an ill-effect. Hazard on the other hand, is a relative term; it includes an element of risk or probability and defines the likelihood of a toxic effect occurring under the conditions of use of the material. Hence the method of use and the properties of the material are relevant to its hazard. There is little to choose between hydrogen cyanide and sodium cyanide as far as toxicity is concerned, but sodium cyanide, being a solid material, is far less hazardous in use.

HYGIENE PRACTICE

The essence of the practice of occupational hygiene is summed up in the three words in the definition quoted – recognition, evaluation and control. Virtually any problem in the sphere of hygiene can be resolved by application of these three stages.

Recognition

Recognition that a hazard may exist depends upon a knowledge of the properties, chemical, physical and toxicological, of the substance in question or of the physical phenomenon concerned. In order to be aware of the possible problems, the hygienist must be conversant with the reference literature available and with its significance. There is an ever-increasing amount of published information on hazards to health associated with work; much of it is repetitive presentation of the same data.

The hygienist must also be able to recognize potential future problems for the sphere of industrial activity with which he is concerned. The current literature, and his contacts with other professional hygienists will draw attention to areas of concern in allied fields.

Evaluation

Having recognized that a hazardous situation may exist or develop, an evaluation of the position is required. This normally involves the application of measurement techniques to establish existing intensities of contamination of the environment and comparison of the results with standards of acceptability. It may, on occasion, be necessary first to develop an appropriate method of measurement.

Control

Having recognized the possibility of a hazard and evaluated its extent, it becomes necessary to recommend appropriate methods of controlling the situation to prevent undue exposure of personnel. This may be achieved in a variety of ways; the options range from substitution of the hazardous agent by a less hazardous one, through segregation of the operations involving the hazard, or enclosure of the process within a booth or by effectively applied ventilation, to the use of protective equipment to isolate the operators from the hazard. Normally the method of choice should allow continuous operation of the process without need for extensive use of protective equipment.

TYPES OF HAZARD

The environmental factors which give rise to hazards may be divided into three main classes: chemical, physical and biological. The chemical hazards include gases, vapours, mists, fumes and dusts of substances in the atmosphere or within process operations where they may have to be handled. They may gain access to the site of their activity by three routes, and it is only after having broken into the body that a hazardous substance can exert its toxic effect. The three possible routes of absorption are by *ingestion*, either directly or as a contaminant of foodstuff or smoking material, by *penetration of the skin* following contact of a liquid or solid with the skin (significant skin penetration of a vapour is very rare), and, most commonly, by *inhalation* of a vapour, mist or dust.

When the hazardous agent is in particulate form, the extent of its activity is often influenced by the size of the particles. For the more inert dusts, which are capable of inducing fibrosis of the lung tissue, but have little or no other toxic property, particle size is most important. Only small particles are capable of penetrating in significant numbers into the depths of the lungs, and any evaluation of the hazard from such dusts therefore necessitates determination of the amount of fine airborne material. Originally particle counting techniques were used, but they are laborious and only give reliable results when done by practised operators. It is now more usual to determine the weight of airborne material of the size capable of penetrating into the alveoli.

The behaviour of particulate matter within the human respiratory system is dependent upon the aerodynamic properties of the particles. Very fine particles remain suspended in air for long periods and only deposit upon the surfaces of the respiratory tract by diffusion processes and Brownian movement. Somewhat larger particles will settle out of still air, or separate out from moving air at places of significant change of direction due to their momentum. It is their settling speed which is important and this is determined not only by their size, or apparent diameter, but also by their overall shape and by their density. It has become usual, however, to classify airborne particles by their 'equivalent diameter'; this is the diameter of a spherical particle of unit density which would settle in still air at the same rate as the particle in question. Particles most likely to settle out in the alveolar region are those of equivalent diameter in the range 0·5 to 5 μm. Such particles form what is known as 'respirable dust'; larger particles settle, or impact higher in the respiratory tract.

For materials having systemic toxicity, the site of deposition is less important, since the material is likely to be absorbed through the mucus linings of the naso-pharanx, or to be swallowed and absorbed from the gut. It has been usual, therefore, to measure the total concentration of airborne particulates when evaluating these hazards. The techniques used tend to rely on open-faced filters and the size of the largest particles caught on such filters is influenced both by their orientation and by the rate of inflow of air into the filter. Recently devices have been proposed which have been shown, in the laboratory, to sample a similar range of particle sizes to that taken into the nose and mouth during normal respiration. It is probable that these 'inhalable' dust samplers will achieve increasing use in parallel with the 'respirable' dust samplers already employed.

The physical group of hazards contains the well-known trio of heat, light and sound, together with the various forms of ionizing and non-ionizing radiations and lasers. They act primarily by impinging on the body surface although their effects may well be manifest in internal organs – occupational deafness and radiation illness being examples. Special problems of the physical aspects of the environment are encountered in work under pressure, in tunnelling work and especially in saturation diving in deep waters.

The biological hazards of occupation, leaving aside the transmitted coughs, colds and 'flu, relate to agricultural, pharmaceutical and micro-biological activities. The most commonplace are the allergy-inducing substances causing conditions such as farmer's lung. Possible developments in the field of genetic engineering, however, present potential problems of environmental control of great significance.

MONITORING OF HAZARD

The evaluation of the extent of these various forms of hazard again has common principles. The objective is to assess the conditions to which the working individual is exposed. In the days when overt disease was induced in people at work, it tended to be in those who stayed in a fixed location throughout the day. The assessment of the environment, and of the effect of any attempts at control, could be made by taking measurements over the working period from a fixed point in the vicinity of the job. Much useful information was derived in this way in mining, lead battery manufacture and other activities; such monitoring is still used to great effect in the assessment of the performance of plant equipment.

There has however been a move towards measurement of the conditions to which the man is exposed wherever he may be. Many individuals move around a complex plant during their working period and even if the average conditions at a variety of locations is known, it is difficult to determine from this, even approximately, an individual's exposure. There has been considerable development of late of various forms of personal monitor which the man wears throughout a shift. The first of these to be widely used were the film badge and dosimeter of the atomic energy industry. These were followed by battery-powered pumps housed in metal cases which could be worn on a harness or belt, at the expense of a modicum of inconvenience. The pump drew a continuous sample of atmosphere through a filter paper or carbon or silica gel absorber located at head height. There has been rapid development of this type of equipment, until there are now available small units which readily slip into the pocket, containing intrinsically safe electrical components – a most important feature in most chemical industry applications, where flammable vapour concentrations may be encountered – sampling at rates of the order of 100 ml/min through small, pre-packed tubes of adsorbent charcoal. For many pollutants it is possible to use chromatographic column support materials as the adsorbent and to displace the adsorbed vapour directly into a detection instrument thermally, thus achieving virtually instantaneous presentation of the result at the end of the sampling period.

A more recent development, of great promise, is the portable diffusion monitor. This is a small device which may be worn as a lapel badge. It is slightly larger than a radiation film badge but has the advantage of being independent of any power supply or pump. The device consists of a layer of carbon or carbon cloth adsorbent under a permeable membrane contained within a plastic holder. Airborne vapour diffuses through the membrane, at a rate dependent upon the atmospheric concentration, and is adsorbed by the carbon. Field trials have shown these monitors to be reliable means of assessing the time weighted exposure of individuals to several organic vapours. Further development is anticipated.

The principle of personal dosimetry has also been applied to the measurement of noise; readily portable noise meters have been designed and produced to monitor, and evaluate in terms of the current acceptable level of 90 dB(A) for 8 hours, the equivalent exposure of the individual over the period for which the instrument has been worn.

The other form of monitoring which is used is biological; it involves determination in blood, urine or breath, of the concentration of the absorbed contaminant or of a metabolite. Phenol in urine is, for example, used to assess exposure to benzene. It is a useful means of assessing the exposure of the individual, or of a group of individuals, in comparison with results of airborne contamination measurement. It does not, however, indicate the source of any exposure and should be used to complement atmospheric monitoring. Its use can prevent the complacent acceptance of the apparently reassuring results of other forms of monitoring which are failing to reveal that the individual, through ignorance or through unauthorized 'short cuts', is receiving an unsuspected and undetected exposure. The results of both static and personal atmospheric monitoring can readily be influenced, for better or for worse, by those determined to provoke a given response; physiological processes, variable though they may be, tend to be more consistent.

STANDARDS

Having carried out the monitoring activity, the results have to be evaluated by comparison with accepted standards. The subject of standards, and of acceptable standards, is currently under active discussion.

The most widely known, and possibly still the least well-understood, set of standard values is the list of Threshold Limit Values (TLVs) published annually by the American Conference of Governmental Industrial Hygienists and reproduced in Britain by the Health and Safety Executive in their series of *Notes of Guidance.* To understand the purpose and precision of the list of TLVs one must return to its origins. It was, and still is, a list agreed annually at a meeting of practising hygienists, of the values which they collectively accept as working guides to achieving acceptable conditions; it was a means of avoiding fruitless disagreement between neighbouring authorities on whether 50 or 100 ppm should be the accepted standard for a particular substance, when all that was known was that 10 ppm was apparently safe and 500 ppm had caused trouble. From its inception it is the entire list and not individual values, which has been approved by vote. The background data on which each value is based are now published in a bound volume, *Documentation on Threshold Limit Values.* Perusal of this book reveals a wide range of precision in the background data, and a wide range of effects which have caused values to be set. Obviously the list, once it was published, was gratefully seized by other hygienists working in the industries which the governmental units inspected and advised, as their own guide. It is in some ways unfortunate that the list, because of its convenience and apparent precision, has tended to be used as the definition of the safe and the dangerous. Health hazards are not amenable to such close definition as are, for example, flammability hazards.

The TLV list had its origins in the days when 'professional judgement' was an acceptable, even a respectable reason for justifying a recommendation. The guidance of the TLV list would be assessed in relationship to the particular application, its duration, its frequence and perhaps even its necessity. Most, if not all, the industrial disease scourges were eliminated through the application of these principles – and doubtless some thoroughly bad practice hid behind them also. The pendulum has now swung to the other side and little credibility is given by some to any professional in the health field, especially one who is employed by industry.

In the search for standards of apparent precision, attempts have been made to increase the applications of existing values such as TLVs. It has been argued that for general population exposures the TLV should be divided by 30. *First* the TLV is divided by 3 because the exposure is for 24 hours and not for 8 hours and *second* the TLV is divided by 10 for additional safety. On the other hand limits for infrequent, short exposures have been proposed, derived by multiplying the 8-hour value by a factor.

These procedures have been proposed for use in the absence of more applicable data, and in these circumstances they do provide a guide. Notice should also be taken of the background against which the original value was fixed. It seems to be far more logical and acceptable to apply this time weighted approach to a value set on the basis of a long-term risk than to one set on the basis of irritancy.

There is really no substitute for standards firmly based on well-collected data. It is unfortunate that far too few such data are available. Where there has been sufficient information on existent environmental levels and associated health records for persons who had worked in those conditions for a significant number of years, good standards have resulted. Those produced by the British Occupational Hygiene Society for asbestos and noise are good examples.

The need to consider the biological action – or pharmacokinetics – of the material when deriving acceptable limits has been studied of late in relationship to both systemic and carcinogenic hazards. The relationship between the biological half-life of the agent and its rate of absorption under various exposure patterns has led to proposals on appropriate levels and on systematic monitoring programmes. The greater the availability of soundly based standards the more will it be feasible to design well-based monitoring procedures; only for those substances for which the basic dose-effect-response data are available, however, is any improvement in precision probable from application of mathematically derived sampling procedures.

Whenever embarking upon monitoring procedures it is important to keep clearly in mind the purpose of occupational hygiene activity and not to get too involved in discussing, obtaining and justifying numbers. The objective remains the provision of a safe and acceptable working environment; TLVs and standards of any other origin are means to achieving this end. The consumption of professional time in statistical manipulation of the results of measurement to prove 'compliance' with an essentially imprecise standard which is apparently exceeded is futile. Effort would be better spent in improving conditions to the point where they are clearly acceptable.

TRAINING

Who then is the hygienist and from where does he come? To be fully effective he must be able to provide a bridge between the engineering and managerial functions of everyday process operation on the one hand and the health and safety functions on the other. Until recently there was virtually no formal training available outside the USA. Postgraduate courses were available there in established academic centres such as Harvard, Pittsburgh and Cincinnati. A handful of British graduates had the opportunity to attend courses in these centres. Others were fortunate enough to work with pioneers of the field in Britain. The British approach had been stimulated by experience in major industries such as coal mining and cotton spinning in the period between 1918 and 1939. The advent of the war in 1939, with its requirements for increased production under enclosed conditions to achieve 'black out' from the air at night, and the requirement for personnel to operate efficiently in hostile climates on ships, on land and in aircraft, stimulated much study of the man–environment interaction. Units were set up jointly between academic centres and the services which persisted after the war and formed the nucleus of the academic training avenues discussed in Chapter 14.

The emphasis in training has, certainly until very recently, been on postgraduate courses. Many of the people taking the courses offered in the United Kingdom have been 'mature students'; they have been seconded from within industry to acquire expertise in occupational hygiene after several years of experience within industrial technology or research. This has meant that they have brought to the course an understanding of the interplay between work and the environment, and of the practicalities of implementing control within operational requirements, from which the less experienced, recently graduated members of the course have benefited. Those involved in teaching postgraduate courses will readily confirm the value of such individuals.

Undergraduate teaching in occupational hygiene has been very limited in both Britain and America; aspects of the subject have been included as options in some engineering and environmental sciences degree courses; one London polytechnic has been running a BSc in Occupational Hygiene for about three years.

This predominance of postgraduate, normally full-time courses at only a limited number of universities has led to frequent queries as to where introductory training may be obtained. A popular addition to the range of courses has recently been initiated by the British Examining Board in Occupational Hygiene – which will be discussed later – in conjunction with technical colleges, leading to the award of a series of Preliminary Certificates in various aspects of occupational hygiene at a level which aims to provide people competent to assess environmental conditions in accordance with prescribed codes of practice.

PROFESSIONAL DEVELOPMENT

Occupational hygiene has been slow to emerge as a distinct profession. Its interdisciplinary origins have resulted in many of the people active in important areas of the subject continuing to be regarded as members of their original professional group – for example chemists or engineers.

The emphasis put on occupational hygiene principles in the Robens Report and the subsequent legislation, together with the obvious need to implement these principles in the control of the hazards from asbestos, vinyl chloride and benzene for instance, have caused many industrial organizations to create management posts in 'hygiene and safety'. These have been administrative posts, co-ordinating the company's response to the requirements and regulations of the legislation; in many instances there have not been available individuals with experience in the broad practice of occupational hygiene, or safety, but only those with limited expertise in the monitoring of particular hazards, often in conjunction with other responsibilities. In Europe as a whole there are still relatively few full-time practitioners of hygiene outside the academic and inspectorial areas; the control of the working environment is often seen as a subordinate activity to the control of occupational disease, the prime emphasis being on clinical surveillance.

The first move towards establishing a separate professional status for occupational hygiene outside America came in 1953 when the British Occupational Hygiene Society was formed. This was, however, instituted as a learned society to serve as a forum where all the disciplines concerned with occupational hygiene, in either its general aspect or in specialized activities, could discuss problems of current interest. From its original 50 or so members the Society has grown to a current membership, drawn from international sources, of over 700. It remains an interdisciplinary Society although it has stimulated several developments of special relevance to professional hygienists. There is no doubt that the Society through its activities, not least of which have been its five-yearly symposia on inhaled particles and vapours, and its hygiene standards, has furthered the practice of occupational hygiene enormously. It has provided, as its original aims intended, a focus to which all the professions concerned have felt able to make a contribution.

In 1967, in response to an apparent demand for a means of accrediting the professional status of practising hygienists, at the same time as a similar requirement was being voiced by health physicists, an examining board was proposed. As originally envisaged this was to be a joint board between hygienists, health physicists and any other environmental science practitioners who wished to initiate professional qualifications. In the event, however, it became The British Examining Board in Occupational Hygiene. The Board offers awards at two levels of competence, the Diploma and the Certificate and, as has been mentioned, the latter has subsequently been subdivided into areas of study each of which is covered by a Preliminary Certificate, which carries similar status to the full Certificate, but within a closely delineated part of the field.

The examinations held by the Board, with the exception of those leading to a Preliminary Certificate, are intended to explore the candidates' competence as practising hygienists; they do not explore their theoretical knowledge in depth so much as endeavour to determine their ability to cope in practice with typical situations in a variety of aspects of hygiene. Applicants are required to demonstrate that they have been in active practice at an appropriate level of responsibility for a minimum period (3 years or 5 years, according to the award envisaged) and that they have achieved appropriate minimum academic standards. The major awards to date have been restricted to persons competent in 'comprehensive practice'; there has been no provision for awards to specialists in particular areas. This has been largely for administrative reasons; the number of people and the time available to organize the system have been small. As with the Society, the Board has been operated by part-time 'volunteers'; it is hoped that as the demand for examination increases, a more formal organization will be practicable.

The Examining Board enjoys almost complete autonomy, except that its members are appointed by the Society. It is, thus, theoretically open to influence by the interdisciplinary Society; this has the advantage of ensuring that its standards conform to an acceptable level in the eyes of fellow professionals. It has the disadvantage of denying the hygiene profession the ultimate decision in its own destiny.

Feelings have been divided, and strong, on this last point. It was felt by some that there was a need for a professional organization, completely independent of any other, for hygienists; other disciplines in occupational health were independent, as well as having a voice in the Hygiene Society, it was argued. As a result, in 1975 the Institute of Occupational Hygienists was formed, with the aims and objectives of promoting and developing the profession of occupational hygiene, advancing public and professional education in the subject, and holding or supervising examinations for awards in any or all aspects of occupational hygiene and allied subjects.

It is apparent that these objectives overlap significantly those of both the Examining Board and the Society. Membership of the Institute is restricted to those who can show qualification and experience in comprehensive occupational hygiene. The most obvious yardstick of such status has been the Examining Board's awards, although other criteria have also been applied. It has seemed to some unfortunate that the constitution of the Institute made quite detailed provision for it to pursue activities of a not strictly professional nature, but of relevance to occupational health practice as a whole, since the facilities in general are limited and should not be diluted by diversification.

However, an issue has arisen within the European Community of concern to all branches of the occupational health field which has served to bring the various bodies into co-operation: this is registration of professional personnel. The first area in which this was required of persons not already holding an officially registered qualification was in the nuclear energy industry under the provisions of Euratom. This requirement must be expected to spread into other activities also. The issue has provided an opportunity for the Society, which has the national and international status to be accepted as a registration authority, and the Institute, which independently represents many of the professional practitioners of occupational hygiene in Europe, to combine. Discussions between the two organizations and the Examining Board have led to the proposal that a new Board, drawing its members equally from the Society and the

Institute, should be created to combine examining and registering functions in a British Examining and Registration Board in Occupational Hygiene, which will be unique within Europe.

OCCUPATIONAL HYGIENE SERVICES

The number of occupational hygienists is still relatively low. The organizations which employ hygienists are correspondingly few and tend to be the large concerns whose activities pose major health hazards to their employees. A large proportion of industry therefore has to rely on outside advice and assistance.

This is available through a variety of channels. On a purely advisory plane, various industrial associations, such as the Chemical Industries Association and the Institute of Petroleum, have advisory committees which consider problems of current interest and will advise their members on appropriate means of controlling potentially hazardous situations. The extent to which they can assist individual firms with specific problems is clearly limited.

The Health and Safety Executive has expanded considerably the laboratory facilities initially created by the Factory Inspectorate. Central and regional laboratories are now in existence, primarily to supply a service for inspectors and field investigators of the Executive. They are normally able to offer practical advice, especially on new or unusual hazards. Queries should be routed through the appropriate inspectorate.

Some university departments operate occupational hygiene services which undertake investigations for clients. They are able to accept requests to study particular problems, to provide a routine surveillance programme or to carry out specialized analysis of samples taken by the client and sent in to the service. Such services are located in London (The TUC Centenary Institute of Occupational Health, London School of Hygiene and Tropical Medicine), Newcastle upon Tyne (The North of England Industrial Health Service, Department of the Industrial Health and Hygiene), Cardiff (The Department of Community Medicine, Welsh National School of Medicine) and Dundee (The Scottish Occupational Health Laboratory Service, Department of Social Medicine). A service of similar origin but now operating independently (while maintaining close liaison with the Department of Occupational Health in the University) is the National Occupational Hygiene Service at Manchester. The Institute of Occupational Medicine in Edinburgh, a joint organization between the University and the National Coal Board also offers a service to other industry, especially for the assessment of hazards from airborne particulates.

Specialist services in individual aspects such as the control of noise, or air pollution, and the provision of ventilation systems are also available.

EXTERNAL ENVIRONMENTS

Any attempt to define a boundary between the problems of the occupational environment and those of the general environment has always been difficult; one man's occupational location may well be another man's highway. The increasing pressures upon producers and suppliers to accept responsibility for advising on the safe use of their products have further blurred the division. The hygienist must become involved in the evaluation of potential hazards for the user of products and the general community; these hazards may be of a completely different order or nature from those involved in manufacture. For example, most solvents are manufactured in closed systems, often by distillation from a hydrocarbon mixture. Exposure to the vapour is unlikely under normal operating conditions. Solvents in use, however, have to escape by evaporation from the location of application and hence the potential for airborne exposure is much increased. In other instances the hazard produced by the product in use may not be associated with its manufacture; noise and vibration may accompany use of a device which has been made in relatively quiet conditions. Noise and air pollution are two areas where occupational hazards re-appear as nuisance factors in the general environmental scene. The techniques of assessment are similar; the standards of acceptability are of a completely different order. The hygienist must concern himself with these problems in conjunction with management and local authorities.

SOURCES OF INFORMATION

For guidance on acceptable environmental conditions for occupational activity the annual list of TLVs is invaluable. In its original form, published by the American Conference of Governmental Industrial Hygienists (P.O. Box 1937, Cincinnati, Ohio 45201) it contains values for chemical and physical hazards. In its reprinted form, as *HSE Guidance Note EH15,* it contains only the chemical values.

For the proper use of the TLV list, the volume of *Documentation of the Threshold Limit Values for Substances in Workroom Air,* from the same source as the complete list, is essential.

The ACGIH also produce a compendium on *Industrial Ventilation – A Manual of Recommended Practice,* obtainable from their Committee on Industrial Ventilation (P.O. Box 453, Lansing, Michigan 48902).

The book most generally referred to on chemical hazards and their evaluation is *Industrial Hygiene and Toxicology* in two volumes, edited by F. A. Patty and published by Interscience Publishers.

The International Labour Office Encyclopedia on Occupational Health and Safety is also a wide ranging source of reference.

Current information and conference reports are to be found in the *Annals of Occupational Hygiene* – the international journal of the British Occupational Hygiene Society, published quarterly by Pergamon Press, and the *Journal of the American Industrial Hygiene Association,* published monthly by the association (66 S. Miller Rd., Akron, Ohio 44313).

Several useful guides on hygiene practice have been published in America by the National Institute for Occupational Safety and Health (NIOSH) and are obtainable from the US Government Printing Office, Washington DC at modest cost; they include the *NIOSH Manual of Sampling Data Sheets; NIOSH Occupational Exposure Sampling Strategy Manual; NIOSH Manual of Analytical Methods; The Industrial Environment – its Evaluation and Control.*

Problems associated with the thermal environment are well discussed in Thomas Bedford's classic volume *Basic Principles of Ventilation and Heating,* published by Lewis of London.

The Guidance Notes of the Health and Safety Executive cover many prevalent hazards.

The TUC Centenary Institute of Occupational Health also offers an information service based upon its access to the published literature on occupational health and hygiene, in addition to the more active forms of investigational service already mentioned.

Further information on the professional organizations mentioned may be obtained from their honorary secretaries: The British Occupational Hygiene Society, Mr J. T. Sanderson, Esso Research Centre, Abingdon, Oxon.; The Institute of Occupational Hygienists, Dr J. R. Belbin, Commonwealth Smelting Ltd, St. Andrews Road, Avonmouth, Bristol; The British Examining and Registration Board in Occupational Hygiene, Mr K. L. Knight, London School of Hygiene and Tropical Medicine, Keppel Street, London WC1.

13. NURSING AND OCCUPATIONAL HEALTH

Dorothy Radwanski

Occupational health practice involves different specialists and some generalists in places where people work. One of the specialists is the trained occupational health nurse. There is discussion and argument in other fields of nursing about the need for specialist nurses. In occupational health practice the need for specialism is evident.

Sadly, the majority of nurses practising in workplaces have not had specialized training before they take up post and are therefore unable to practise as they might. In situations where teams of nurses are employed, junior members of the team may be given, by trained senior colleagues, sufficient in-service training to allow them to function well in that particular organization. Specialized training is needed so that nurses are able both to undertake their work with authority in any workplace, and to adapt it according to the needs of the organization. They must be able to liaise with other specialists and make a respected contribution. The lack of occupational health nursing advice is likely to diminish any scheme devised to contribute to workers' health and safety.

As well as being specially trained, the occupational health nurse requires other qualities and background. She* needs to be independent and well motivated, open minded and discreet. This specialty is not for the faint-hearted and not for the poorly trained and inexperienced. It is also not the job of choice for nurses who either prefer to be concerned with the care of patients during their cure or to practise prevention in purity, without the interference of emergencies and the giving of treatment.

THE WORK SITUATION

There are about 9000 nurses in workplaces in the United Kingdom which probably amounts to about 3 per cent of the total number of nurses employed in the country. Most of these practise outside the National Health Service. It would be unlikely, in any country, that the occupational health nurses formed more than a very small proportion of the total. They are employed in all sorts of factories which make everything from cars to washers, from beer to whisky, from perfume to artificial fertilizers. They work in office blocks, airports, construction sites, department stores. They

*For the sake of simplicity, 'she' is used throughout in reference to the nurse.

may practise in group services looking after small workplaces, in hospitals or at universities.

As the understanding of the need for health care at work spreads, it is likely that some occupational health nursing input will be thought valuable in most working situations. What is true about all these workplaces is that the first concern of management will usually be the product or the result.

The organization of occupational health services varies and it is evident that there is need for improvement. Sometimes national undertakings have head doctors and nurses who make the policy and undertake a greater or lesser degree of surveillance of other professional staff. The staff may be distributed throughout the country or occasionally around the world. Almost invariably there is a great deal of local autonomy. Sometimes there are no occupational health leaders within an organization and no real structure within a company or group of companies. Commonly, the occupational health nurse has no professional line of responsibility away from her local situation. It follows that she has to ensure that the conditions in which she works are appropriate for the skilled practitioner to be able to do her best. This is very different from other fields of nursing where the situations are agreed by senior colleagues before a nurse takes up post. The time for the occupational health nurse to ensure that the conditions are right is before she takes up post and not at some hoped-for later date when it will all be very much more difficult.

Another reason for specialized training is so that the nurse will not, in good old fashioned nursing style, try to do everybody else's job. In large occupational health units, there will be other specialists. Where she is the sole health care practitioner, she should be able to look after around 1500 people. It is obvious that variables such as shift work or particular hazards make this figure a very rough guide. Where she is the sole health practitioner, she will assess how much she can manage herself, how much she is competent to do well and stop at that, calling for advice from other specialists where necessary. Nursing resources are not limitless and because we expect occupational health nurses to be adequately rewarded it follows that they should be used and use themselves with care. Nurses ought to recognize when they are underemployed (as well as when they are overworked) and not just stretch the jobs to fill the time.

This field has fewer opportunities for promotion to different posts than other nursing fields of work. This has happily not stopped high calibre nurses choosing this most interesting specialty. It should be recognized by employers and medical colleagues that the occupational health nurse requires to have opportunities for career enhancement like any other professional.

Most occupational health nurses – the majority – work without the constant support and advice of a medical practitioner and even those who do will not expect the doctor to be there at all times. So the occupational health nurse has to be an independent and confident practitioner, able to rely to a considerable extent on her own judgement. Nurses who would like to try this field of work can take temporary jobs, working in teams of nurses where they can still utilize skills they already have, to see if they like it. They can then decide whether to undertake enough training to make the work worthwhile as a career.

Some nurses are now offered, during their basic training, the opportunity to learn about occupational health and these nurses will be able to undertake specialist training at the end of their basic course if they wish to choose this specialty. Every nurse, during her basic training, should be given some idea of the problems faced by people at work and what can be done about them. They should also understand the importance that work has in the life of every human being. The patient is not given optimum care in a hospital ward, as an out-patient or by a district nurse at home if he is not shown understanding about his work.

Men and women are equally acceptable in occupational health nursing, but the majority are women. Since the day of the dedicated spinster (in nursing) has passed, we expect most of our nurses to be busy with family problems between the years of 25 and 45. Since this is a specialty that is particularly attractive to nurses over 25, most practitioners are likely to be married. It is, of course, a job that is attractive to married people who would wish to be at home at the usual social times. It is not necessarily wrong for nurses to try to be at home with their spouses but it is desirable that a real interest in the work is added to the social convenience.

Thus it seems sensible for girls to be advised to undertake their specialist training before they begin to have families, so that at the end of this period in their lives they are equipped, with the aid of a refresher course, to take up appropriate and satisfying posts. Married ladies who wish to return to work must have comparable skills to offer before they can be considered with the other professionals.

Occupational health nurses are involved in a range of duties many of which differ from those in other nursing specialties and which are different from any they have encountered already in their careers. They are more in control of the organization of work than in many other circumstances and must be able to plan and use the resources they have. There has lately been recognition that they are able to do this in the Health and Safety Executive's consultative document on occupational health services *The Way Ahead*, published in 1977, which suggested that nurse-based, small occupational health services run by nurses should be tried. Many nurses have been in sole charge of an occupational health nursing service in one factory. It seems surprising that so little experiment has been carried out in nurse-based group services.

Very few nurses work within a team containing all the specialists associated with occupational health. It is clearly not practical for every workplace to have its own complete team. There are many variations in the constitution of the team and many situations where the nurse works as the sole health practitioner. The exact composition of the team is of little importance provided it is appropriate for the work that has to be done.

The nurse required to set up a service without the benefit of other specialists must know when to take specialist advice. It would therefore be true to say that while a nurse can monitor an environment using the simpler tools of occupational hygiene, she will usually require to have the help of an expert hygienist in the first place. While she can assess the problem she may need expert advice on solving it.

Before the actual content of the job of the occupational health nurse can be considered, there needs to be an assessment of what other resources there are in the work situation already that can be used for health and safety matters. The occupational health nurse, with her training and background, is likely to be able to liaise well, perhaps best, with all the others. She is acceptable to both management and workforce and has to ensure that this acceptability is justified, by keeping abreast of developments in the specialty to ensure optimum service at all times.

The practice of occupational health nursing has sometimes been hindered because the nurse was not careful enough to settle the question of accountability before she took up post. There should always be a nursing assessor on the interviewing panel for occupational health nurses to ensure that the candidate has professional support in the requirements for the job. It may be appropriate in one situation for the nurse to be responsible to the personnel manager, and unthinkable in another. The nurse to doctor responsibility is no longer accepted unquestioningly. The nurse who reports to the safety officer seems to have a situation quite impossible to sustain. It will depend on the individual circumstances of the post who is the most appropriate person to be the nurse's reporting authority.

Where an appropriately trained medical adviser is employed, he is most likely to be the leader of the occupational health team. This usually works well and is unexceptional. In all other cases, the occupational health nurse requires to have a suitable reporting authority, that is, one who understands the principles of occupational health, including confidentiality and the right of the nurse to determine her own work content. It will be impossible for her to set about her work properly if the reporting authority is unsuitable.

Where the occupational health nurse is the sole health practitioner she obviously cannot report to another nurse and this is not essential, but whoever it is must be senior enough to be able to influence policy and to give support when necessary. The trained occupational health nurse should be able to recognize an acceptable situation.

THE WORK CONTENT

Some of the duties recognized as being part of the role of an occupational health nurse will be more emphasized in one place than in another or even be done by other people. This is unimportant provided that the jobs are well done. The occupational health nurse must convince herself that all the duties which might be hers are being done well and after that she need not mind whether she does them or somebody else does. The list of duties first issued and constantly updated by the Royal College of Nursing is familiar but it has been shown that nurses still do not always recognize the particular duties that might constitute part of their jobs. Some nurses have thought they should stick to the duties common to nurses in any situation. Other nurses have claimed expertise in a wide range of duties without really understanding what they all involve. The job must contain elements of prevention and the nurse should concentrate most on the aspects of the work in which she is expert. It is equally true that the arrangements for first aid and treatment should be in the hands of the nurse and it is probably wise if she is practically involved. Most occupational health nurses are involved in treatment at different levels as part of their work.

Even in very highly organized occupational health services it is essential to have a number of first aiders in the workplace. They may be used in a major emergency, for standing in in the absence of the nurse or for supplying routine first aid. They should be considered as an important extension of the occupational health service and come under the control of the nurse. These first aiders will enjoy her influence during training and practice as well as her direct supervision. She will not achieve the complete confidence of the workforce if she does not have skill in first aid practice, teaching and organization. In planning a treatment service, it is wise for the nurse to decide on a level of treatment which can be carried out safely at all times, rather than stretch the programme beyond the safe level. If she is required to stitch a wound only twice a year, she is better not to do it at all. On the other hand, if the industry is likely to encounter special problems such as foreign bodies in the eyes, the occupational health nurse must become skilled and competent in their removal.

The workforce is likely to accept advice relating to prevention more easily from the nurse who meets his need for skilled and immediate treatment. Everybody can appreciate speed, care and comfort in treatment and in the work situation it is almost impossible for the nurse to be respected if she is used in a purely preventive role. For most nurses, too, the desire to help care for people is not satisfied merely by giving advice and teaching.

The occupational nurse has a knowledge of the workers that is one of the greatest assets to health care. It also means that she is well known to the workers. She risks boring them away from her good influence if she launches into a health education attack at every opportunity. There may occasionally be opportunities for health education to groups of workers, for example apprentices during their first month at work or workers who are beginning new jobs with new hazards; but there will probably be far more opportunities on a face-to-face basis where the nurse can allay fears and also give some advice.

Problems such as alcoholism, obesity and smoking are not subjects peculiar to the work situation. In some neighbourhoods these subjects for health education are not dealt with by other agencies and so it is sometimes necessary to launch a programme to advise about these dangers. More often, what is available locally should be drawn to the workers' attention.

The occupational health nurse need not assume competence in all these difficult and complicated areas but she must concentrate on matters peculiar to the work situation, such as care of the skin or eyes. It is very much her responsibility and should be within her field of competence. She must seek opportunities and skills to communicate on matters such as these on which she is expert. A time of failure when all the education and safety measures have not prevented an accident and when the worker is injured is a fruitful time to try a little gentle advice.

Communication at work

The giving of general advice or more specific advice about health at work is different from the communication of necessary information to management and workers. In most occupational health situations, the nurse is paid by the employer. It is well recognized and accepted that this does nothing to alter the confidential nurse/worker or nurse/client relationship but it does mean that management holds the money needed for improvements. The nurse should be able to show to management the problems that require attention so that finance can be obtained.

Workers' representatives, notably safety representatives, as well as management will wish to know the facts about dangerous substances or occurrences. There is plenty of opportunity nowadays for them to be given the facts at work. If this is not done, in their own working situation, they may receive training from their parent union. In Great Britain, employed persons may also seek advice from the Health and Safety Executive.

Care is needed in explaining to workers exactly what is happening to them or may happen to them in relation to the materials they use. They must not be misinformed, or kept in ignorance but should not be unnecessarily worried. This is sometimes a difficult balance to achieve. The good nurse has always believed that giving advice was part of her duty and is therefore less nervous of militant questioning than those who are less well prepared. She often has to try to explain the facts to workers returning from hospital appointments unsure of what they have been told, and has plenty of practice in interpretation of this kind.

The skills of communication are essential to the occupational health nurse whose success will depend upon them. Some nurses may confuse communication with over-communication and soon debase this currency.

Good communicators try to learn the acceptable methods of communication for a particular situation. Matters of general importance to health may be better covered on television or radio programmes than by the nurse at work, but she should be prepared to follow up and help workers to relate advice to their own situation.

Documentation

The nurse is sometimes required to set up a record-keeping system and this should be undertaken with control. Strange record systems have been set up in a great many occupational health services – some people seem quite unable to accept anybody else's record system and like to devise more complicated ones, using more paper and taking more time to systematize than anyone has to spare. When asked the reason for all this, they will say that it is always helpful in health supervision of the workers, for medical reasons and legal reasons or to make it easier for cross-reference and for research. Usually these reasons are not good enough to justify the result. It is high time that record systems in occupational health services at least could be compared with each other. We have heard a great deal about the need to keep records confidential and this is essential. In fact, some of the record systems are so obscure and complicated that confidentiality is the least of the problem. It is really quite difficult to use the information when necessary.

The nurse working on her own will know the statutory requirements and decide carefully how much more needs to be undertaken. When this is decided by an assessment of priorities, it should be accurately completed at all times. An important part of care is attention to accuracy and careful completion of every task. It is terrifying for clients to believe that the nurse can't find the note, didn't know what happened the last time and appears likely to be about to make a mistake. Therefore the occupational health nurse setting up a record system should devise the simplest possible, eliminating as far as she can too much writing or the possibility of error.

Workplace visits

A great deal of nonsense has been talked about the role of the nurse in environmental control. Encouragement has been given to her to go striding about the workshops, busily making measurements. This has naturally been resisted by some employers who have suggested that the nurse should stay in her own department awaiting clients. The truth, as so often, lies between the two. The nurse and usually a considerable number of other people in any workplace, notably safety representatives, are capable of noting during a walk through the works whether the guards are on the machines, whether there has been oil spilt on the floor, that the fire exits are free, that the exhaust ventilation is turned on when necessary and that the lighting is good. There is no mystique about such observations – almost anybody can be trained to make them.

A nurse can and should learn to use the minor tools of the hygienist to monitor environmental changes. She is not a hygienist unless she chooses to become one by further training, but she, among other practitioners, can draw attention to a hazard. The important thing about having a nurse walking about the workplace is that she, probably better than anyone else can observe changes in individuals, keep a friendly eye on those who never seek attention even when they should and familiarize herself with the actual work done by each individual. It is really by her knowledge of the workers in their work situation that the nurse makes her contribution to occupational health and safety. By understanding their work, she is able to help people. She will know when they are unfit to carry on with their jobs and when they require to change jobs after illness or injury. She will be able to relate their work to them and thus care for them to optimum standards.

A friendly liaison kept up with all sections of the workforce has to be maintained at an acceptable level – never spilling into familiarity or retreating into isolation. This situation makes it easier for workers to take advice and it is part of the delight of the job, that the delicacy in relationships makes for success or failure.

The health department

The management of the occupational health department is usually in the hands of the nurse. This department may be called by any of a number of titles and what it is called seems to be of little importance in practice. There are wide varieties in size and extremely wide varieties in equipment, according to the content of the work of the particular occupational health service, the budget allowed and the personal preferences of the personnel. The temptation to air preferences without any eye to cost or utility should be resisted.

There are a number of essentials which should be kept in mind. The department must be clean, which involves the arrangement of regular competent daily cleaning. Clients must be treated in a dignified manner, that is, there must be privacy. Conversations must not be overheard. The records of individuals must be kept out of sight of prying eyes. Materials should be appropriate to the treatment given – sterilized where necessary, regularly supplied and maintained and nothing should be lying about which could cause danger in untrained hands.

The nurse's office must never be allowed to degenerate into a sloppy visiting parlour for special friends to drop in to chat. It should be easy of access to those who need it and forbidden to those who do not. This is true of all health departments whether in occupational health departments or in hospital. The clients must feel that the place exists for them and their needs and that they are not a subsidiary nuisance to friends of the nurse who are being entertained. The constant client should not be greeted more effusively than the seldom attender who is less well known to the nurse.

It is easy to work to high standards when observed by fellow professionals and much more difficult in isolation. On the other hand, many independent practitioners enjoy working to self-imposed standards which would be difficult for colleagues anywhere to better.

The occupational health nurse will not always have the chance of ensuring that her department is on the ground floor with a very easy access to everybody, has proper waiting space, the most up-to-date equipment or exactly what she would want. It is within her scope to maintain the highest standards in the situation she has accepted. For the best occupational health nurses, one of the satisfactions of their work is the fact that the vigilant correcting eye is their own.

Liaison with other health agencies

The occupational health nurse liaises with a number of people outside the workplace in which she finds herself. The local hospital is an obvious example. She must make it clear to the accident and emergency department personnel what actually happens in the workplace. Hospitals and other health practitioners cannot be expected to take on trust a nurse whom they do not know, whose functions they cannot imagine and who practices in a place beyond their experience. Hospital practitioners often do not know very much about other people's working situations, and do not realize that the nurse in the workplace may, without the advice of a doctor, treat as many casualties as a nurse in an accident and emergency department. The patients may not be in such severe condition but may be in larger numbers.

Depending on the area, it may or may not be easy to get to know the general practitioners. In large places such as London, where workers scatter to homes in widely different areas, it is more difficult than in a smaller town where they are all known. It is particularly useful when general practitioners have part-time occupational health appointments because this does something to increase their awareness of what happens at work. Nurses, on the whole, do not make enough use of each other in different specialties, although nurses at work are rather better at this because it is more important for them. From time to time health visitors, school nurses and hospital nurses are a necessary extension from the work situation. A worker who has problems in coping with illness within his family may be able to continue at work because the occupational nurse is able to help him to rally all the aids available to him.

Visits to workers who are off sick in their homes are sometimes undertaken by occupational health nurses. In most situations it is more sensible to liaise with the health visitor or the district nurse or the other practitioners responsible for care in the home. There is no guarantee that the worker who sees the nurse in a friendly fashion at work wishes to see her in his home.

Invitations to visit the place of work should be offered, after clearing this with management, to other health care practitioners, so that they can see the circumstances in which the occupational health nurse works. If the nurse at work is too ashamed of her working situation to invite other health practitioners to see it, it is clearly not good enough for the workers to use.

Screening procedures

Most nurses at some stage in their career are involved in carrying out some screening procedures. This is true from the earliest days in training when student nurses occupy rather a lot of their time testing urine. In most situations, these are carried out as part of a diagnostic process, as part of a medical examination or as progress monitoring. Nearly always the need for screening is established by a physician. There is nothing mystical about screening procedures and almost anybody can be trained to undertake parts of this work. Nowadays, when screening procedures are fashionable and frequently carried out, more and more are undertaken by nurses. There is no harm in this, even if it is an unprecedented extension of the nurse's role, provided the following conditions apply:

1. That she is thoroughly trained in the procedure, including an assessment of competence other than her own.
2. That the physician who has delegated the procedures is satisfied of her competence.
3. That she feels confident and is satisfied that undertaking the procedures constitute no breach of her conditions of employment and that she is protected in case of error.
4. That she is given in this, as in all other procedures, opportunity for updating and refreshment.
5. That screening procedures do not take up too much of the time available for health supervision and other areas of her work.

The nurse on her own may decide that she wishes to instigate preplacement health interviews with screening procedures. She should stop and think before trying to set up a complicated system just like the one she left at her last job. If no good reason can be put forward for instigating any procedure, it should be discarded. It is unpleasant for workers or potential workers to be given a series of tests without much explanation, rather like an obstacle race with ever-changing rules. Whatever procedures are adopted, it is necessary to carry them out with full explanation to the client and considerable delicacy in practice.

THE NEED FOR SPECIALISM IN OCCUPATIONAL HEALTH NURSING

Some sort of occupational health nursing has been going on for about a century and it has been a misunderstood and maligned specialty, not even recognized as such for many years. There are a number of reasons for this.

A small proportion of nurses has been employed in this work and an even smaller number were excellent. Those who were employed were and are likely to be independent people, not requiring the shelter of hospital or tightly structured nursing service.

People in general, and the health professionals in particular, have tended to admire more the nurse who offered obvious tender loving care, coupled with technical competence in the dramatic situations of serious illness and recovery. Specialized training in this field has been difficult to come by, but is becoming easier nowadays. Financial and other sacrifice has often had to be made by nurses who pursued a career in occupational health nursing because they themselves recognized the need to be trained. The minority who, through all sorts of hardship, managed to become trained considered themselves to be an elite. Since the first aim of an elite is seldom to enlighten the masses, specialized training did not become as easily accessible as it should. Those in practice, other than the trained minority, thought that specialized training was not necessary or out of reach, mainly because they were acceptable without it.

The unique thing about occupational health nursing is that the nurse observes the same population for all her working life in any particular place. Patients go home from hospital, district nurses visit only when there are problems and health visitors visit, on the whole, at specific times in the life of a family. The occupational nurse's knowledge of individual workers is enormous. If she is accepted she will know about their home backgrounds and indeed about their joys and sorrows. She uses her understanding of the firm's fortunes, the possible dangers of the process and the changing of social conditions to give an optimum caring service. Seldom can health care practitioners have more knowledge, sometimes spread over many years, of the client's background, health and social pattern than the occupational health nurse. She may not indulge in grand scale counselling but her well-informed attention is valuable.

A part of any caring process is to ensure, if possible, that the person being cared for can eventually take care of himself. Nurses have tended, in many situations, to take away the right of patients to determine for themselves. It should be for the occupational health nurse to pursue the encouragement of self-help. If workers are in full possession of the facts, and providing that self-determination will not hurt other people, much should be left to them. Where it is impossible for individuals to care for themselves or to have their own way, the nurse will be there to comfort and support.

Legislation concerned with health and safety at work is increasing. Less has been said about caring for workers who don't have optimum health in any case and where the job, though safe, is monotonous, drab, boring and non-essential. Where workers do not, in these circumstances, feel important to anybody, the occupational health nurse should aim to encourage them to care for themselves in a positive fashion by making them aware of the facts, providing explanation where necessary, comfort and interest always and a sound repair job when all else fails.

FURTHER READING

Health and Safety Commission (1977) *Occupational Health Services: The Way Ahead.* (Prevention and Health series.) London, HMSO.

Permanent Commission and International Association on Occupational Health (1969) *Report of the Nursing Sub-committee on the Nurse's Contribution to the Health of the Worker 1966–1969.*

Permanent Commission and International Association on Occupational Health (1973) *Report of the Nursing Sub-committee on the Nurse's Contribution to the Health of the Worker 1971–1973: Report No 2: Education of the Nurse.*

Royal College of Nursing (1975) *An Occupational Health Nursing Service: A Handbook for Nurses and Employers.* London, Royal College of Nursing.

14. TRAINING IN OCCUPATIONAL HEALTH AND SAFETY

Suzette Gauvain

The concept of professional training in occupational health and safety is relatively new. The professional disciplines described in this chapter are: doctors, nurses, occupational hygienists and safety professionals. In many cases they are fighting for acceptance amongst other professionals, managements and unions. Usually little is understood of what it is aimed to achieve. A team approach to their work and to training is required.

The purpose of professionals in occupational health and safety is to try to achieve and maintain a safe and healthy working environment for the workers concerned. The products manufactured by industries should be safe for the users. Those who live in the neighbourhood of the factories should not be affected by pollution. To achieve these objectives training in occupational health and safety is essential.

The functions of each professional group in the team need clarification. The structure and content of training programmes need constant re-assessment. Two main elements are essential in training. Practical instruction 'on the job' and academic training in a university department or departments with adequate resources, in terms of qualified instructors and equipment, commensurate with the task.

The degree of professional expertise in all disciplines may be considered in three layers: (1) consultants or specialists who may either head a team or become advisers to the organization or organizations concerned; (2) members of the team or heads or directors of small teams who may require less highly specialized training than the first group; (3) members of the team who need only basic training.

In addition to these groups there may be individuals or groups who require even more specialized training in particular aspects of occupational health and safety at an even higher level in such topics as epidemiology, toxicology, clinical occupational pulmonary disease, clinical occupational dermatology or, for example, in acoustic or ventilation engineering.

Training may be provided by industries and employing organizations on an in-service basis on introductory, continuation and special courses; by professional societies; and by academic departments of occupational health and safety, who themselves require highly trained professional staff.

The pattern of training required will obviously vary, but the aim should be to ensure that the training should be appropriate to the functions of the individual professional disciplines and the level of the job in the team.

The organization of academic training may be on a full-time basis, for a fixed period; part-time on a modular basis (blocks of days, weeks or months) or on a day-release pattern.

Historical development in Britain

Legislative action, largely influenced by enlightened reformers, has done much to improve the health of workers in Britain. Action started with the Health and Morals of Apprentices Act of 1802, and a further step forward came in 1833 with the first Factory Act when the first four Factory Inspectors were appointed. The Factories Act of 1844 permitted Superintending Inspectors of Factories to appoint surgeons to certify that children starting work in textile factories had the appearance and development appropriate to the age of 9 years. In 1898 Thomas Legge was appointed as the first Medical Inspector of Factories.

Industrial medicine was a very late development in the medical field. Industrial medical officers, in some instances, were originally employed not necessarily to prevent illness or to protect the health of the employees, but to protect employers from legislative claims against them from workmen under the Workman's Compensation Act of 1897.

The certifying surgeons, who were later called Appointed Factory Doctors had certain statutory duties, but as a result of the recommendations of the sub-committee of the Industrial Health Advisory Committee in 1966 were 'replaced by a much smaller number of doctors with a wider range of duties and more expertise in occupational health matters'. This small group of doctors with more expertise were formed from the Medical Inspectors of Factories who had become the medical staff of the Medical Services Division of the Department of Employment and provided the basis for the Employment Medical Advisory Service in 1973.

In 1899 the first Engineering Specialist and in 1902 the first Electrical Specialist were appointed to the Factory Inspectorate. The total number of Factory Inspectors has now increased to many hundreds and specialist inspectors have been recruited in different specialties such as construction, fire, mechanical, civil and electrical engineering.

In 1972 the Employment Medical Advisory Service Act received the Royal Assent and the report of the Robens Committee was published. As a result of the recommendations of the Robens Committee, the Health and Safety at Work etc. Act was laid before Parliament and received the Royal Assent in 1974. Under the Health and Safety at Work Act, the Health and Safety Commission was formed with its executive, the Health and Safety Executive, in which all the Inspectorate have been brought together and are represented on the Management Board of the Health and Safety Executive with the Employment Advisory Service as the medical arm. This brought official recognition of the multidisciplinary needs for an occupational safety and health team.

Present situation

Following this brief historical introduction, this chapter is designed to provide current information concerning the training of professional staff in occupational health services with particular reference to the United Kingdom and to indicate changes that are likely or should, in the opinion of the author, influence developments in the future.

The professional staff whose training in occupational health will be discussed are doctors, nurses, occupational hygienists and safety professionals – engineers, members of the inspectorates and safety advisers. Information on the training available for ergonomists, psychologists, bio-medical engineers and background information on the training of other professionals already mentioned can be obtained from *Occupational Health, a Guide to Sources of Information* (Gauvain, 1974).

FUNCTIONS

When discussing training it is essential to relate this to the functions of the professional disciplines undergoing training.

The doctor in industry

The functions of doctors have been defined by the British Medical Association (1975) in their policy document, *The Doctor in Industry*, which described the duties which doctors holding appointments in occupational medicine may have to perform as follows:

1. The effect of health on work
   - *a.* Advice to employees on all health matters relating to their working capacity.
   - *b.* Examination of applicants for employment and advice to their placement.
   - *c.* Immediate treatment of medical and surgical emergencies occurring at the place of employment.
   - *d.* Examinations and continued observation of persons returning to work after absence due to illness or accidents and advice on suitable work.
   - *e.* Health supervision of all employees with special reference to (i) young persons, (ii) married women, (iii) elderly persons and (iv) disabled persons.
2. The effect of work on health
   - *a.* Responsibility for the nursing and first aid services.
   - *b.* The study of the work and working environment and their effects on the health of the employees.
   - *c.* Periodical examinations of persons exposed to special hazards in respect of their employment.

d. Advice to managements regarding:
   i. The working environment in relation to health.
   ii. Occurrence and significance of hazards.
   iii. Accident prevention.
   iv. Statutory requirements in relation to health.

e. Medical supervision of health and hygiene of staff and facilities, with particular reference to canteens, kitchens etc. and those working on the production of foods or drugs for sale to the public.

f. The arranging and carrying out of such educational work in respect of the health fitness and hygiene of the employees as may be desirable and practicable.

g. Advice to those committees within the organization which are responsible for the health and safety and welfare of the employees.

The Employment Medical Advisory Service

The Employment Medical Advisory Service which has a staff of 140 occupational health doctors and occupational health nurses defines its work and functions in an introduction to the Employment Medical Advisory Service, as follows:

The Employment Medical Advisory Service (EMAS) is an organization of doctors and nurses whose job is to give advice about occupational health. It was set up in 1973 as part of the Department of Employment, and in 1975 became part of the Health and Safety Executive (HSE). The legislation governing EMAS is the Health and Safety at Work etc. Act 1974, and the Factories Act 1961 as amended by the Employment Medical Advisory Service Act 1972.

Working conditions can cause ill health or make it worse. Employers, work people and the self-employed have a duty under the Health and Safety at Work etc. Act 1974 to see that illness caused by work is kept to a minimum. Any employed or self-employed worker, trade union representative or employer can look to the Employment Medical Advisory Service for help with an occupational health problem.

The two main functions of EMAS are

1. Helping to prevent ill health caused by work;
2. Advising people with health problems about the type of work which suits them or which they should avoid on health grounds.

In carrying out these functions EMAS is responsible for:

1. Advice to the inspectorates and other policy divisions of HSE on the occupational health aspects of health and safety regulations and codes of practice;
2. The regular medical examination of persons employed on processes known to be hazardous. Where these examinations are prescribed by health and safety regulations, they must either be carried out by EMAS or delegated to doctors specially appointed for the purpose.

Where regular examinations are not prescribed, EMAS may undertake them if there is a known risk, and other satisfactory arrangements cannot be made;

3. Other medical examinations, investigations and surveys of workers in connection with their employment;
4. Advice to the inspectorate and other policy divisions of the Health and Safety Executive and to employers, trade unions, employees and others concerned on the occupational health aspects of poisonous substances, immunological disorders, physical hazards (such as noise, vibrations, ionizing radiations and dust) and mental stress. This advice involves, amongst other things, taking part in setting standards of exposure to particular substances and physical hazards;
5. Occupational health research – identifying and assessing health hazards, planning and mounting population and other studies, commissioning studies from the Medical Research Council and other bodies and co-operating in studies mounted by industry;
6. Advice on the provisions of occupational, medical, nursing and first aid services;
7. Advice on the medical aspects of rehabilitation for employment and of training for and placing in employment, principally to the Employment Service Agency, Training Services Agency and Careers Service.

EMAS does not provide medical treatment. People found to be in need of treatment are referred to their own doctors or, where appropriate, direct to hospital.

Occupational health nurses

The Royal College of Nursing supply the following list of duties which fully trained occupational health nurses could perform:

1. Health assessment in relation to an individual worker and the job to be performed.
2. Noting normal standards of health and fitness and any departure or variation from these standards.
3. Referring to the doctor such cases which in the opinion of the nurse require further investigation and medical as distinct from nursing assessment.
4. Health supervision of vulnerable groups.
5. Routine visits to and surveys of the working environment, and informing as necessary the appropriate expert when a particular problem requires further specialized investigation.
6. Employees health counselling.
7. Health education activities in relation to groups of workers.
8. The assessment of injuries/illness occurring at work and treatment or referrals as appropriate.

9. Occupational health nurses also assume responsibility for the organization and administration of occupational health services, and the control and safe keeping of non-statutory personal health records.
10. Where a full-time medical officer with occupational health training and management experience is employed, the doctor assumes overall responsibility for the leadership and organization of the occupational health service. As a matter of principle in such organizations nursing staff organized in hierarchies work to one nurse leader who is responsible for the overall organization and administration of the occupational health nursing services. The most 'senior' nurse should work in close partnership with the doctor in charge.
11. Nurses also adopt a teaching role in respect of the training of first aid personnel, and the organization of emergency services.

It can be seen that some of the functions, defined as appropriate to these two professional groups, occupational physicians, (doctors in industry or occupational health doctors) and occupational health nurses, overlap. If these definitions and functions are accepted, training must aim at the fulfilment of these functions.

Occupational hygienists

Hall (1974) defined occupational hygiene as the measurement, evaluation and control of health risks in working environments. He stated that: 'Hygienists have to utilize knowledge from the fields of chemistry and physics, toxicology and applied physiology and engineering (particularly industrial ventilation). A fully qualified occupational hygienist is usually a science or engineering graduate with wide experience and a higher qualification in the subject. Some hygienists specialize in one particular field, not necessarily restricted to occupational environments, e.g. acoustic engineers, health physicists (dealing mainly with ionizing radiations), or aerosol scientists. An occupational hygiene assistant is a technician or trainee, often with a technical rather than an academic qualification.'

In other words, though an occupational hygienist when fully trained is a highly skilled scientist, there is no standard basic training requirement as there is for doctors and nurses who must be fully registered practitioners in their own disciplines before embarking on specialized postgraduate training in occupational health either as a doctor or a nurse.

A hygienist may have been trained originally in one of a variety of different scientific disciplines, but he or she must have attained an academic standard of sufficient distinction to be admitted to a postgraduate training course.

Safety professionals

Safety professionals include members of labour inspectorates, and, in the case of the United Kingdom, inspectors in the Health and Safety Executive, safety engineers and safety advisers.

Inspectors

Robens (1972; para 201) stated, 'Inspectors at various levels assist in framing and revision of legislation; undertake investigations, surveys and research; participate in the preparation of advisory literature; liaise with manufacturers of plant and equipment; sit on various kinds of technical committees; deliver lectures; and participate in conferences at home and overseas. But the main day-to-day activity of the majority of inspectors is the inspection of work places'.

He summed up his recommendations as follows for the planned unified inspectorates, now in being in the Health and Safety Executive:

1. 'That the new inspectorate should be geared to an explicit policy which has as its prime objective the prevention of accidents and ill health and the promotion of progressively better standards at work through the provision of information and skilled advice to industry and commerce.'
2. 'That the provision of advice and the enforcement of sanctions where necessary, should continue to be regarded as two inseparable elements of inspection work'.

He recommended that in addition to in-service training more resources should be devoted to training which should include management techniques, industrial psychology and ergonomics and that selected inspectors should attend an academic diploma course on health and safety at the Department of Safety and Hygiene at the University at Aston.

Safety engineering

Atherley (1974) states: 'Safety engineering encompasses a number of well-established specializations in engineering:

a. Safety Technology; one example is the highly specialized inspection of pressure vessels done by certain insurance companies.
b. Safety and Reliability Engineering; this involves making predictions about failure in plant and machinery and has been developed to a considerable degree of specialization by the UKAEA Safety and Reliability Inspectorate.
c. Safety Design Engineering; there is a growing body of engineering knowledge with specific applications in safety. Examples are the design of primary safety in motor cars; the design of fail-safe mechanisms; and tamper-proof mechanisms in guarding.'

He defines occupational safety as advice to management on the design of plants, processes and equipment; the specification of safe systems of work; attention to legal requirements; committee work and joint consultation on safety matters; safety training for management and workers; investigation of accidents; and generally the advancement of all aspects of accident prevention.

General inspectors, like occupational hygienists, may be recruited from a wide variety of academic backgrounds in the arts and sciences. Specialist inspectors will be recruited from those who are particularly qualified either as civil, mechanical, mining, electrical or other specialist engineering backgrounds or other appropriate scientific backgrounds such as physics or chemistry.

Safety advisers to industrial organizations may be engineers or other professionally trained personnel selected from without or within the organization, either already trained in safety, or selected for further training in this specialty.

From these definitions of the functions of the members of the occupational health and safety team it is clear that occupational health and safety in all these professional disciplines is a postgraduate study. Is this necessarily right? Should education on the basic concepts of health and safety begin at the undergraduate stage of training? The situation may be altered in the future. A factor which may influence this may be, that, as a consequence of the Health and Safety at Work Act 1974, 8 million 'new entrants' comprising workers in hopsitals, universities, schools and the self-employed come under the legal provisions of the Act. In the future, education in health and safety may well become part of the curriculum in schools and universities; for undergraduate medical students in hospitals more emphasis may be placed on teaching occupational medicine, so that they may, at least, have a basic introduction to the subject at this period (Gauvain, 1970). The functions of the members on the occupational health team having been defined, it is important to consider the actual work being undertaken by occupational health services in Britain.

Survey of occupational health services by the Employment Medical Advisory Service 1976

The Employment Medical Advisory Service undertook a survey of a stratified sample of industries to obtain a general view of the current situation regarding the provision of occupational health services in Britain and to provide a framework for the planning of future research. The survey revealed that the most frequent activity undertaken was the treatment of acute emergencies, minor illnesses and injuries, and the next most frequent activity was pre-employment, pre-placement medical examination/screening procedures, but that in general there was less emphasis on prevention or epidemiological investigations. Reasons for this are likely to be that management requires an immediately available treatment service. If the industry is some distance from a hospital out-patient department there may be added need to provide an efficient emergency service on the spot. However, it is worth considering whether more emphasis on prevention might lessen the need for treatment services. A conclusion from the findings of the survey was that properly planned studies were needed to obtain objective information about the relative benefits and costs of providing for the treatment of occupational injuries within the occupational health services and within the National Health Service.

The survey also showed, after correction of sampling bias that about 85 per cent of all firms in the survey, employing about 34 per cent of the workforce, had no occupational health service other than first aiders employed for less than 10 hours a week.

Small firms (up to 250 employees) usually did not have any medical or nursing service. Large firms mostly had some form of medical and/or nursing service and very large firms (over 1000 employees) usually employed both doctors and nurses.

The sample included 3383 firms. Of the 106 doctors employed full-time, 42 per cent had specific additional occupational medical qualifications (diplomas or degrees); 98 per cent of these doctors were in charge of their own services. Of the 612 doctors employed part-time, 13 per cent had similar specific occupational medical qualifications; 81 per cent were in charge of their own services. Of the 764 registered nurses employed full-time, 20 per cent had the occupational health nursing certificate; 21 per cent were in charge of their own occupational health services. Of the 203 registered nurses employed part-time, 17 per cent had occupational health nursing certificates and 23 per cent of the part-timers were in charge of their own services. More than 25 per cent of the state enrolled nurses appeared to be in day-to-day charge of their own occupational health services.

The specially qualified doctors and nurses tended to work together and the less well qualified nurses tended to be working with less well qualified doctors or indeed without any regular medical supervision.

For those who are familiar with occupational health services in Britain these findings will cause little suprise; but as a result, a number of recommendations have been made in the discussion document, *Occupational Health Service; The Way Ahead* (Health and Safety Commission, 1977a) in which the results of this survey are published. The recommendations include suggestions that epidemiological surveys and other studies designed to identify and measure the effects of occupational hazards should be pursued with more participation by doctors and nurses employed in industry; that occupational health services of large firms should be extended to smaller firms and that the joint provision of specialized occupational health services for firms within the same industry should be considered. A further suggestion was that a project to evaluate the practicability of entrusting the organization and provision of local occupational health services to fully qualified occupational health nurses should be set up.

These are all practical suggestions for improving occupational health services within the country. However, to be effective it is suggested that professional staff who have not already had training in occupational health may require this.

Need for training

Managements and professional staffs in industry may be influenced on their own need for training in health and safety by proposed new legislative measures, which include the Safety Representatives and Safety Committee Regulations 1977. These regulations have been set up by the Health and Safety Commission under the Health and Safety at Work etc. Act 1974 and became operative on 1 October 1978. In addition to the Regulations they have provided a Code of Practice on Safety Representatives and Guidance Notes. The Safety Representatives have a number of important functions amongst which are the investigation of potential hazards and dangerous occurrences and the causes of accidents in the workplace; the investigation of complaints by an employee that the Safety Representative represents relating to that employee's health, safety or welfare at work and attendance at meetings of Safety Committees in connection with any of the functions which have been listed in the publication of the Health and Safety Commission (1977b). The Medical Advisory Committee of the Health and Safety Commission has set up a sub-committee on first aid, the terms of reference of which are: 'to review the existing statutory and other arrangements for occupational first aid and, in particular, the arrangements relating to training, and to formulate in consultation with organizations concerned recommendations for the future.' The recommendations of this sub-committee, when they are published, are likely to have a far-reaching effect on the training of first aiders and on the responsibilities of occupational physicians and occupational health nurses in this respect.

Approximate numbers of occupational health and safety professionals

When discussing the work of occupational health services, it is useful to have an estimate of the numbers of doctors, nurses, occupational hygienists and safety professionals employed in occupational health and safety. Unfortunately, it is only possible to make approximate estimates. It is believed that there are between 400 and 500 doctors working full-time in occupational health services and university departments in the United Kingdom and between 3000 and 4000 doctors working part-time, most of whom are general practitioners. The Society of Occupational Medicine had a total membership of 1293 on 1 October 1977 of which 1056 were ordinary members. In the United States of America it is believed that there are 2000 doctors working full-time in occupational medicine and 10 000 part-time. Estimates suggest that there are 9000 registered and state enrolled nurses working in occupational health services in the United Kingdom and that there are approximately 150 to 200 occupational hygiene graduates in the United Kingdom and upwards of 1500 in the United States. It is known that there are approximately 1500 Inspectors in the Health and Safety Executive, of which approximately 700 are general inspectors, 170 specialist inspectors respectively in the

Factory Inspectorate. The numbers of other safety professionals are unknown.

TRAINING IN OCCUPATIONAL HEALTH AND SAFETY

In Great Britain five university departments as well as the Institute of Advanced Nursing Education are known to provide academic training for occupational health and safety professionals. However, the professionals taught, and the courses of training provided, differ between the universities. Information concerning the relevant syllabuses of training should be sought by potential trainees from the university registrars or the heads (professors or directors) of the departments concerned, unless otherwise stated.

1. The University of Aston in Birmingham, Safety and Hygiene Group, Gosta Green, Birmingham B4 7ET.

The Safety and Hygiene Group provides courses for safety professionals. *First*, a one year Master of Science degree course lasting four terms full-time in occupational safety and hygiene, and it is proposed to provide a part-time Master of Science course over 4 years. Enquiries should be made of the course tutor. *Second*, a Diploma in Safety and Hygiene lasting 2 terms (6 months) and run twice a year. Enquiries should be made to the diploma course tutor.

In addition to the safety professionals attending the diploma course, it may be possible for doctors and nurses to attend parts of this course which is run in modular format.

2. The University Department of Community and Occupational Medicine, the Medical School, Ninewells, Dundee DD1 9SY Scotland.

The University Department provides the following courses in the Wolfson Institute of Occupational Health in the University of Dundee:

	Course	Duration		Frequency
1.	Diploma in Industrial Health course	(10 weeks)	–	Annually
2.	Certificate in Industrial Health course	(10 weeks)	–	Annually
3.	Occupational Health Nursing Certificate course	(6 months)	–	Bi-annually
4.	Occupational Health Nursing Refresher course	(1 day)	–	Annually
5.	Basic Occupational Health Nursing course	(4 weeks)	–	Annually
6.	Medical Training Course for Divers	(2 weeks)	–	Bi-annually
7.	Recent Advances in Occupational Health course	(1 week)	–	Annually
8.	Environmental Health course	(3 days)	–	Annually

3. The Department of Occupational Health, University of Manchester, Stopford Building, Oxford Road, Manchester M13 9PT.

The Department of Occupational Health provides courses for doctors and for occupational hygienists; an 18 month part-time day-release course to doctors leading to a diploma in Industrial Health and for occupational hygienists a part or full-time course lasting one or two years leading to a Master of Science degree in occupational hygiene.

4. The Department of Occupational Health and Hygiene, 21 Claremont Place, University of Newcastle upon Tyne NE2 4AN.
The Department of Occupational Health and Hygiene runs a part-time day-release course for doctors leading to a Diploma in Industrial Health and a Master of Science Degree course (one calendar year full-time) for occupational hygienists.

5. The TUC Centenary Institute of Occupational Health, The London School of Hygiene and Tropical Medicine, Keppel Street (Gower Street), London WC1E 7HT.
The following postgraduate courses are available:

Occupational Hygiene M.Sc degree course	–	Full-time over one calendar year (Sept-Sept) Part-time over 2 years (commencing Sept).
Diploma in Occupational Hygiene	–	Day-release over 2 years (commencing Sept).
Occupational Medicine M.Sc degree course in Occupational Medicine	–	Full-time over one academic year (Sept-July) Part-time over 2 years (commencing Sept).
Diploma in Industrial Health course	–	3 months full-time (Sept-Dec) One academic year full time (Sept-Jul) Day-release over 15 months (commencing Sept).

Higher degree courses are also available in Occupational Medicine. Occupational Hygiene and Occupational Health. The Institute offers training programmes leading to the Ph.D. and M.Phil. for science and medical graduates, occupational health nurses, occupational psychologists and occupational therapists who hold the equivalent of a first or second class honours degree.

6. The Institue of Advanced Nursing Education, the Royal College of Nursing of the United Kingdom, Henrietta Place, Cavendish Square, London WIM 0AB.
The Institute of Advanced Nursing Education provides courses leading to the Occupational Health Nursing Certificate (OHNC), a full-time course

lasting 6½ months, consisting of part 1 (1 month, a foundation course) and part 2 (5½ months, certificate course); day-release courses are also available. In addition to day-release two blocks of up to 5 days full-time attendance are required over an 18 month period for part 1 and part 2 (OHNC). Courses are also run in a number of centres outside London. State enrolled nurses are able to take the part 1 course.

A one academic year course is in preparation for the Occupational Health Nursing Teacher Certificate of the Royal College of Nursing of the United Kingdom.

Courses available in Britain provide training facilities for doctors, nurses, occupational hygienists and safety professionals, but the geographical location of training facilities is widely scattered and the facilities are limited in each training centre.

The definitions provided of the functions of the Health and Safety Professionals clearly indicate some overlapping of these functions and therefore of their training needs. Are the facilities available distributed most effectively and most economically? It may be far more economical and effective in the use of teaching time to devise modular training courses – that is modules of days or weeks devoted to certain topics of common interest that may be attended by all or some of the groups of professional trainees. The TUC Centenary Institute of Occupational Health in its teaching programmes for doctors and occupational hygienists has created modular training programmes at Master of Science and Diploma levels based on the common needs of both professional groups, but safety professionals and occupational health nurses are not eligible for this training programme. The aims of training courses for each professional group need careful definition (Gauvain and Schilling, 1973). Provided that these aims are adhered to and achieved there should be no disadvantage to combined training, certainly at a common level of knowledge. More specialized training needed by particular professional disciplines is probably best taught separately. This, also, can be in modular format devoted to the individual disciplines concerned; the disciplines dividing for their own specialist interests.

Future needs must however be considered for *all* professional disciplines in occupational health and safety under three main headings which are categorized by grades defined as follows:

Grade 1: Training as a consultant or specialist adviser to the highest academic and practical level attainable either in a broad or narrow specialist field of expertise in a particular occupational health and safety discipline.

Grade 2: Training to an efficient academic diploma level with a good general and some special knowledge in whatever particular occupational health and safety discipline is appropriate.

Grade 3: Basic training in occupational health and safety in whatever professional discipline is practised.

Grade 1 training

Grade 1 training may be catered for by providing higher degree training (M.D., D.Phil., or M.Phil.) or more generally by Master of Science (M.Sc.) degree courses in all the occupational health professional disciplines and, as indicated in the preceding section on training available on occupational health and safety in Britain, there are Master of Science degree courses in occupational medicine, occupational hygiene and in occupational safety and hygiene. No such Master of Science courses are available for occupational health nurses, though Ph.D. and M.Phil. courses are open for them to follow, if they hold an equivalent of a first or second class honours degree, at the TUC Centenary Institute of Occupational Health.

The value of 'team training' should not be underestimated. Because the numbers requiring such highly specialized training are likely to be small, training could probably be more economically concentrated in one or perhaps two centres. A possible solution might be a national institute of occupational health and safety. Such a centre would be suitable for full-time training and for part-time training for those living in the vicinity of the centre. However, this would not solve the problem of day-release or part-time training for those living at a distance.

As things are at present universities might be willing to second their students to other universities with special expertise in particular aspects of training. For example to or from the University of Aston, on a modular basis, in order that all the professional disciplines might come together and fill gaps in training where the particular expertise is not available in the parent university department.

In occupational medicine the realization of the need to produce 'specialists' has been recognized by the medical profession. The training envisaged is of a rather different type and similar to Higher Specialist Training in other medical disciplines. The training includes a period in a university department and rotational training options in industry, the Employment Medical Advisory Service, research institutes and the National Health Service. The training given in the rotational posts would be practical as well as theoretical and would be under the supervision of a specialist in occupational medicine.

Higher specialist training

The Joint Committee on Higher Medical Training (JCHMT) of the Royal College of Physicians has set up a Specialist Advisory Committee (SAC) in Occupational Medicine with the following functions:

1. To recommend to the JCHMT those training posts which should be approved for Higher Specialist Training.

2. To recommend to the JCHMT those trainees who have satisfactorily completed a training programme for accreditation as specialist in occupational medicine.
3. For an initial period to recommend to the JCHMT occupational physicians with appropriate experience and expertise for retrospective accreditation as specialists.

The trainee in occupational medicine should undertake general professional training (after the pre-registration year) which is normally 3 years primarily in general medicine and usually leading to an M.R.C.P. (UK). (In some circumstances an appropriate alternative qualification may be accepted by the JCHMT on the recommendation of the SAC in individual cases.)

Higher Specialist Training is normally 4 years' training in approved and supervised posts in industry and research establishments with formal training in a university department. Before recommendation for accreditation as a specialist, account is taken of the programme, reports of the supervisors, publications and academic attainments. The tentative plan for the sponsorship of Higher Specialist Training is for payment to be that of a Senior Registrar in the National Health Service; contributions to the payment of Senior Registrars will be sought from industry and other sponsoring organizations and the Health and Safety Commission. The co-ordination of payment is planned through the Health and Safety Executive. Future careers for specialists are expected to be in posts in research, the Employment Medical Advisory Service, the National Health Service, industry and in academic departments of occupational health.

In order that doctors already working in occupational medicine may obtain recognition as specialists, criteria for retrospective accreditation as specialists in occupational medicine have been recommended to the Joint Committee on Higher Medical Training by the Specialist Advisory Committee in Occupational Medicine. These are that during the transitional period, (which would be for 5 years in the first instance), the Specialist Advisory Committee would require that applicants for accreditation:

1. Should be fully qualified medical practitioners.
2. After full registration should have adequate experience, during two or three years in other branches of medicine.
3. Should normally have had 12 years' full-time experience in the practice of occupational medicine of which not less than 3 years have been in a responsible post analagous to that of a consultant in sole charge.
4. Additional qualifications, specialist experience (e.g. research experience, university appointments or service in HM forces) and published work would also be taken into account.

Because of the varied nature of occupational medical practice the Specialist Advisory Committee recognizes that it may have to exercise judgement in individual cases before recommendation is made to the Joint Committee on Higher Medical Training.

Faculty of Occupational Medicine

The Royal College of Physicians has (April 1978) set up a Faculty of Occupational Medicine which has its own consitution and will be likely to set up criteria for fellowship, membership and associateship of the Faculty. A Faculty of Occupational Medicine had previously been established in Ireland.

Professional recognition of occupational medicine must increase the prestige of the discipline and improve standards of training and should ensure that occupational medicine is recognized as a clinical medical discipline.

Grade 2 training

Courses leading to diplomas in the professional occupational health and safety disciplines are available in one or more of the university departments, with the exception of diploma courses for Occupational Health Nurses. However, in Dundee there is a considerable amount of joint teaching for doctors and nurses, who are preparing for the Occupational Health Nursing Certificate.

'Team training' is as desirable at this level as for the specialist, but many of those preparing for diplomas may be more experienced in industry so that this cross-contact may be less vital, though even more rewarding. However, for general practitioners on day-release courses, who may have only had occupational health experience in one industry, this can be of immense importance.

Outside the universities, Diploma in Industrial Health examinations are held for doctors by the Society of Apothecaries of London and the Conjoint Board of England set by the Royal College of Physicians of London and the Royal College of Surgeons of England. Regulations and the syllabus of training are obtainable respectively from The Secretary at The Examination Hall, 8–11 Queen Square, London WC1 and The Registrar, The Society of Apothecaries, Black Friars Lane, London EC4 V62. The University of Glasgow also holds an examination, in two parts, for their own Diploma in Industrial Health. Diploma training is most suitable for members of the occupational health and safety team who do not necessarily aim to achieve specialist recognition, but who, nevertheless, wish to have a whole or part-time career in occupational health and safety.

Grade 3 training

Basic training is the most pressing need facing all who are concerned about the efficiency of occupational health services. The findings of the survey undertaken by the Employment Medical Advisory Service, already referred to, indicates how few doctors and nurses are in possession of Diplomas of Industrial Health or Occupational Health Nursing Certificates. Though basic (foundation) courses, part 1, are well established for nurses working in occupational health services in many parts of the country, similar courses are not available for doctors. Because so many doctors and nurses without occupational health training are in charge of, or working in occupational health services, much greater effort needs to be made to ensure that training is provided. The organization of basic training courses has been attempted in the past by the Society of Occupational Medicine and by University Departments.

The Department of Community and Occupational Medicine, the Welsh National School of Medicine, Heath Park, Cardiff, CF4 AXN, though it does not run postgraduate academic courses, teaches undergraduates and graduates on short courses and some of the university departments of occupational health do run courses annually for short periods, but a far more comprehensive plan on a regional basis needs to be made.

The professional societies and many of the larger industries have the expertise to set up such courses, which could be organized on a modular (day, days, week or weekend basis). At present there are no professional or legislative requirements for training. The new Faculty of Occupational Medicine may make a requirement for some form of certificate of competence before admitting associates. If, as appears probable, 3000 to 4000 part-time doctors are working in occupational health services, many are unlikely to have had any training, though a number of them may be working under the guidance of full-time occupational physicians, and some may have had considerable practical experience. Perhaps there is an opportunity here for the professional societies in occupational medicine, occupational hygiene, occupational health nursing and safety to form a committee to try to mount joint or individual specialist courses on a pilot plan to fill this need. No doubt assistance could be sought from university departments, but it would appear that their role is far more important in grade 1 and grade 2 training.

Further, continuing education or refresher courses

Courses of this type need to be specialized. For members of professional societies, many of the societies' meetings fill this need.

Individuals who wish to have further education in some special aspect of occupational health and safety should make their requirements known to the respective professional societies; if they are medical to the Post-graduate Medical Federation or to any of the university departments already mentioned. Such requests are likely to be sympathetically received.

Content of teaching programmes

If the concept of combined training common to all professional groups is accepted, the policy must be defined. Each professional group in whatever grade of training requires a tutor experienced in that particular discipline to guide and decide on the training courses which should be common and which divergent.

The primary role of all health and safety professionals is to know how to investigate and assess hazards. A basic need is therefore a knowledge of epidemiology and statistics and an appreciation of how to investigate, measure and evaluate these hazards. The particular skills of measurement, environmental and biological monitoring, will require common, but more detailed teaching depending on the level of training it is aimed to achieve and on the professional groups taught.

To gain experience in investigation, projects to test the understanding of the trainees followed by seminar presentations contributed to by all members of the group and chaired by a leader experienced in research methods provide an opportunity to test the effectiveness of teaching. The tutors should themselves undertake research and be familiar with research methods.

Prevention and control of hazards is the ultimate aim, but the major responsibility for prevention and control is the province of the occupational hygienist and the safety professional, who will have more specialized teaching in this aspect than the other members of the team.

There is no intention here to go into detail on the content of courses. Syllabuses are available from the relevant university departments and the relevant examining boards. The syllabus of training and aims of teaching for what is being classified in this chapter as grade 1 and grade 2 training, for occupational hygienists and doctors have been defined by the TUC Centenary Institute of Occupational Health; the University of Aston has similarly defined its policy for safety professionals. The Institute of Advanced Nursing Education defines the syllabus for the Occupational Health Nursing Certificate.

As has already been stated, courses are not as yet available for all occupational health and safety professionals in the same centre.

The importance of eliciting student opinion on the courses provided should not be under-estimated (Gauvain, 1968). Every attempt should be made to modify the course content and the type of teaching provided in the light of student (consumer) opinion.

DEVELOPMENT IN OTHER COUNTRIES

In considering developments in other countries most attention will be given to occupational physicians and the emphasis will be on the differences and similarities between the different countries and Britain.

The Standing Committee of Doctors of the EEC with the sponsorship of the Commission of the European Communities, held a workshop on Occupational Health Services in Europe in 1977. Table 14·1 summarizes the information on training schemes for doctors in industry, provided by the delegates to the workshop in the nine countries of the EEC.

Table 14.1 A survey of the variety of training schemes for industrial

	Industrial medicine in the basic training	Statutory	Training carried out by. . .
Belgium	None	Arrêté Royal of 5.3.1970	5 universities
Denmark	None		
France	+ Yes	Arrêté of 16.5.77 Secretary of State for Univ. and Pub. Hlth	17 universities
Ireland	None		4 British universities
Italy	± Optional	?	13 universities
Luxemburg			
Netherlands	± Optional	Regulations of the Royal Medical Association	4 universities
Federal Republic of Germany	+ Yes	?	2 universities
UK	± Optional	1975 report of the JCHMT	4 universities

physicians in the nine countries of the European Economic Community.*

Specialist training required for the practice of industrial medicine	Duration of the specialist training	Examination on completion of studies	Specialized post-university training
+ Yes	1) Diploma: 1 or 2 years 360 hours of courses + 8 sem. in-service training. 2) 'Licence': 1 year, thesis	+ Yes	+ Yes
	2 years (in preparation)		in preparation
+ Yes	2 years	+ Yes	+ Yes
			in preparation
	16 weeks teaching (over 1 or 2 years) + 7 months in-service training	+ Yes	+ Yes
			Belgian and French training recognized
For certain services	3 months basic course + 6 months (321 hours) 2/5 theoretical and 3/5 practical exercises + 2 years supervised practice	Declaration of the institute only	+ Yes
	2 years internal medicine 2 years industrial medicine	Declaration of the institute only	+ Yes
	1 or 2 years depending on university in question	+ Yes	+ Yes

* After Champiex and Hentz document number 3995/77 EN.

Considerable differences are apparent. Many of the differences are due to dissimilar developments in occupational health services in the different countries, often due to dissimilar legislation. A background paper describing the present status of occupational health services in the nine EEC countries (CP 77/113) is available from the office of the Standing Committee of Doctors of the EEC, Kristianagade 12A, 2100 Copenhagen, Denmark. The original sources of information on which the paper is based are listed in the references at the end of this chapter.

In the Federal Republic of Germany specialist training in occupational medicine lasts 4 years; specialist training for the supplementary title 'industrial physician' lasts 2 years. In both cases, the theoretical part of this specialist training (3 months) is provided at the academies of occupational medicine in Berlin and Munich (Wagner, 1978). Table 14.2 gives an estimate of the number of occupational physicians in the EEC Member States (Wagner, 1977).

Realization of the need to provide far more comprehensive and intensive training of occupational health professionals has been expressed in the United States. Eckardt (1976) has described the Occupational Health Safety Programmes Accreditation Commission (OH/SPAC) which consists of the American Academy of Industrial Hygienists (AAH), the American Academy of Occupational Medicine (AAOM), the American Association of Industrial Nurses (AAIN), the American Conference of

Table 14.2 Number of occupational physicians in the EEC member states. (Source: Amongst others, Compilation by Thomas Kennedy, Executive Secretary, Standing Committee – Wagner R. (1977) – V/Lux/221/78e.)

State	Number and type of occupational physicians		Year
	Full-time	Part-time	
Belgium	825		1974
Denmark	6	94	1976
France	2119	3084	1976
Federal Republic of Germany	1500	4500	1977
Ireland	10	100	1974
Italy	2000 altogether		
Luxemburg	7	3	1977
Netherlands	400	40	1973
United Kingdom	800	2000	1976

Governmental Industrial Hygienists (ACGIH), the American Industrial Hygiene Association (AIHA), the American Occupational Medical Association (AOMA), the Health Physics Society (HPS), and the American Society of Safety Engineers (ASSE). The development of a standards committee coincided with the Occupational Safety and Health Act 1970 which created the Occupational Safety and Health Administration (OSHA) and the National Institute of Occupational Safety and Health (NIOSH). The Commission plans an accreditation programme for Occupational Health and Safety which will involve site visits.

Suskind (1977) describes his 2-year residency programme and his mini-residency programme for part or full-time doctors working in occupational medicine and his programme for medical students. He believes interest in professional and scientific careers in the occupational health disciplines is increasing substantially.

Block (1977) states than NIOSH estimates a need for 2000 occupational health physicians defined as duly licensed physicians who are certified or who are qualified to become certified by the American Board of Preventive Medicine, and 28 000 industrial physicians, defined as duly licensed physicians who have had specified short postgraduate courses in occupational health and safety and who maintain competence by continuous postgraduate educational courses. He states that since 1955 the American Board of Preventive Medicine have only certified 707 physicians as competent in occupational medicine. There has been a decline in membership of the AOMA from 4069 in 1959 to 3684 at the end of 1975. The Occupational Health Institute (OHI) created by the Industrial Medical Association some years ago (now the AOMA), contracted in 1975 with the Human Resources Research Organisation (HUMRRO) to examine alternative educational delivery systems and to develop a plan for the establishment of a postgraduate school of occupational health. They agreed on four educational objectives:

1. To instruct physicians regarding skills, techniques and knowledge related to occupational medicine.
2. To prepare physicians for board examinations.
3. To prepare those already certified by the ABPM for re-certification.
4. To provide a variety of instructional experiences which would meet the needs of those concerned with relicensure.

Discussing the evidence for the need for such training Block states that the results of the certifying examinations of the ABPM in occupational medicine over the previous 5 years showed that those who had academic training had a 78 per cent success rate, and those with experience, but without academic training, had only a 39 per cent success rate. The requirements for certification in occupational medicine have been published (Seltser, 1977).

The most significant appreciation of the need for training in Occupational Safety and Health has come from the Department of Health, Education and Welfare, Public Health Service, Center for Disease Control which has provided programme guide-lines for Grants for Occupational Safety and Health Education Resource Centers (Finklea, 1977). The National Institute of Occupational Safety and Health is implementing 'a new national competition for training project grants to support a limited number of Occupational Safety and Health Educational Resource Centers. It is proposed to establish by 1980, subject to the availability of funds at least 10 centres – at least one in each Department of Health, Education and Welfare Region. . . . The objective of this competition is to provide a mechanism for combining and expanding existing activities, and arranging for coordinated multidiscipline and multilevel training and continuing education in occupational safety and health, under a single grant servicing a geographic region. The Program is intended to afford opportunity for full and part-time academic career training, for cross training of occupational safety and health practitioners for mid-career training in the field of occupational health and safety, and access to many different and relevant courses for students pursuing various degrees. Further, the combination of these should result in cross fertilization among the various disciplines and levels of occupational safety and health practice.'

Grants to a number of centres have already been made. Suggestions for a similar pattern of training suitable for health and safety professionals in the United Kingdom have already been made in this chapter.

In Canada particular interest has been shown in the training of occupational safety and health professionals in Ontario, where an Act respecting the Occupational Health and Safety of Workers is before the Ontario Legislature.

The Universities of Toronto and McMaster are interested in providing training programmes. The Department of Preventive Medicine and Biostatistics of the Faculty of Medicine and the Department of Chemical Engineering of Toronto University are anxious to organize joint programmes for doctors, nurses, occupational hygienists and safety professionals at specialists M.Sc. Grade 1 and diploma, Grade 2 level. A diploma course in industrial health has been organized annually at the university for many years. The Royal College of Physicians and Surgeons of Canada has been asked to recognize the specialty of occupational medicine and other provinces in addition to Ontario are also interested in organizing undergraduate medical and postgraduate training programmes in occupational medicine.

A number of universities in other countries provide courses for diplomas or M.Sc. degrees in occupational medicine. These countries include Australia (the University of Sydney), New Zealand (the University of Dunedin), South Africa (the University of Witwatersrand), and the University of Singapore.

In the USSR and the East-block countries training and the planning of medical services differs considerably from Western nations, and much more emphasis on training in preventive medicine is usually provided in the undergraduate period. It is not proposed to discuss this here but further information can be sought from the World Health Organisation.

CONCLUSIONS

The need for training of occupational and safety professionals is now gaining recognition, but many countries still do not have the facilities to provide their own training.

Training should be related to the functions of the professionals concerned, and have been divided in this chapter into three grades: specialists (M.Sc. or Higher Degrees), diplomas and basic training.

Emphasis has been placed on the importance of the 'team approach' to training, at all grades, and to work in occupational health services.

To obtain trainees of the right calibre, career prospects, both in the terms of financial reward and work satisfaction, must be seen to be available.

REFERENCES

An Act Respecting the Occupational Health and Safety of Workers, 1977, Bill 70 1st Session, 31st Legislature Ontario, Canada.

An Introduction to the Employment Medical Advisory Service, London. Health and Safety Executive (1977).

Atherley G. R. C. (1974) Health and safety inspectors, safety advisers, safety engineers. In: Gauvain, S. (ed.) *Occupational Health – A Guide to Sources of Information,* Chapter 8. London, Heinemann.

Block D. L. (1977) The quest for confidence. *J. Occup. Med.* **19,** (5), 315–318.

British Medical Association (1975) *The Doctor in Industry.* London, British Medical Association.

Eckardt R. E. (1976) Occupational Health/Safety Programmes Accreditation Commission. *J. Occup. Med.* **18** (12), 822–824.

Finklea J. F. (1977) Grants for Occupational Safety and Health Educational Resource Centers. Division of Training and Manpower Development, National Institute for Occupational Safety and Health, Robert A. Taft Laboratories 4676 Columbia Parkway, Cincinnati, Ohio. 45226 USA. Category of Federal Domestic Assistance Programme No. 13.263. Occupational Safety and Health Training Grants.

Gauvain Suzette (1968) The use of student opinion in the quality control of teaching British. *Br. J. Med. Educ.* **2,** 55.

Gauvain Suzette (1971) Analysis of answers to questionnaires sent to 24 medical schools on the teaching of occupational medicine to medical students. In: *Symposium at Royal College of Physicians on Occupational Health for the Undergraduate Medical Student.* 1. London, Society of Occupational Medicine.

Gauvain Suzette (ed.) (1974) *Occupational Health – A Guide to Sources of Information.* London, Heinemann.

Gauvain Suzette and Schilling R. S. F. (1973) Education in occupational health. In: *Occupational Health Practice,* Ch. 22. London, Butterworth.

Hall S. (1974) Occupational hygienists. In: Gauvain S. (ed.), *Occupational Health – A Guide to Sources of Information,* Ch. 3. London, Heinemann.

Health and Safety Commission (1977a) *Occupational Health Service: The Way Ahead.* London, HMSO.

Health and Safety Commission (1977b) Safety Representatives and Safety Committees (S11977 No. 500). *Health and Safety at Work.* London, HMSO.

Health and Safety Executive (1977) *An Introduction to the Employment Medical Advisory Service.* London, Health and Safety Executive.

Robens Report (1972) *Safety and Health at Work.* Report of a Committee. Cmnd 5034. London, HMSO.

Royal College of Nursing (1975) *Occupational Health Nursing Services: a Handbook for Employers and Nurses.* London, Royal College of Nursing.

The Royal College of Physicians (1975) *Second Report of the Joint Committee on Higher Medical Training.* London, Royal College of Physicians.

Seltser R. (1977) Requirements for certification in occupational medicine. *J. Occup. Med.* **19,** (12), 847.

Suskind R. R. (1977) Perspectives in education: occupational medicine graduate training. *J. Occup. Med.* **19,** (3), 211–214.

The Present Status of Occupational Health Services in the 9 EEC countries Background Paper: CP77/113, Kristianagade 12A, 2100 Copenhagen, Denmark.

Sources as follows:

1. Commission of the European Communities Directorate General for Social Affairs, *The Training of Industrial Medical Officers in the 9 European Community Countries* (document number 1109/74).
2. Danish Medical Association (1976) *Minutes of the Occupational Health Subcommittee of the Standing Committee of Doctors of the EEC, Copenhagen, 13 March 1976* (document 235–24/76). Copenhagen, Den Almindelige Dansek Laegeforening.
3. de Boer L. (1973) Occupational health in the Netherlands. *J. Soc. Occup. Med.* **23,** 79–83.
4. Forssman S. *The Place of Occupational Health in the Public Health Services,* 25th Session of the World Health Organisation Regional Committee for Europe Technical Discussions, Algiers, 2/6 September 1975 (W.H.O. Document EUR/RC25/Tech Disc./1, 24 June 1975).
5. Standing Committee of Doctors of the EEC (1977) *Minutes of the Occupational Health Sub-committee, Brussels, Belgium, 10 March 1977* (CP 77/29), Copenhagen Standing Committee of Doctors.
6. Standing Committee of Doctors of the EEC (1976) Questionnaire prepared by Professor J. Champeix (France): *Le But de la Medecine du Travail dans les 9 pays de la CEE* (CP 76/43) and responses from the national medical associations of Belgium (CP 76/65), Denmark (CP 77/95), France (CP 76/51), Germany (CP 76/44), Ireland (CP 77/81). London and Copenhagen, Standing Committee of Doctors.
7. Standing Committee of Doctors of the EEC (1977) Questionnaire prepared by Professor J. Champeix (France): *Formation du Medecin du Travail* (CP 77/76) and responses from the national medical associations of Germany (CP 77/86), Ireland (CP 77/96), Italy (CP 77/79), Netherlands (CP 77/85), and United Kingdom (CP 77/87). London and Copenhagen, Standing Committee of Doctors.
8. Standing Committee of the EEC (1977) *Comments from the Netherlands on EEC Commission Document on Training of Industrial Medical Officers in the 9 European Countries* (CP 77/14). Copenhagen, Standing Committee of Doctors.
9. World Health Organisation Regional Office for Europe and International Labour Organisation (1974) *The Teaching of Occupational Health and Safety* (Document 5203). Copenhagen, W.H.O. Regional Office for Europe.

15. STANDARDS OF FOOD HYGIENE

J. L. Kearns

THE NATURE AND EXTENT OF THE PROBLEM

The simplicity, contemporary validity and commercial sense evident over five thousand years ago in the control of food poisoning is a challenge to all those concerned with the provision of wholesome clean food today. The major problems to be tackled in our time range between the extremes of ignorance and an overwhelming amount of detailed theroretical knoweledge. That being so, it is not suprising that the part played in the control of food hygiene is not clear to all of the parties involved.

In recent times, attention to the medical examination of the food handler has been emphasized at the expense of distracting attention from the disciplined control of the raw or cooked material. This imbalance has led to misleading assumptions that an individual found fit to handle food on one particular day remains so for a further 364 days until re-examined perhaps by a second doctor who may not apply the same standards as the first!

This state of affairs is the more deplorable when food is perhaps the most widespread hazard to which every member of the population is exposed several times a day throughout a lifetime. Whether at home, work, school or play, everyone has an opportunity to be harmed by food contaminated by himself or someone else, or to contaminate someone else's food.

It is because food is a vehicle for harmful substances that it is a hazard. Ancient royal houses used poisons to speed up the rate of succession, and crude tests were carried out by unfortunate tasters who were the laboratory animals of the time. Nowadays the preparation of some kinds of food and drink in metal receptacles, with which ingredients may react, causes accidents from time to time. Occasionally, neglect leads to the gross contamination of food (Kepelman et al., 1966).

In most countries where food is produced or processed on a large scale, quality control of wholesomeness and acceptability to the consumer is of major commercial importance. When thousands or even millions of individual items are marketed daily the producer or retailer is constantly aware of the appearance and condition of the food sold or served. Fortunately, with a few crucial exceptions, the appearance, taste or smell of a faulty product become unacceptable some time before there is a risk of actual harm to the consumer. Examples of this type of contamination are the moulds which seriously affect the keeping qualities of various foods. Even when a meal is actually being served, the presence of a hair can be disgusting, although it would be unlikely to do any actual harm if it were swallowed. Gastric acid is certainly strong enough to kill most organisms so long as they are not in massive numbers.

Perhaps it would be useful to emphasize the meaning of the word 'vehicle' when it refers to food. There are few circumstances in which food is contaminated with a sufficiently large quantity of chemical or bacterial agents to cause immediate harm. It is the length and circumstances of the journey of the food between contamination and the consumer which gives its 'passengers' the opportunity to double every 20 minutes. The fundamental factor in a practical and effective approach to food hygiene is the prevention of such an increase in numbers of bacteria. From the raw state, food passes through several stages of preparation, the last of which is most frequently in the home of the consumer. Sometimes a large number of people have an opportunity to contaminate it by carelessness or ignorance. Someone who does not contaminate the food himself may allow the few germs deposited by someone else to multiply in favourable conditions of temperature and moisture, until they reach numbers sufficient to overwhelm the defences of the very young or the weak, or to produce enough heat stable toxin to kill even a healthy adult.

It has been both satisfying to the status of the doctor and reassuring to the layman to consider that food hygiene is a predominantly medical problem. In fact it would be more accurate, though less flattering, to regard the food handler as a larger species of vermin, who is nonetheless capable of understanding some very simple rules which could protect the food he or she handles from any harmful bacteria or parasites, or even from bodily debris shed onto the food. The responsibility for both the training and control of standards rests with those in authority, whether in the home, restaurant or the food factory. The doctor is but one of several technical resources who add a degree of expertise to the prevention or solution of specific problems. Neither the doctor, the nurse, the food technologist, nor the controller of vermin can be effective in the absence of adequate hygiene discipline among all food handlers.

THE FOOD HANDLER

From time to time outbreaks of food-borne infection occur even in those countries which have the good fortune to have temperate climates, effective disposal of sewage and clean water supplies. When outbreaks occur, they either expose a fault in hygiene standards or provide a stimulus to the improvement of existing standards. To have sold an article of food which is known to have caused an outbreak of food poisoning can be a commercial disaster to a factory or a restaurant.

One such episode occurred in Aberdeen, Scotland, in the mid-sixties.

Three important features of that episode are relevant to the topic of this chapter. *First,* the typhoid infection was carried not only by the original batch of corned beef, but was transferred to other meats sliced by the same implements. It was not *someone* who contaminated the meat personally, but *something* which was used incorrectly. *Second*, a schedule for screening people in various jobs was prepared which ranged from a simple questionnaire to a full battery of more than 20 laboratory investigations on a particular individual over a period of several weeks. *Third,* people working in a food factory were categorized in terms of the risk which they might have represented to the product (Deans Weir, 1965).

Some years later, a problem arose in the selection of those students embarking upon a several-year-long university course and a subsequent career in catering. On that occasion a young man was found to have an infection of the ear, causing it to discharge from time to time. Could he be allowed to enter for that course, or should he be directed towards another career in which his condition would not be a risk to others? His case provoked a careful analysis of the multiple factors involved, which in turn led to broad agreement upon a large number of issues among the medical officers who look after large food companies in the United Kingdom.

It is worthwhile to consider the definition of a food handler and its implications for hygiene control. Food is handled in every household, but few serious cases of food poisoning originate in the home. This is partly because the food is bought in good condition and partly because it is cooked and eaten almost immediately. Countless thousands of people prepare or serve simple articles of food in offices, hospital wards and workshops where the time interval necessary for gross contamination does not elapse. Those circumstance in which eating or drinking is forbidden in the workplace protect the unwary from eating toxic inanimate materials. If one excludes that huge number of theoretical but insignificant food handlers, there remains the population which is of most interest because it comes into contact with food in bulk. If the vehicle for infection is traced from the raw to the finished article, food may be at risk at one or more of several stages, either directly from people or from the implements they use. Its journey takes it past the research worker who may be testing products for quality and replacing them on the production line. Evidently all those who process or serve the food have an opportunity to maintain or improve quality, or through neglect to damage it. Where food is set out for display, demonstration or sale, further opportunites to cause disaster occur. At several points along that chain, and in the home of the consumer, the conditions in which the food is stored may be of vital importance.

In the course of its journey one article of food may come into contact with other potentially dangerous foods. Thus in a meat preparation department, the raw meat may be so rich in salmonellae as to be a hazard to the people handling it, rather than the other way round. Certainly, raw meat products must not come into direct or indirect contact with food that has already been cooked. That is why raw meat, even in a domestic refrigerator, should be stored below other foods to prevent accidental spillage. Even the implements used on raw meat must be confined to that purpose alone.

From all that has gone before, it follows that a food handler may be defined as one who touches:

1. The food itself.
2. The implements or machines with which it comes into contact.
3. The materials in which it is packed.

Conversely, the fork lift truck driver who moves pallets containing cartons of boxes in which products are sealed in plastic film cannot be considered to be a food handler.

The practical implication of that definition is that a large proportion of people who represent a potential risk to food can be identified clearly and another section of workers who pose no risk at all can be excluded from any screening programme. There are a few people in an indefinite group between the two, who have access to food production departments in the course of the day. The clerk sent to check attendance records, the electrician going to change a bulb, the visitor passing through, do not represent a significant hazard, but as a precaution they should wear adequate, clean, protective clothing whenever they enter a food department. While the risk they pose to the product is minimal, the awareness of food hygiene demonstrated by the wearing of protective clothing encourages discipline among those who work in that department all the time.

PROTECTIVE CLOTHING AND CLEANLINESS

There are some factors in the maintenance of food hygiene which have little to do with infection as such. The presence of a hair in food has been quoted as an example of something unappetizing, and it is a useful starting point in the discussion of the appropriate appearance of the food handler. Personal appearance is a particularly important factor when the waiter, shop assistant, or manager, is in the direct view of the public. Standards of health apart, the consumer expects that body debris like hair, dandruff or flaking nail varnish is either absent because of careful and proper grooming, or is covered adequately. Those who wait at table may not need protective clothing in the strict sense. Very often there is a traditional or even a contemporary uniform, but it must always be changed as required for cleanliness and not merely because another week has passed! Occasionally in the public gaze is the chef de cuisine, who has worked a long and hard apprenticeship to gain the privilege of white tunic, blue striped trousers, and a high hat, the latter being utterly inadequate to cover the long hair worn by many chefs today. Either the hair must be very well kept despite the hot, steaming atmosphere of a kitchen, or a hair net should be worn. It is not easy to persuade a young long-haired man to wear a hair net in a food preparation department, much less in his own kitchen, but then Lister had quite a task persuading his colleagues to refrain from surgical operations while clad in top hat, dark coat and pin stripe trousers! The possibility that the very length of the hair in the soup is more likely to attract protest is often sufficient to stimulate the constructive pride of an otherwise reluctant chef.

In 'the front of the house' where the customer awaits his meal, whatever the quality of the food, the elegance of the china, or even the gleam of the silver, all will be rendered worthless by the poor appearance of the hands and fingernails which place the meal before him. A mixture of tradition and practical experience has led to our acceptance of 'ordinarily' dressed waiters and waitresses. In the time between the food being ready to serve and its actual consumption, there is very little opportunity to contaminate it seriously, with one major exception. Cold dishes, particularly meat and cream, must either be kept at a low temperature or used so fast that they are not at ambient temperature for long enough to allow multiplication of germs to a significant and harmful level. This point deserves emphasis because on more than one occasion a technically competent but unrealistic official has suggested that a sweet trolley be refrigerated. If the load of contents is controlled carefully so that they are used up within an hour or two of coming out of refrigerated storage or display, they are safe on an ordinary trolley. Refrigeration of such a trolley poses difficulties of weight, wiring and enclosure, and there is no guarantee that its temperature could be accurately maintained in a restaurant in which the ambient temperature varies from place to place.

In food production departments in factories, protective clothing is nearly always required. Two major factors should determine the design of such overalls. Hygiene requires that the ordinary clothing of the worker should be protected from the flour, jam or meat and vice versa. If this concept of two-way protection is emphasized, it is easier to make sure that the individual wears clean adequate overalls in good repair. Safety requirements are sometimes of additional importance and require that some members of staff wear one-piece boiler suits without belts. These are suitable for maintenance engineers in food departments. In addition to these two main groups there are some situations in which there is a need for additional clothing to protect against sharp hand-implements. Examples are the butcher's apron; the waterproof aprons used in the preparation of fish; and warm protective clothing for those who have to work in cold stores (Andrew, 1963).

In production departments the most important item of head-dress is a hair net. This applies to every man or woman who does not have a 'short back and sides' hairstyle. In addition, caps of linen, paper or plastic may cover such a hairstyle thus protecting the hair from particles of foodstuff.

Nothing is, however, more ridiculous than an inadequate head-dress perched on top of a mass of hair in a food department. In particular, nothing discredits hygiene standards more effectively, than a nurse striding through a food production department with 'her own' hospital's head-dress secured with hairclips. Such a garb is no more appropriate than it would be when leaning over an open abdomen in an operating theatre!

Solid foreign bodies are unacceptable in food whether they are sharp or not. For this reason hairclips, ear-rings, other than sleepers for pierced ears, and false eyelashes cannot be worn in food departments. Commonly wrist watches and jewellery other than wedding rings are banned for the same reason. There are those who would not permit even wedding rings. Certainly in the event of accident any ring is a potential danger, either because it will tear off a finger or because it will constrict the finger if it is squashed.

Most users and suppliers of overalls in the food industry seem to expect that all outdoor clothing above the hips should be covered. Irrespective of sex, an overall coat may be adequate. Ideally, openings should be at the back, since zips, buttons, press-studs and 'Velcro' type fasteners all have disadvantages in that they tear, pull off, or wear out very quickly. A one-piece overall of about knee length is ideal, particularly if it is slipped on over the head, with the high collar fastened at the back of the neck.

Either sex may prefer to wear a shorter tunic and trousers. These have obvious advantages if there are multiple steps or bridgeways in the work-place. However, trousers have the disadvantage of resting on the floor of toilets from time to time!

In practice, it is still common for women to wear the adequate protection of knee-length overall, and a cap completely covering the hair. Meanwhile, men wear either tunic and trousers or simple white coats, with an often bewildering variety of 'status' hats of little hygienic adequacy.

The length of sleeves depends upon several factors. In wet, dirty jobs it is common to provide detachable lower sleeves which can be changed more frequently than the overall as a whole. Sometimes it is easier to have short sleeves and bare forearms. In other circumstances, long sleeves are necessary for warmth as for example in a meat preparation room which is cool but not cold enough to require more than ordinary warm clothing. Overalls *must* cover cardigan and jumper sleeves completely. In cold rooms and freezers, insulated clothing is necessary, and has been described in detail by Andrew (1963).

Footwear, more often than not, is of the ordinary outdoor type. There is a tendency to wear worn-out or comfortable slip-on shoes in food factories. This should be discouraged because the commonest accidents in the food industry are slipping and falling. Even in the few instances where safety shoes are necessary, they are most effective only in the protection they afford to toes. The need for easy cleaning means that food factory floors tend to be slippery, particularly when fat is an ingredient. Only limited success has been attained in finding a combination of a composition shoe sole which compliments the non-slip character of the various types of factory floor.

It is important that there should be no pockets above waist level and that those pockets and pouches which hold handkerchiefs, purses, pencils, watches, should be inside the overall and not of the external patch type. Only then can the contents of pockets be regarded as unlikely to fall into the food. Finally, the use of gloves is of doubtful value. Gloves are of use in protecting hands against detergents and may be an appropriate protection in some of the dirtier operations in preparing food for consumption. However, they are not necessarily beneficial in ensuring clean food. When gloves are in use one often sees the operator removing them, leaving them on the bench, and going to wash hands. Impermeable gloves nearly always result in as much moisture from sweat inside the glove as there is moisture from the product outside. Furthermore, since the use of antiseptic unscented soap and water at reasonable intervals throughout the day maintains virtually sterile skin (Leading Article, 1970), there seems little point in risking inadequate cleaning of gloves, or the possible excoriation of moist hands inside them. Gloves may be nipped dangerously by machinery, or have small pieces torn off which go into the product.

Once the major criteria set out above have been satisfied, decisions about the material, cut, colour and design of overalls may be discussed with those who wear the overalls. It makes no sense to consult staff in a totally free frame of reference, because the primary purpose of protective clothing in the food industry is to protect the product and the person without risk to either, not to clothe employees in irrelevant sartorial elegance.

BIOLOGICAL FOOD POISONING

The most frequent causes of bacterial food poisoning in temperate industrial countries include staphylococci, salmonellae, group A streptococci, shigellae and the vibrios cholerae and haemolyticum. More rarely, but with potentially devastating effects, clostridial toxin strikes the unsuspecting. There are also a number of parasites which flourish in tropical countries where effective sanitation is lacking. Bacteriological details are available in any good textbook and only the major features which have practical significance to food hygiene will be dealt with here.

Staphylococci are germs which are frequently recognized by the layman as causing the formation of pus in spots and boils. They are very common and inhabit the skin of up to 15 per cent of the population. Furthermore, they can be imagined as having similar dietary preferences to humans. They grow readily in cream and meat products. Furthermore, they produce a waste product which is both heat stable and intensely irritant to the intestine. The staphylococcus itself is killed by cooking but the toxin it leaves behind causes vomiting and diarrhoea within a few hours of being eaten. In most cases the degree of irritation is such that the toxin is expelled within about 24 hours.

Typically, someone with perhaps only a small infected cut or boil inoculates an article of food which rests at room temperature for several hours. Then the food is served either cold or reheated and within hours someone is ill, more often than not being able to identify the likely article of food that caused the misfortune. It is rare that any of the food is left to establish the cause definitely, and since there is no germ to culture, the causative organism is hardly ever identified positively. Nevertheless, in commercially damaging terms a short, sharp, extremely unpleasant bout of illness is attributed without doubt to a particular meal or product. The customer, even though he may not report the episode, does not allow the vendor a second chance.

The second important group of organisms is the salmonellae which cause typhoid, paratyphoid, and several other diseases which affect the intestinal tract. In contrast to the staphylococcus, the salmonella may take days to cause trouble and weeks to clear. Even if the patient does not die, he often cannot be cured and a carrier state is established in which he becomes a source of disease to others in his family or elsewhere.

Typically in such an episode a meat product is inadequately cooked. The right temperature maintained for sufficient time would kill all salmonellae and render the food harmless. However, it is not unusual to take meat out of the refrigerator, thaw it inadequately, and cook it at such a rate that the centre still contains sufficient live germs to overcome the defences of the body. Barbecued chickens are a notorious source of such infection (Semple et al., 1968).

The third major group of bacteria is the clostridia which form toxins which poison the nervous system. Unlike either of the previous examples, these germs are capable of resisting heat. When the temperature falls they resume reproduction, producing plentiful toxin in the absence of air, even inside a tin.

In addition to those three major groups of bacteria, there is a virus which causes infection of the liver and results in jaundice. One form of this disease may be food-borne hepatitis, but it is characteristic of the disease that the virus is being spread during several days of an incubation period before the patient himself either becomes ill or is jaundiced. While there may be theoretical advantages in attempting to screen against this virus, those investigations that are possible can only be done after the incubation period in which spread has already occurred.

Since food is not a means of transfer of the human pulmonary tuberculosis bacillus, there can be little justification for routine chest radiography of food handlers. If such an investigation is undertaken, one should be aware that it is for the protection of fellow workers and not a food hygiene measure.

In various countries other bacteria are the object of interest among enthusiastic hygienists. In some cases diarrhoea is actually induced by the use of enemata, and it is not unusual in the United States to be screened for veneral disease as well. Meticulous attention to detail arising from sincere conviction may well have led to these investigations being adopted, but they have no place in the protection of food, unless there are some bizarre local recipes which can be shown to require such vigilance!

Characteristic of the food industry is the large number of migrant workers who move from one country to another. When emigration spans continents, and particularly when workers move from tropical to temperate climates, there is frequent anxiety about the parasites which may be reimported into countries where they have been eradicated by effective public health measures. The maintenance of high standards of sewage disposal and the provision of clean water supplies effectively breaks the natural life cycle of most parasites. Again, the appropriate use of unscented soap and water with a nail brush is a further barrier to the dissemination of harmful organisms (Leading Article, 1970). As an example of the organisms which may be expected in a population moving from a tropical to a temperate zone, McGirr published the following Table in 1968 (McGirr, 1969).

Table 15.1 Analysis of 100 unsatisfactory stool samples.

Giardia intestinalis	63
Entamoeba histolytica	14
Salmonella typhimurium	4
Trichuris trichiura	4
Strongyloides stercoralis	3
Hookworm	3
Enterobius vermicularis	2
Ascaris lumbricoides	2
Shigella sonnei	1
Clonorchis sinensis	1
Hymenolepis nana	1
Untraced specimens	2
	100

Before leaving this topic, it is worth while to emphasize the effectiveness of hand washing. Many modern factories have hand washbasins at the entrance to food production departments at which everyone entering must wash his or her hands. It is widespread practice to encourage the washing of hands after visits to the toilet, and is also surely appropriate today to encourage additional hand washing by food production workers from time to time during a shift. It has been shown that there is a natural balance of bacteria on the healthy skin, and on healthy skin there are insufficient dangerous bacteria to cause trouble unless the food is allowed to incubate and multiply them. The too frequent use of detergents removes protective fat, and the over-zealous scrubbing of skin with a nail brush causes mechanical damage (Leading Article, 1970). The aim must be to strike a balance between reasonably clean hands and those with reddened sore skin more vulnerable to infection. Since deep glands in the skin begin to repopulate the surface bacteria after half an hour, washing three to four times in the course of the day, particularly but not exclusively after having been to the toilet, would seem to be an adequate frequency,

PLANT AND PREMISES

The environment in which food is processed, stored, transported and served is obviously of great importance. Contamination of food is possible not only from the people who handle it, but from the organic or inert dust and dirt which can fall into the food, or be dropped into it by animals. A thorough review of architecture, fixtures and fittings is not appropriate here, but some underlying principles are outlined to suggest desirable standards to be achieved and maintained.

Rooms or departments in which food is prepared should be used only for that purpose. Clothing should be changed and stored in separate areas, and such cloakroom and toilet facilities as are provided should be isolated from the food preparation area by a lobby or corridor. The food preparation/storage area should be animal-proof, with no access for mice around pipes, nor for birds and insects through windows. One of the most difficult areas to deal with is the kitchen, where humid heat must be dispersed without causing uncomfortable draughts. Moreover, the condensation of fat both in flues and in exhaust ventilation ducts must be regularly cleaned to avoid a serious hazard in terms of both of hygiene and of the spread of fire.

Equipment is generally of adequate standards in large enterprises, but in small cafés and canteens much of it is old and worn. If the wear and tear of surfaces permits the accumulation of food, that surface becomes a culture medium for potentially harmful organisms. Even modern equipment may contain inaccessible hollows or angles in which bacteria or vermin may settle and multiply. Often faultless equipment is sited so that it is impossible to clean under or around it. An example is the hand washbasin (never to be used for implements!), which is loosely secured to a tiled wall, leaving a gap in which dirt accumulates. Such cracks appear in or between tiles and require immediate repair or replacement. Tiles are durable and easily cleaned, but modern hard plasters covered with polyurethane paints may serve just as well. A common material hazard in a food area is glass. Windows crack, light bulbs are broken and containers fall. Wired glass, shielded light fittings, and the use of plastic containers go some way to prevent glass particles being lost in food. The removal of wrist watches in food departments is a common practice to prevent watch glasses being broken. While such awareness and discipline has psychological value, most watches are nowadays cased in plastic. Many people wear glass spectacles, and fittings such as glass-covered fire alarms are necessary risks.

Whatever the state of plant and premises, they must be kept clean. Operatives themselves may 'clean as they go', or hygiene teams may be appropriate. Neither will be effective unless there is a clear schedule and procedure to be observed. Who is to clean what, how often and with what? Most important of all is the written record of *what* is to be done, and *whether* it has been done. Since authority is fundamental to discipline, it is essential that someone of appropriate rank should demonstrate responsibility by appropriate checks. Mechanical maintenance and repair requires equally meticulous attention if bits of machinery are to be kept out of the food.

In some countries legislation lays down temperatures appropriate for the preparation, storage, transport and display of foodstuffs. For similar reasons, the speed with which food should pass through those stages of its journey has sometimes been determined by 'dating' the product not only in the shop, but in easily understood terms for the guidance of the housewife in the use of her domestic refrigerator.

SCREENING

On the assumption that medical screening is of prime importance in protecting food, medical examination of food handlers by doctors has been advocated as an initial measure as part of selection, and subsequently at various intervals. Debate continues, and sometimes it has been suggested that those working in the food industry should report their movements on holiday to medical staff, who will then 'clear' them to return to work! The mystery of such an approach surely exceeds that of inspired training and discipline dating from the third millenium BC, for it is not realistic to expect individuals to report their holiday intentions. It is even less reasonable to suppose that foremen, the crucial leaders, could record, analyse and react appropriately to the plans of the scores of food handlers in their command.

The crucial episode upon which everyone's attention should be focused is the bout of sickness or diarrhoea, wherever and whenever it occurs. By adequate training, all can understand that a germ has caused sickness, and that withdrawal from food handling is necessary. Moreover, when the illness has passed, soap and water are effective in preventing transfer to others. To encourage responsible behaviour, the financial penalty for withdrawal from work must be minimized for both employer and employed. Temporary transfer to a non-food-handling job, or if none is available, total exclusion from the workplace on pay is necessary if epidemic spread is to be avoided (Deans Weir, 1965). At least *three* stool cultures are necessary to clear an individual whose history demands laboratory investigation. It is not economically justifiable to bar a food handler from his job for several days unless there is such a specific need.

To restrict him for only one stool culture achieves nothing positive, although there may be some false reassurance in the meaningless ritual. It takes 48 hours to examine and report upon a single specimen of faeces, and there are few scientists who would attempt to demonstrate that a single faecal examination is of value. Conversely, those who can argue a sound scientific basis for rectal swabs would not survive the abuse of the first prospective food handler expected to adopt the posture of an oven-ready chicken!

In *Men under Fire,* General S. L. A. Marshall of the US Army, argues that success in battle depends on structuring the army into small groups. In recent decades, lessons of war and insurgency have emphasized the need to win the 'hearts and minds' of the people. So it is with food-borne infection. A simple message often repeated is the key to the successful production and service of food. To the doctor or nurse that message is to look out for the patient who is a food handler suffering from:

1. Inflammation of the ear.
2. Inflammation of the eye.
3. Persistant or recurring skin conditions subject to infection, or persistent gross disease on the exposed skin or scalp.
4. Persistent upper or lower respiratory disease producing copious phlegm (this is the patient likely to spit).
5. Oral sepsis.
6. A positive history of intestinal disease.

To the food handler, the message must be to report any episode of diarrhoea or sickness, and to have any infected cut or spot covered with a waterproof dressing which will activate metal detectors. Even when no disease is present, careful cleanliness must be maintained *all the time.* Spitting is absolutely forbidden, but nails bitten by a dirty mouth never seem to attract criticism, although they deposit spittle *on* the food or plate!

To the manager at whatever level, the message must be that leadership and constant example in personal appearance and protective clothing is crucial. It is the team leader who should select, train and maintain his staff. A simple questionnaire can be couched in everyday terms to identify the potential risk not immediately apparent in the slovenly appearance of an applicant for a job. A well-trained medical orderly or nurse can monitor the effectiveness of such a questionnaire administered by a manager, and can carry out hygiene inspections on doubtful candidates, or on those who give a positive answer to a question.

A full scale medical examination is necessary only if there is a clinical indication to justify the deployment of expensive skills. Where no doctor is retained by the employer, a card similar to that in Table 15.3 may be useful in attaining consistent relevant standards when seeking the help of the employee's own doctor.

Table 15.2. Model questionnaire to be used by a trained manager. (A positive answer requires the opinion of medical staff.)

1. Have you ever had an illness or accident, causing you to be off work for a period of two weeks or more?	YES/NO
2. Have you ever attended an out-patient's clinic, or ever had a course of treatment (tablets, injections or physiotherapy) lasting one month or more?	YES/NO
3. Are you *now* receiving medical treatment for any condition (e.g. physiotheraphy, tablets, injections, diet)?	YES/NO
4. Are you suffering, or have you suffered, from:	
Fits/epilepsy	YES/NO
Diabetes	YES/NO
Nervous trouble	YES/NO
Any bowel trouble, e.g. typhoid or recurring diarrhoea	YES/NO
Skin disease or dermatitis	YES/NO
Any earache/ear infection?	YES/NO

Table 15.3. Model card for use by employee's own doctor.

Dear Doctor,
Please examine this patient for fitness to work in food production. Conditions to be borne in mind include:

Otitis media/externa.
Conjunctivitis/blepharitis.
Chronic or recurring skin conditions subject to staphylococcal contamination.
Chronic gross skin disease on the exposed skin or scalp whether subject to staphylococcal contamination or not, is undesirable in some jobs in the food industry.
Chronic respiratory disease producing sputum in working hours.
Chronic oral or dental sepsis. This condition would have to be under adequate treatment before acceptance.
Typhoid, paratyphoid, enteritis or dysentry.

side 1

Patient's NAME:
ADDRESS:

This patient is fit to work in food production.
Signed: DOCTORS NAME
or Stamp: ADDRESS
Please return to:
NAME & ADDRESS
OR STAMP OF
ENGAGING MANAGER

side 2

It is quite probable that doctors and nurses will be accused of abdicating responsibility when they point out the pre-eminence of the manager's duty. However, once the doctor or nurse has re-examined his own rôle, he will have an understanding of how to help the manager to confront the problem posed by the burden of responsibility which has been obscured hitherto by ambiguity and confusion. Far from washing *their* hands of the problem, medical staff must demonstrate that the washing of hands is the most effective barrier to the transmission of infection.

Acknowledgement

The material contained in this chapter is derived from practical experience in the J. Lyons Group of Companies, from colleagues in various parts of the British food industry and from the work of others in international, governmental, professional and trade bodies.

REFERENCES AND FURTHER READING

Andrew G. H. (1963) Work in extreme cold. *Trans. Assoc. Ind. Med. Offrs.* **13**, 16–19.

Association of Public Health Inspectors (1972) *Towards Cleaner Food.* Report of the Working Party on Food Hygiene, Association of Public Health Inspectors, London.

Deans Weir R. (1965) The problems of typhoid screening in the food industry. *Trans. Assoc. Ind. Med. Offrs.* **15**, 65.

Food Manufacturers' Federation Inc. (1975) *A Guide to Health and Safety in the Food Industry.* Food Manufacturers' Federation Inc., London.

Hobbs Betty C. (1968) *Food Poisoning and Food Hygiene,* 2nd ed. London, Arnold.

Kepelman H. et al. (1966) The Epping jaundice. *Br. Med. J.* **1**, 514–516.

Leading Article (1970) The surgical scrub. *Br. Med. J.* **3**, 418.

McGirr O. (1969) Screening of food handlers. *Proc. R. Soc. Med.* **62**, 601–602.

Semple A. B. et al. (1968) Outbreak of food poisoning caused by *Salmonella virchow* in spit-roasted chicken. *Br. Med. J.* **4**, 801–803.

World Health Organisation (1970) *The Requirements for Food Hygiene and Food Handlers.* Report of the Seminar on Food Hygiene, Warsaw. Geneva, W.H.O.

*This publication includes a considerable list of sources of further information.

16. TRAVEL BY AIR, SEA, ROAD AND RAIL

Frank S. Preston

'A journey of a thousand miles begins with one step.'

Old Chinese Proverb

INTRODUCTION

This chapter is concerned with the medical aspects of travel by air, sea, road and rail and how the individual copes with the health problems that travel presents.

The whole concept of transportation is changing and in fact has probably been changing since the dawn of time when man took his first tentative steps at travel and exploration of his world.

At first he was limited by the distance he could walk; later he looked to the animal kingdom for help, taming and harnessing the camel, the elephant, buffalo and horse. Each in turn were to present their own problems and special techniques. Later he began hollowing out logs and venturing on the great rivers of the world and eventually having invented the sail, which was to last a thousand years, he explored the seas and oceans of the world. In the early nineteenth century sail gave way to steam about the time the first steam trains were appearing on land. But we go too fast – the wheel was probably man's greatest invention as far as land travel was concerned and was known to the Ancient Britons and certainly to highly developed nations such as the Romans and the Greeks. The wheel and the haulage animal were to last for centuries and are still with us.

Air travel is a late arrival on the scene, following the Wright Brothers' first flight at Kitty Hawk in North Carolina in 1903 and the rapid strides made in aviation in two World Wars.

It was not until the late 1950s, with the arrival of the turboprop and turbojet engine, that mass air travel became an established entity. In 1977, 650 million passengers were flown by the world's airlines, excluding the airlines of the USSR and China.

Transportation by every means continues to develop. In the last decade, we have seen man in orbit round the earth and walking on the moon. Interplanetary flight would seem a distinct possibility in the next half-century at the present state of our knowledge and technical development.

PREPARATION FOR THE JOURNEY

Whatever means one chooses to make a longish journey inevitably requires some preparation, be it, on the one hand, adequate rest before setting out, suitable clothing and material provisions, to proper inoculation against endemic diseases and accurate knowledge of the country through which or to which one is proceeding.

The requirements for vaccination and inoculation against disease are contained in the International Health Regulations published by the World Health Organisation based in Geneva. This agency, one of many set up by United Nations is the international watch-dog on endemic diseases and issues a weekly epidemiological bulletin on disease states round the world. Most nations of the world subscribe to these regulations which give advice on the protection of individuals against diseases such as smallpox, cholera, typhoid fever, poliomyelitis and yellow fever. Airlines, travel agents and immunization centres will advise travellers of current requirements for the countries they intend visiting.

Fortunately, most of these diseases including smallpox and cholera are on the wane. Smallpox has largely been beaten but small pockets of the disease still exist in countries such as Bangladesh and Ethiopia, and a fair number of countries still demand evidence of recent vaccination against smallpox and cholera. Vaccination against smallpox must have been carried out within 3 years and cholera within 6 months of travel.

There is no doubt that smallpox vaccination has largely removed this scourge from the world but it has been so successful that in some communities we are beginning to see a largely unvaccinated population which bodes ill for any introduced infection.

Cholera vaccine is usually given in two injections of 0·1 ml intradermally, 7–14 days apart and this gives something like 60 per cent protection to the individual provided he takes reasonable hygenic precautions against the drinking of untreated water, eating of unwashed fruit and so on. The inoculation is valid for 6 months and has to be repeated at the end of this time.

Yellow fever carried by the mosquito *Aedes aegypti* is still endemic in equatorial regions of the world particularly in Africa and South America. Inoculation is demanded by many countries bordering these areas and is given in the form of a single injection which is effective for ten years.

Other protective inoculations may be advised for certain areas but are not obligatory under the International Health Regulations. Amongst them are inoculations against typhoid, paratyphoid A, B and C which can be given together in two separate injections or combined with tetanus serum in the form of TABT.

In certain parts of the world including India, Nepal and Kashmir, it is advisable to have protection against infective hepatitis. This is given in the form of gamma-globulin 2 ml intramuscularly and gives a fair degree of protection provided that sensible hygienic measures are taken during the journey and in these areas.

Acute poliomyelitis is still endemic in many parts of the Near and Middle East and it is strongly advisable to be protected against this crippling disease. It can be taken very easily as the Salk vaccine by mouth.

Vaccination against smallpox and inoculation against yellow fever should either be carried out at the same time or given 3 weeks apart. Smallpox vaccination should not be given to pregnant women, to sufferers from eczema, skin allergies or to those receiving treatment with steroids. An internationally recognized exemption certificate can be issued. Yellow fever vaccine is usually prepared on an egg medium so anyone allergic to eggs should not be given the vaccine.

Table 16.1. Vaccinations and inoculations.

Type	Required by	Validity	Duration
Smallpox	Countries in Near, Far East, Africa, South America	8–10 days after primary Immediately after re-vaccination	3 years
Cholera	India, Pakistan and other designated areas	7 days after injection	6 months
Typhoid (TAB, TABC, TABT)	Advisable except North Europe, North America, United Kingdom	4 weeks 2 injections	1 year
Typhus	Advisable India, Pakistan, South-East Asia	10 days after injection	1 year
Yellow Fever	Parts of Africa, Central and South America	After 10 days	10 years
Hepatitis A (Gamma Globulin)	North and Central Africa, Middle East, Asia, South America	7 days after injection	6 months
Poliomyelitis	Advised for world-wide travel	3 doses of vaccine by mouth at 4 week intervals.	4–6 months Give booster dose in high risk areas

TROPICAL DISEASES

The traveller in tropical areas where diseases are endemic can be particularly at risk to malaria, the dysenteries and other fly and tick-borne diseases. Of these malaria is the most serious and this is carried by the anopheline mosquito where the organism spends half its life cycle. This is completed by its injection into man during the act of biting and feeding by the mosquito. Malaria in all its forms accounts for some 3.5 million deaths per annum and is also responsible for much chronic ill health, particularly if the disease is not promptly diagnosed and treated.

Malaria

In endemic areas which include most of Equatorial Africa, South America, the Indian sub-continent and the Far East, adequate covering of exposed areas of the body is essential during the hours of darkness when mosquitoes normally fly, and the use of mosquito-nets and adequate insecticidal spraying of sleeping accommodation at night is essential. In most air-conditioned bedrooms the use of nets can be dispensed with, provided adequate spraying with insecticide is carried out. All travellers living in or passing through malarial areas must however take anti-malarial tablets when in the area and for 28 days after leaving it. Proguanil hydrochloride (Paludrine) is a suitable anti-malarial taken daily (100 mg) or alternatively chloroquine (Nivaquine) (400 mg weekly). Chloroquine is probably the best drug for treatment and should be reserved for this rather than prophylaxis.

It is essential that any traveller returning from a tropical region and developing a fever tells his doctor where he has been. Failure to do so can result in tragedy because cerebral malaria can develop within 48 hours or so of being bitten by an infected mosquito. Air travel is so rapid that removal of a prospective victim to a temperate climate may not allow time for the disease to manifest itself and when it does it may be missed. Some 1160 cases of malaria were seen in the UK in 1977 alone. This is a marked increase on previous years and the same is true of other countries in northern latitudes who report similar rises in the incidence of malaria.

The dysenteries

These can be classified very broadly as bacterial and amoebic. Bacterial dysentery usually presents in the form of an acute massive infection with violent explosive diarrhoea, abdominal pain and vomiting. Amoebic dysentery due to the organism *Entamoeba histolytica* develops more slowly and progresses with watery loose stools, fever and chronic ill-health. Complications include liver and brain abscesses. Both forms of dysentery are transmitted by faecally contaminated milk, water, ice or by eating uncooked food which has been infected by flies or by unhygienic handling. Treatment of bacterial dysentery is usually fairly easy using antibiotics and antispasmodics but treatment of amoebic dysentery on the other hand is long and tedious, with frequent relapses.

FOOD POISONING AND TRAVELLER'S DIARRHOEA

Food poisoning due to the ingestion of infected food, usually prepared under doubtful hygienic conditions, is a distressing complaint frequently afflicting the traveller. Recent outbreaks have been seen in groups of airline passengers who ingested seafood infected with *Vibrio parahaemolyticus.* This causes an acute form of food poisoning with violent diarrhoea, vomiting and extreme prostration. Other infections have been due to typhoid. One infamous case where 200 airline passengers were affected was traced to a staphylococcus infection in the hand of the airport chef. The catering manager of the firm concerned was so affected that he committed hara kiri! No guesses as to his nationality!

Traveller's diarrhoea can be a most distressing condition which may on laboratory examination show no causal organism – or at least usually none can be traced. In groups of travellers it may be worth treating them with antibiotics prophylactically and in fact this was done in the case of the British Olympic teams over the years. They were given minimal daily doses of Streptotriad with very good results during a number of Olympic games including Rome, Tokyo and Mexico City. They did not get diarrhoea but they did not win any gold medals either – so the minimal dosages used may have affected athletic performance to some extent!

MOTION SICKNESS

Motion sickness is probably as old as man himself when he made his first tentative attempts at travel on land and sea. It was well known to the Ancient Greeks and the word nausea is derived from the Greek *naus* – a ship.

The condition has plagued the traveller throughout the ages, Julius Caesar, Lord Nelson, Charles Darwin and Lawrence of Arabia being a few recorded sufferers of note, the last being particularly subject to motion sickness when riding a camel. Little was done about the disease until World War II when it became necessary to transport large bodies of men by land, air and sea and keep them in a suitable physical condition to go straight into action. The survival of those in rafts and life-boats largely depended on the successful prevention of motion sickness. In the last decade we have seen motion sickness in space amongst American and Russian astronauts and cosmonauts.

The exact aetiology of motion sickness is unknown but it would appear that an intact vestibular apparatus is essential to produce the condition. Motion sickness does not appear in animals where the labyrinthine mechanism has been destroyed by disease or operation.

The eyes, too, seem to play a considerable part in the aetiology of the disease. It is important in ships to remain on deck and focus on the distant horizon or when below decks to keep the eyes closed and the head fixed. Similarly in aircraft, or in trains and cars, gaze should be directed to points well away from the vehicle. Persons subject to the disease are much less prone when given a task to perform thus occupying the mind.

There has been much controversy in the past regarding prevention and treatment. The mechanism by which drugs reduce the incidence of the disease is still obscure, but all appear to have an action on the central nervous system. Drugs include the antihistamines, belladonna, phenothiazines, antihistamines and the barbiturates either together or in combination.

In selecting a drug for an individual it should be remembered that the drug most suitable for the majority may not be the drug of choice for that particular individual, especially if he has to perform a skilled task.

For instance, to give an airline pilot or car-driver an antihistamine with the possible effects of drowsiness and disorientation is to invite disaster. In the same way it would be pointless administering drugs by mouth to an individual who is already vomiting. Using the oral route, it is important to administer the drug before the individual is exposed to the motion. In the survival situation Brand and Wittingham (1970) have shown that the intramuscular injection of hyoscine hydrobromide (0·2 mg) gave good results when given to survivors in life-rafts compared to others who were given a placebo. This single dose controlled symptoms within 15 to 30 minutes and afforded protection for about 4 hours.

Wood (1970) at Pensacola found that hyoscine hydrobromide (0·6 mg) by mouth was still the best for bad-risk cases undergoing short exposures to motion and that promethazine hydrochloride given in 25 mg doses twice daily was almost as good. Both of the above drugs are particularly good for night travel as they also provide sedation. Less effective drugs are meclozine (50 mg twice daily) or cyclizine (50 mg twice daily); the latter should not be given to expectant mothers. Dimenhydrinate (50 mg twice daily) is also effective but produces drowsiness as a side-effect.

Work by Wood and Graybiel (1970) has revealed that combining promethazine (25 mg) with dexamphetamine (10 mg) gives consistently good results which are almost as good as hyoscine hydrobromide (0·6 mg) combined with dexamphetamine (10 mg).

Further evidence by the same authors has shown that promethazine (25 mg) combined with ephedrine hydrochloride (25 mg) was the best preventative against motion sickness. Hyoscine hydrobromide is contraindicated in glaucoma and in cases of urinary retention. Dexamphetamine is contraindicated in cases of high blood pressure. The addictive qualities of dexamphetamine should also be recognized.

The success of drugs in the prevention and treatment of motion sickness depends largely on the susceptibility of the individual and on the duration of severity of the motion. From a technological standpoint great strides have been made in diminishing the harmful accelerations in vehicles. Examples are vibration-free jet engines which enable aircraft to cruise above the weather, the use of stabilizers in ships, hydro-elastic and hydraulic suspensions in road vehicles, welded rails and improved rolling-stock in railroads.

TRAVEL AND THE CIRCADIAN RHYTHMS

Diurnal variations of light, temperature and other environmental cues resulting from the axial rotation of the earth affect all living things including plants, with the exception of those living in polar latitudes where extremes of light and dark are dependent on season.

These variations have imposed on all living organisms with the possible exception perhaps of fish at great depths an internal diurnal cycle which affects many bodily functions. The term 'circadian' (from the Latin *circa* – around, and *dies* – day) was first used by Franz Halberg at the University of Minnesota and he has been instrumental in building up a new science which he has named 'Chronobiology'. Circadian changes are denoted by alternating periods of sleep and wakefulness which impose a background of rhythmic metabolic changes, including body temperature, changes in the chemical constituents of the blood, kidney and gastrointestinal function, liver, endocrine and respiratory systems and in the ability of the individual to carry out skilled tasks.

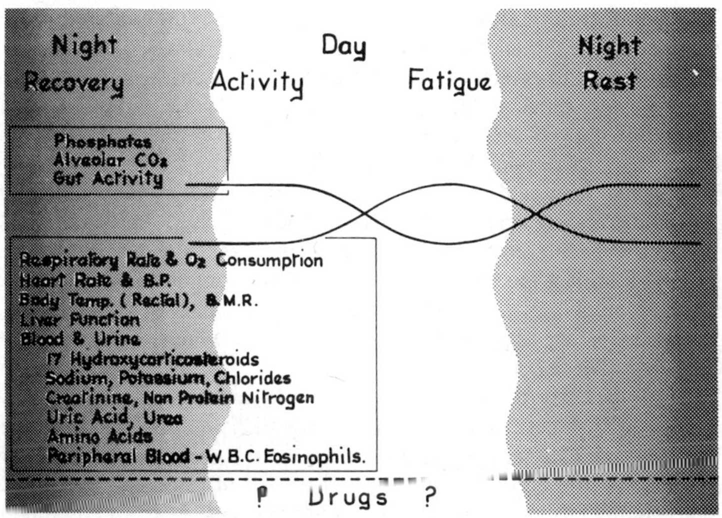

Fig. 16.1. Diagrammatic representation of the ebb and flow of the various circadian rhythms in the body during 24 hours.

Much of the original work on this subject was carried out by Kleitman (1949) on US submarine personnel, but navies have known of these problems for centuries and as a result introduced the 'watch-on' and 'watch-off' some 400 years ago.

In recent astronautic flights both Russian and US crews were kept on local home-based time during space-flight as once clear of the earth's shadow the normal light-dark cycle is disrupted, which interferes with sleep and the individual's ability to perform adequately. Definite work/rest cycles were therefore introduced corresponding to local time back on earth, and in some space-flights hypnotic drugs were dispensed to achieve sleep.

As far as our earthly traveller is concerned, our world is divided into 24 time zones of 15 meridians, each representing one hour of time.

When man travels by surface transport, for instance by train or ship, his rate of time-zone crossing is slow, and so when travelling East or West adjustments can be made by 30–60 minutes per day depending on his mode of travel. No adaptation is required for travel North or South.

The air-traveller however is in a different category when flying East or West either just below the speed of sound or in a supersonic aircraft. He or she may cross five time zones in 3–6 hours depending on the type of aircraft. As a result, established circadian rhythms will be disrupted, especially when the individual attempts to adjust to the new environment and local time at his destination and particularly if he attempts to undertake social or work activities when he should be catching up on sleep.

There is an endogenous control of the circadian rhythms as study of the plasma cortisol levels show a diurnal variation. The effect of such an ebb and flow in adreno-cortical activity reflects changes in the cardiovascular, respiratory and renal systems. Flink and Doe (1969) showed that the excretion of the 17-ketosteroids in the urine takes something between 5 and 9 days to re-establish after a flight from the US to Japan. Other workers have suggested the importance of the pituitary-adrenal cortical system in the maintenance of circadian rhythms.

It has also been shown by Imrie et al. (1963) that the normal circadian exaction of urinary potassium can be abolished or modified by the experimental blocking of ACTH by prednisolone. This is promising as it may be possible in the future to produce drugs which could abolish or modify circadian rhythms.

To sum up, therefore, the individual would appear to possess an endogenous or hormonal 'clock' which is essentially hormonal in nature. This 'clock' is influenced by external cues via the central nervous system, principally by the changes from light to dark and vice versa but also by ambient temperature variations and other sources such as community noise. There is also remarkable accord between plasma cortisol and changes from day-to-night and night-to-day ensuring that the individual prepares for sleep at night and for activity on the return of daylight.

The traveller

Where does the poor traveller fit in to all this? First of all, if he is transported rapidly across time zones he will have trouble in achieving adequate sleep in his new environment, at least for the first few days. In work carried out on pilots and cabin crew in British Airways, Preston (1973) found that individuals could become very sleep-deprived, particularly if early retiral to bed is not practised on arrival, and that there was an inability to re-establish a satisfactory sleep pattern for several days with resultant diminution of physical and mental performance.

In addition, due to the very dry cabin atmosphere experienced in most jet-transport aircraft the individual can become very dehydrated in flight. Our experience has been in non-humidified aircraft that after 90 minutes' flight at high altitude the relative humidity (RH) may have fallen to 20 per cent or less.

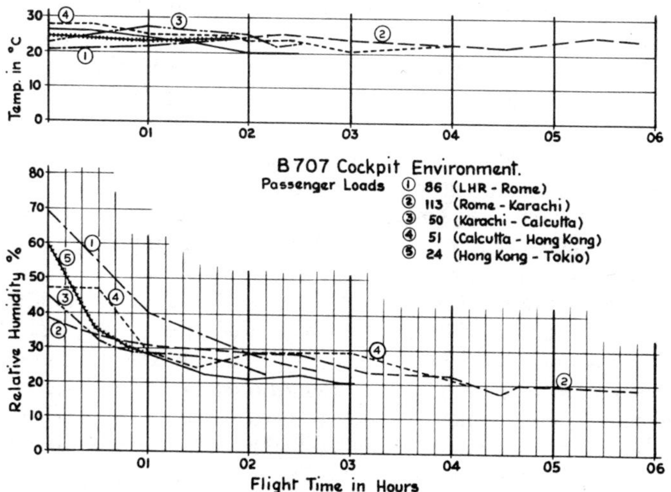

Fig. 16.2. Aircraft temperature and humidity levels during flight. Note how relative humidity levels fall markedly during the first hour and then level off.

Prolonged exposure to these levels will produce dryness and brittleness of the hair, cracking of the nails and reduction of urinary output together with drying of the skin and mucous membranes. We have always advised our crews and passengers to drink between four and five pints of fluid daily when flying to combat these effects.

Alcoholic drinks, particularly spirits, and beverages such as tea and coffee may in themselves produce further dehydration since the first may draw fluid into the gastro-intestinal tract and the others have a direct diuretic action.

Water and squash-type drinks are certainly the best as far as fluid replacement is concerned. Most airlines provide water-fountains and have stringent regulations on the potability of drinking water. Carbonated drinks should be avoided as they can cause abdominal distension and flatulence at altitude.

Airlines and shipping companies tend to overload the innocent traveller with food and he may tend to eat anything that is offered, often out of sheer boredom. There are no medals given for completing every gastronomic presentation and the result may be disastrous to the individual.

It has been known for many years that there are changes in the output of the digestive juices both in character and output during the normal 24-hour cycle. Johnson and Washeim noted as long ago as 1924 that there is a rise in gastric acidity during sleep, together with a fall in volume and that the secretion appears to be more before 02·30. There are also circadian rhythms in serum bilirubin, urobilinogen and in the formation of bile. The pancreatic rhythms were noted by Pfaff as long ago as 1897, excretion being highest in the early afternoon and falling to a minimum at night. Colonic activity is reduced or ceases entirely between 22·00 and 04·00 and a resumption has been noted between 04·00 and 06·00.

To eat large, rich and often unaccustomed meals at such times is simply asking for trouble and although offered by the airline, refusal should be the order of the day. Remember of course that the airline has a problem in that the joining passenger must be fed. His circadian rhythms may well be in a different phase from yours.

Smoking in the rarified cabin atmosphere of transport aircraft which may be at an altitude of between 5000 and 7000 feet is to be discouraged as the carbon monoxide in the inhaled cigarette smoke combines directly with haemoglobin to form carboxyhaemogloblin. This further reduces the individual's 'ceiling' which has already been depleted by the fall in the partial oxygen pressure. At sea-level this falls from 160 mmHg to 126 mmHg at 5000 feet.

ARRIVAL AT DESTINATION

In planning long trans-meridian flights it is advisable to arrive as near one's bedtime as possible and having arrived, go straight to bed. Even better, plan to arrive in the early evening of the new environment, refusing all offers of entertainment and retire. This is the situation where a mild hypnotic for the first few nights will ensure adequate periods of sleep. Much work has been done at the RAF Institute of Aviation Medicine at Farnborough on the use of hypnotics in aircrew over the last few years. Their recommendations are that diazepam (Valium) is probably the best hypnotic for this purpose as it has little or no long-term effects on mental performance which many other hypnotics including the barbiturates exhibit to varying degrees and often for prolonged periods (Ministry of Defence, London, 1977).

Business meetings should be avoided for at least 24 hours after arrival. As you are not at your best, wrong decisions may be made and there is certainly very definite physiological evidence that reaction time, short-term memory and general mental efficiency can be lowered for two or three days. The body is slow to adapt to new time zones, possibly between

5 and 9 days, longer in the older person – so that the individual should make every effort to take things easy during this period, making every effort to catch up on his sleep deficit which will certainly be present.

LONG RAIL JOURNEYS

With the exception of perhaps the Trans-Siberian Railway very few really long railway journeys exist in the world today. It is now no longer possible to cross Canada by rail but it is possible to travel by rail from New York to Los Angeles.

I have had no experience of the Trans-Siberian railway, but I have spoken to travellers who have made the journey. The main problem appears to be the necessity to provide oneself with adequate supplies of food and water for the journey as dining cars appear for certain sectors and then disappear for others. Food and beverages can be purchased at stations *en route* but the language barrier may present problems. Supplies of soap, towels, toilet paper are essential on all USSR trains. Choose the de luxe class of travel as they have let-down bunks at night which allows the weary traveller to stretch out horizontally. First class in Indian trains still tends to be good with air-conditioned sleeping compartments and conductor-service.

Rail travel in the United States is generally of a high standard, AMTRAK providing a nation-wide service with sleeping cars, restaurant cars and good personal service.

Take plenty of reading matter, card-games and other distractions if you plan a long train journey.

LONG ROAD JOURNEYS

In the United Kingdom where distances are short no particular problems arise on our motorways except for the fact you should not start out when tired, for instance at the end of a working day. Motorway driving demands a high state of attention and concentration. Two hours' high-speed driving is long enough. Stop at a suitable service station, walk around, remember the inner man and keep up the blood glucose level.

Increasing numbers of travellers are now undertaking long overland journeys to the Far and Middle East either as tourists or for business purposes. In addition there is now a great deal of long distance road-haulage traffic to the Balkans, the Near East, the Persian Gulf, Iran and India on an almost regular and daily basis. Commercial drivers on these routes are highly professional in their driving standards and behaviour, and although they are not governed by the Road Traffic Acts for commercial drivers when overseas, nevertheless they may be subject to individual national regulations *en route.* Relief drivers, adequate sleeping facilities in the driver's compartment, heating and cooling facilities are essential. In addition adequate supplies of safe drinking water and above-suspicion food supplies are necessary.

In the Balkans and Middle East it is not advisable to camp at the road-side. Commercial vehicles would never dream of doing so, preferring security-patrolled vehicle compounds. Stealing of loads, vehicle parts and hold-ups are the order of the day in some countries. The tourist is therefore well advised to stick to official camp sites where he is assured of some security for his vehicle and its occupants.

If travelling by road, record-breaking attempts and long journeys during the hours of darkness should be avoided. Plan your journey by getting the best advice from the motoring associations and the national tourist organizations of the countries you plan to pass through.

Circadian rhythm changes when journeying by road or rail are slow compared to those in air travel and it may be necessary to put the clock back or forward 30–60 minutes per day if travelling east or west. No changes in local time are necessary for north or south travel.

For those susceptible to motion sickness adequate medication as previously described should be given, remembering that the driver or drivers require special consideration due to the adverse side-effects produced by some drugs.

REFERENCES

Brand J. J. and Whittingham P. (1970) Intramuscular hyoscine in the treatment of motion sickness. *Lancet* **2,** 232.

Flink E. B. and Doe R. P. (1969) Adrenal studies in long trans-ocean flights. *Proc. Soc. Exp. Biol. Med.* **100,** 498.

Imrie M. J., Mills J. N. and Williamson K. S. (1963) The renal action of small doses of cortisol at night. *J. Endocrinol.* **27,** 289–292.

Johnson R. L. and Washeim H. (1924) Studies in gastric secretion II. Gastric secretion in sleep. *Am. J. Physiol.* **70,** 247–253.

Kleitman M. (1949) *The Sleep-wakefulness in Submarine Personnel.* National Research Council (USA) Factors in Undersea Warfare. Baltimore, Waverley Press, 329–341.

Ministry of Defence, London (1977) *Hypnotics and Sedatives for use by Aircrew.* MOD. MA2 (RAF), Clinical Memorandum 3/77. Tavis House, London.

Pfaff F. (1897) Some observations in a case of human pancreatic fistula. *J. Boston Soc. Med. Sci.* **2,** 10–18.

Preston F. S. (1973) Further sleep problems in airline pilots on world-wide schedules. *Aerospace Med.* **44,** 775–782.

Wood C. D. (1970) Selection of an anti-motion drug. *J. Louisiana State Med. Soc.* **122,** 95.

Wood C. D. and Graybiel A. (1970) Evaluation of anti-motion drugs; a new effective remedy revealed. *Aerospace Med.* **41,** 932.

17. ALCOHOL-RELATED DISABILITIES

Marcus Grant

The title of this chapter is also the title of an unusually far-reaching, if also rather confusing, World Health Organisation publication (Edwards et al., 1977). That publication argues that the expression 'alcohol-related disabilities' has a wider and more pragmatic appeal than, for example, the term 'alcoholism' which has, over the years, become surrounded with a host of separate, and sometimes contradictory, shades of definition. It is, of course, unlikely that 'alcoholism' will become an obsolete label in the forseeable future. Nevertheless, the change of emphasis implied by the W.H.O. publication is of particular importance in the sphere of occupational health.

Alcoholism as such will certainly be discussed in this chapter but so will a range of drinking difficulties which, though clearly less severe than would be suggested by so extreme a clinical label, nevertheless demand serious attention by the occupational health specialist. The burden of evidence suggests that where early intervention takes place (Cartwright et al., 1975) and where good communication exists between the relevant practitioners (Edwards and Grant, 1977) people with alcohol-related disabilities, which may exist in a variety of different life areas, can be helped significantly so that more severe alcohol problems, which would have been likely to occur, can be avoided. This is precisely the position of occupational health specialists where the high observability profile of the potential patient population, the ease of access to identified patients and the manipulability of the health care and allied services combine to produce a situation in which a rational approach to alcohol problems is likely to be particularly effective.

Traditional objections to alcoholic patients have been shown (Wilkins, 1974) to bear little relation to the real world. There is no particular evidence that those with alcohol-related disabilities are less treatable, more time-consuming or have a worse prognosis than many other kinds of patients. Indeed, the experience of running alcoholism recovery programmes in industrial (Von Wiegand, 1972) or service (Gwinner, 1976) settings, makes it clear that, under favourable circumstances, very high recovery rates can be anticipated. Not only are occupational health specialists particularly well placed in terms of access, therefore; they are also known to be particularly effective. It is important to emphasize this point here, since there certainly still exist a number of practitioners who believe that the most appropriate treatment for those whose drinking causes problems at work is to dismiss them. Or, as if humanity existed merely in softening fatal body blows, to retire them prematurely on medical grounds. It is assumed in this chapter that the functions of occupational health are to prevent problems occurring and to cure existing problems rather than to erect, however well-intentioned, a fabric of denial and camouflage.

DEFINING ALCOHOLISM

Certainly, a word can sometimes take on unfortunate overtones. Alcoholism is probably one such word and the W.H.O. re-classification is an attempt to set the record straight. It is important to state here that alcoholics are not necessarily those pathetic figures in dirty raincoats with bottles of methylated spirits in their pockets. Such vagrants account for less than 5 per cent of the alcoholic population of most civilized countries and they are the ones, by and large, least likely to become involved in occupational health programmes.

Even having abandoned false stereotypes, however, it is still difficult to arrive at a definition of alcoholism which could win universal approval. It is often convenient to think of alcoholism as a disease. Such a view is clearly preferable to considering it as a sin or moral weakness. At the same time, however, the disease model can prove less than satisfactory since it can offer the alcoholic the opportunity to use the sick role to diminish his responsibility for his condition or its cure (Robinson, 1976). Similarly, it can lead to the attractive and popularly held view that alcoholism is a kind of allergy and that there are predetermining factors, either of a biochemical or personality nature, which are present in alcoholics prior to the onset of harmful drinking. It is only fair to say that exhaustive research (reviewed by Shields, 1977) has so far failed to provide convincing evidence of such predisposing characteristics.

Recognizing the difficulties posed by the present multiplicity of definitions, Davies (1974) has attempted to reduce them to their basic elements. He suggests that alcoholism can reasonably be defined as 'the continuous or intermittent consumption of alcohol leading to dependence or harm'. He explains that dependence can be either physical or psychological and that harm can be physical, psychological or social.

Most alcoholics drink heavily every day. The problem, since what is defined as heavy drinking varies considerably between cultures or between classes within cultures (O'Connor, 1978) is to set some objective criterion for determining a threshold beyond which the likelihood of damage is significantly increased. De Lint (1974) has suggested that a daily intake of 15 centilitres of absolute alcohol represents such a threshold.

Some alcoholics do not drink every day. There is a striking case relating to a lighthouse keeper who, during his four-week stints of duty on the lighthouse, was totally abstinent. On his periods of shore leave, however, having given his landlady the rent for the whole period, he would spend his entire wages in becoming and remaining totally drunk until his next spell of duty, when he would revert to total abstinence. Clearly, the drinking pattern as a whole must be considered when a diagnosis is being made.

Davies (1974) lists the consequences of excessive alcohol consumption as 'dependence or harm'. Whether one accepts his distinction between physical and psychological dependence or whether one prefers the notion of the alcohol dependence syndrome which is described by Edwards (1977), it is clear that dependence is not an all or nothing state and that any individual's level of dependence must be measured against some kind of notional scale. One's own drinking habits are not really a sufficiently objective scale and it is the tendency of some practitioners to rely too heavily upon their own consumption levels that has led to an alternative definition of an alcoholic as 'somebody who drinks more than his doctor'.

It is important to remember that dependence does not presume harm and that there is growing evidence (Clare, 1977) to suggest that there is a significant spontaneous remission rate from alcoholism. Harm is, however, the most significant part of the definition in that it is usually because some harm has been occasioned by his drinking that the alcoholic first comes to notice. Harm can be either to himself or to his family or colleagues. For the purposes of this chapter, special emphasis will be placed upon the effects of alcohol on work, but it should be recognized that it will also affect other aspects of social functioning and the total physical and mental health of the drinker.

EFFECTS OF ALCOHOL ON WORK

For practical purposes, it is important that those involved in occupational health should distinguish between the short and long-term effects of alcohol consumption. Acute alcohol intoxication is certainly likely to cause problems. Most organizations, however, have clearly defined procedures for dealing with drunkenness among employees and it is likely that, where only a single incident is being considered, the pattern of the employee's previous work record will be taken into account. Legislation relating to employment protection should be taken into consideration as well (Osborne and Gordon, 1978) since the decision is likely to be of a disciplinary rather than a medical nature.

Clearly an employee who is drunk is likely to show reduced efficiency and loss of fine motor skills. The evidence has been reviewed by Hore (1977a). It is seldom, however, that the occupational health specialist will be involved in such isolated cases, except where called in to determine whether an employee is indeed drunk. On such occasions, considerable caution must be exercised since no really satisfactory criteria for establishing objective standards of acute intoxication exist. It will usually prove better to suggest that the decision as to whether an employee is drunk and therefore unable to perform his task relates most directly to the nature of the work in which he is engaged, and that it is therefore more properly a managerial decision to be made by his immediate supervisor.

Where, however, there is evidence of repeated drunkenness, the nature of the problem is very different. Any of the effects listed below might, of course, occur in relation to a single episode of drunkenness and, depending upon the seriousness of the consequences, might require action by the organization. It is when they form part of a demonstrable pattern of behaviour that the occupational health specialist has a special role to play because it is then that the problem moves from questions of discipline to questions of health and continuing safety.

Hore (1977b) has also reviewed evidence relating to rates of absenteeism and industrial accidents amongst employees who drink heavily. The number of days loss of work is shown to be as high as 70–85 per annum with a corresponding tendency towards frequent late arrival for work. It should be noted that episodes of absence will often be explained most convincingly by the employee and that vague complaints such as gastritis and back trouble will be blamed for the time away from work.

The evidence on accident rates is just as convincing, even if the figures are rather less dramatic. Studies in the United States and in France have indicated work accident rates of twice or three times the normal. The differential rates are particularly apparent amongst young and middle-aged employees. The majority of alcohol-related work accidents occur in the afternoon.

In summary, therefore, although the effects of excessive alcohol consumption make themselves felt in all aspects of physical, mental and social functioning, those items which are most directly relevant to the employment situation relate to loss of efficiency, absenteeism and increased likelihood of accidents. The practical implications of these will be discussed in greater detail in the section of this chapter concerned with recognition.

OCCUPATIONAL FACTORS

There is a considerable body of evidence from a range of sources which makes it clear that different occupations have very different rates of alcoholism. The OPCS has reviewed the evidence and, using male liver cirrhosis mortality as the best available indicator of relative alcoholism prevalence rates, has drawn up the following table (Table 17.1).

Four factors (Plant, 1977) appear to influence most strongly the drinking habits of different occupations and to link, in general terms, the high-risk occupations shown in the table below.

Without doubt, the first and most potent factor of all is the availability of alcohol. In some occupations alcohol is available easily during working hours. It may even be provided free or at a reduced price. This factor is of particular relevance to those engaged in the production, sale and distri-

Table 17.1. Occupations with the highest mortality from cirrhosis of the liver. (From *Occupational Mortality, 1970–72, England and Wales, Office of Population Censuses and Surveys, HMSO London, 1978*). *Crown Copyright.*

Occupation	Rank in top 20	All deaths SMR
Publicans, innkeepers	1	1576
Deck, engineering officers and pilots, ship	2	781
Barmen, barmaids	3	633
Deck and engine room ratings, barge and boatmen	4	628
Fishermen	5	595
Proprietors and managers boarding houses and hotels	6	506
Finance, insurance brokers, financial agents	7	392
Restaurateurs	8	385
Lorry drivers' mates, van guards	9	377
Cooks	10	354
Shunters, pointsmen	11	323
Winders, reelers	12	319
Electrical engineers (so described)	13	319
Authors, journalists and related workers	14	314
Medical practitioners (qualified)	15	311
Garage proprietors	16	294
Signalmen and crossing keepers, railways	17	290
Maids, valets and related service workers	18	281
Tobacco preparers and products makers	19	269
Metallurgists	20	266

*Standardized mortality ratios are calculated taking into account the age composition of an occupational group. The average standardized mortality ratio is expressed as 100.

bution of alcoholic beverages, but it is also important to those who are accustomed to entertaining business contacts over a drink.

It relates to the second factor, which can best be described as the social pressure to drink. Some occupations exert distinct and persuasive encouragement towards an acceptance of a heavy drinking pattern. Those who spend their life on board ship, members of the armed forces and commercial travellers could all be seen as being subject to increased social pressure to drink.

Third, occupations which involve a high degree of mobility and which divorce workers from the stabilizing influence of home tend to show higher rates of heavy drinking. In some cases, this may relate to the frustrations caused by the absence of acceptable sexual outlets; in others, the unfamiliarity and lack of stable social context caused by frequent travelling.

The final factor is that of relative freedom from supervision. Those who are less closely supervised have more opportunity to drink during working hours. It has been suggested (Murray, 1975) that this factor may be of particular importance with regard to senior workers such as company directors and medical practitioners.

Vulnerability here, as elsewhere in the sphere of occupational health, is the key to understanding the problem. In the past, there has been a tendency to polarize the man and the bottle and to assume that the vulnerability was a measure of the weakness of the man. Equally, of course, last century it was thought to be a measure of the strength of the bottle. What is becoming clear now is that vulnerability is a measure of the relationship between the man and the bottle and that, if that relationship is to be improved so that vulnerability is reduced, then both the man and the bottle (or, at least, the availability of the bottle) may require manipulation.

PREVENTION AND EDUCATION

It has been pointed out by Grant (1977) that one of the main advantages of adopting a preventive approach to alcohol problems in employment is that such an approach does not presume the necessity to identify individuals. Given that alcoholism – or even the renamed alcohol-related disabilities – carries still a sense of social stigma, it must be obvious that one of the reasons for the difficulties which are encountered in persuading sufferers to come forward to receive treatment, is that they are often ashamed of the label which they would thus be accepting. In a delicate union–management situation the suggestion that a particular employee was an alcoholic could easily be seen as an accusation rather than as an offer of help.

A broadly based preventive approach may, therefore, forestall unnecessary confrontations. It is also in keeping with general trends in occupational health practice. The prevention of alcohol-related disabilities can proceed in two distinct, though closely linked, ways: through controls and through education.

It is perfectly legitimate for an employer to control the availability of alcohol to his employees. It is also sensible for him to seek support on health grounds for such controls as he wishes to implement. It has already been established in this chapter that the ease of availability of alcohol is a most potent factor in determining consumption rates. Thus, though the employer may not wish to remove alcohol totally from the place of work (though some employers have indeed done just that), he may well wish to monitor, for example, the flow of Scotch through his export manager's drinks cabinet or the average *per capita* lunchtime beer consumption in the works canteen.

Employees who display evidence of clear drunkenness are likely to be subject to some kind of disciplinary procedure. This is, however, a control system which only comes into operation once the offence has been committed. More effectively, an employer can make the availability of alcohol conditional upon certain prerequisites, the foremost of which can be that specific limits are set upon the actual amount of drinking which people are allowed to do while at work.

There are some categories of employees who should be the subject of special controls. These categories include those who are known to be particularly vulnerable and those, such as drivers, pilots and supervisors, whose job involves responsibility for the safety of others. For such people, the special controls can take the form of regular monitoring by the occupational health staff so that, for example, routine liver function tests can serve as an additional safeguard. Suitable procedures are discussed in detail by Pollak (1978) and will be reviewed further in the next section of this chapter.

Rational control policies should provide a context within which primary preventive education can be expected to be rather more effective than if no such context existed. The aim of primary prevention is to increase general awareness so that people choose to alter their behaviour to decrease the number of disadvantageous consequences. There is no one way of approaching such a complex problem and no clear evidence that particular approaches always yield good results. What is most important is that the medium and the message which are adopted should be consonant with the overall management style of the company. The question of the prevention of alcoholism requires each company to decide for itself the most effective way in which to communicate the relevant information within the context of existing practice with regard to staff training, occupational health, safety regulations, disciplinary procedures, personnel management and the use of leisure.

In the United Kingdom, the Alcohol Education Centre and the Scottish Health Education Unit have produced a sophisticated multimedia resource pack to assist companies in this task. Of crucial importance, however, is the extent to which the individual employee perceives the information and advice offered as having direct relevance to him. To this end, it is useful to introduce the concept of self-monitoring as an aid to health. This can be achieved through the operation of a quantity/frequency guide coupled to a key indicators questionnaire. The quantity/frequency threshold identified by de Lint (1974) is clearly inappropriate for this subclinical approach and a more useful method of quantification is set out in Table 17.2.

Precise equivalents in terms of centilitres of absolute alcohol will, of course, vary between countries, depending upon both the alcoholic strength and the common measures of beverage alcohol available. The effect of such a self-monitoring system, which can also of course be used as the basis for a clinical interview, is that it focuses attention on the actual quantity of alcohol consumed. Many drinkers are unaware of how much they do in fact get through in an average week, and are certainly surprised to see how quickly the odd drinks add up to a substantial total.

A key indicators questionnaire can easily be compiled using the information given in the next section and wording the questions so that they appear unthreatening and exploratory.

Table 17.2. Estimation of total alcohol consumption for last week.

The basic scoring unit will be 1 centilitre of alcohol. The values shown are approximate.

1 glass of wine	=	1
1 single tot of spirits	=	1
1 glass of sherry or port	=	1
1 pint of beer or lager	=	2
1 can of special strength lager	=	3
1 pint bottle of wine	=	7
1 litre bottle of wine	=	10
1 bottle of sherry	=	12
½ bottle of spirits	=	15
1 bottle of spirits	=	30

	Beer	Wine	Fortified wine	Spirits	TOTAL
Monday					
Tuesday					
Wednesday					
Thursday					
Friday					
Saturday					
Sunday					
				TOTAL	

If the total for any single day is more than 10 or if the total for the week is more than 50, then the subject is drinking heavily.

If the total for any day is more than 15 or if the total for the week is more than 70, then the subject is probably experiencing some problems already.

EARLY RECOGNITION

As with many other conditions, early recognition of alcoholism leads to improved prognosis. Indeed, where alcohol-related disabilities are identified before they become associated with severe dependence, it will usually be possible for the individual to learn to modify the way he drinks in order to eradicate the harm without having to eradicate the pleasures of alcohol from his life.

A variety of screening and early detection instruments have been reviewed by Murray (1977) whose conclusion is that they have a real, though limited applicability, particularly when used to scrutinize distinct rather than diffuse occupational groups. In addition, the notion of at-risk factors (Wilkins, 1974) which include life areas other than those which are most evident in the place of work, is clearly too important to ignore, although it will not always be easy for the occupational health specialist to have access to as much information as would ideally aid such diagnosis.

It must also be admitted that many people, out of a misplaced sense of loyalty, will tend to cover up for the problem drinker and to make excuses for his poor performance. The excess of tolerance, which leads to remarks such as, 'There's no use asking Harris for a decision after lunch' but to no positive action, has the effect of delaying recognition and thus leads to a deterioration in the prognosis. Since alcohol is a drug of dependence, where the problem is ignored or colluded with, it will tend to become worse. Part of the solution relies, of course, upon education so that people come to recognize that in covering up for their drinking colleagues they are doing them no kindness; but equally, there is a pressing need to improve diagnostic skills.

The three areas identified above as showing in an employment context the clearest evidence of the damaging effects of excessive alcohol consumption were loss of efficiency, absenteeism and increased likelihood of accidents. It is important to note here that all three relate directly to the effectiveness of the individual as an employee. Often, people who do drink too much will resent questioning which focuses on their drinking behaviour and will put forward the argument that how much a man drinks is his own affair and that the questioner is poking his nose into private matters which are no legitimate concern of his. Since, however, excessive drinking has adverse effects upon matters pertaining directly to the individual's employment as well as to more general issues of physical and mental health, the argument is specious. In the case of employees whose job involves potential hazards, such as the operation of machinery, the necessity for preventive action on occupational health grounds is all the more pressing.

Hore (1977b) suggests that absenteeism is probably the first item which should alert one's suspicions. Of particular importance is a pattern of Monday morning absenteeism, which may well relate to the after-effects of very heavy weekend drinking sessions. The commonest reasons for absences which are in reality alcohol-related are given as psychiatric disorders, digestive, respiratory, muscular-skeletal disorders and accidents. Hore (1977b) also quotes from the work of Maxwell (1972) who describes physical changes (redness of eyes, tremulousness of hands, flushing of face) personality changes (nervousness at work, edginess and irritability, sensitivity to others' opinions about drinking, intolerance of fellow workers) and behavioural changes (putting off jobs, more spasmodic work performance, avoiding boss or associates, neglecting details, making mistakes, lower quality or quantity of work). It is, of course, the overall change in the behavioural pattern which should alert one rather than single manifestations of unconnected symptoms. Nor are the diagnostic skills required particularly arcane. Maxwell himself states (1972) that 'in spite of the great efforts which are generally made by alcoholics to conceal the changes in their behaviour, most fall, in fact, into the observable class'.

If, therefore, suspicion has been alerted because of a work-related incident and if simple observation would tend to confirm the diagnosis, it is important to check the individual's work and sickness records and to discover if, for example, he has been seeing the industrial nurse for a number of minor accidents.

Of blood tests, the most useful is probably the gamma GTP (gamma glutamyl transpeptidase). Other tests where a raised count would tend to confirm the diagnosis include aspartate aminotransferase, cholesterol and glutamate dehydrogenase. If investigation of the blood film reveals macrocytosis, this can also add to the burden of evidence.

It is important to emphasize, however, that useful as such tests are, their purpose will generally be to confirm a diagnosis which has already been made on grounds directly relating to the work performance of the individual. They are not in themselves screening techniques which are in any way reliable with a total workforce.

TREATMENT

The extent to which any occupational health department feels confident in undertaking the task of treating those suffereing from alcohol-related disabilities will depend both upon the severity of the disabilities and, very likely, the availability or lack of availability of outside referral points. The modern view of alcoholism treatment is certainly that it is best undertaken in a multidisciplinary context. It is only fair to add, however, that there is a wide variety of standards of care on offer so that it is of crucial importance, where outside help is being sought, that the occupational health specialist should satisfy himself as to the competence of the agency and should go out of his way to explain to that agency the special circumstances which will make industrial referrals rather different from other patients or clients. Ideally, of course, there should be access to a sufficient range of treatment options so that each case can be assigned to the combination of agencies most likely to prove effective. Care should certainly be exercised in avoiding inappropriate referrals. Alcoholics Anonymous, for example, can prove a total salvation to one individual and a total disaster to another.

Given the probability that those identified at work will be less advanced in their alcohol dependence than if they had emerged in the community, it is wise to accept the necessity for a range of treatment goals. For most alcoholics, the outcome of a successful treatment programme is total abstinence from alcohol. There is now, however, growing evidence (Hodgson, 1977) to suggest that a proportion of alcoholics can return to what is often called 'normal social drinking'. It may be that this goal will prove particularly relevant to the better motivated and more supported individual, who may well emerge in the employment context. The function of an occupational health programme in the area of alcohol-related disabilities is, after all, to restore the individual to full, effective functioning. This may or may not be the same thing as stopping his drinking.

Policies and programmes

There is no doubt that preventive and therapeutic efforts are most effective within the context of a written statement of policy which has been produced by a company and has been agreed by both unions and management. The most productive terms for such a statement of policy have been reviewed by Grant et al. (1978) but a number of central issues are crucial. These include:

1. That the employee, once identified, is offered appropriate treatment.
2. That refusal to accept treatment returns the handling of the case to the disciplinary procedures of the company.
3. That the employee's job is kept open while treatment is being undergone.
4. That the policy applies equally to all employees.

The advantages of such a policy hardly require enumeration. If, instead of being dismissed or covered up for, alcoholics are successfully treated, then this is good for the economic health of the company just as it is good for the personal health of the drinking employee. The pivotal position of the occupational health department in the creation and implementation of an alcoholism policy is reinforced by the growth in most countries of legislation relating to the protection of the health and safety of employees. It is, therefore, the responsibility of the occupational health specialist not merely to offer the most effective diagnostic and treatment service possible, but equally to co-ordinate a broadly based programme of preventive education.

REFERENCES

Cartwright A. K. J., Spratley T. A. and Shaw S. J. (1975) *Designing a Comprehensive Community Response to Problems of Alcohol Abuse.* Report by the Maudsley Alcohol Pilot Project to the Department of Health and Social Security.

Clare A. W. (1977) How good is treatment? In: Edwards G. and Grant M. (ed.), *Alcoholism: New Knowledge and New Responses.* London, Croom Helm.

Davies D. L. (1974) Implications for medical practice of an acceptable concept of alcoholism. In: Kessel N., Hawker A. and Chalke H. (ed.), *Proceedings of the 1st International Medical Conference on Alcoholism.* London, Edsall.

de Lint J. (1974) The epidemiology of alcoholism: the elusive nature of the problem, estimating the prevalence of excessive alcohol use and alcohol-related mortality, current trends and the issue of prevention. In: Kessel N., Hawker A. and Chalke, H. (ed.), *Proceedings of the 1st International Medical Conference on Alcoholism.* London, Edsall.

Edwards G. (1977) The alcohol dependence syndrome: the usefulness of an idea. In: Edwards G. and Grant M. (ed.), *Alcoholism: New Knowledge and New Responses.* London, Croom Helm.

Edwards G. and Grant M. (1977) Introduction. In: *Alcoholism: New Knowledge and New Responses.* London, Croom Helm.

Edwards G., Gross M. M., Keller M. et al. (ed.) (1977) *Alcohol Related Disabilities.* W.H.O. Offset Publication, No. 32. Geneva, World Health Organisation.

Grant M. (1977) Preventing alcoholism in industry. In: Grant M. and Kenyon W. H. (ed.), *Alcoholism and Industry.* London, Alcohol Education Centre and Merseyside, Lancashire & Cheshire Council on Alcoholism.

Grant M., Isles G., and Kenyon W. H. et al. (1978) Responding to alcohol related problems in employment. In: *Resource Pack for Industry.* Alcohol Education Centre and Scottish Health Education Unit.

Gwinner P. D. V. (1976) The treatment of alcoholics in a military context. *J. Alcoholism* **11,** (1), 24.

Hodgson R. (1977) Behaviour therapy. In: Edwards G. and Grant M. (ed.), *Alcoholism: New Knowledge and New Responses.* London, Croom Helm.

Hore B. D. (1977a) Alcohol and alcoholism: their impact on work. In: Grant M. and Kenyon W. G. (ed.), *Alcoholism and Industry.* London, Alcohol Education Centre and Merseyside, Lancashire & Cheshire Council on Alcoholism.

Hore B. D. (1977b) Alcohol and alcoholism: the impact on work. In: Edwards G. and Grant M. (ed.), *Alcoholism: New Knowledge and New Responses.* London, Croom Helm.

Maxwell M. A. (1972) Alcoholic employees, behaviour changes and occupational alcoholism programmes. *Proceedings of the 30th International Congress on Alcoholism and Drug Dependence.* International Council on Alcohol and Addictions, Lausanne.

Murray R. (1975) Alcoholism and employment. *J. Alcoholism* **10,** 1, 3.

Murray R. (1977) Screening and early detection instruments for disabilities related to alcohol consumption. In: Edwards G. and Gross M. M., Keller M. et al. (ed.), *Alcohol Related Disabilities.* W.H.O. Offset Publication, No. 32. Geneva, World Health Organisation.

O'Connor J. (1978) *Ethnic Origin and Drink.* London, Tavistock. In the press.

Osborne J. and Gordon J. (1978) The law, alcoholism and employment. In: *Resource Pack for Industry.* Alcohol Education Centre and Scottish Health Education Unit.

Plant M. A. (1977) Occupational factors in alcoholism. In: Grant M. & Kenyon W. H. (ed.), *Alcoholism and Industry.* London, Alcohol Education Centre and Merseyside, Lancashire & Cheshire Council on Alcoholism.

Pollak B. (1978) Guide for the assessment and management of alcoholism in industry. In: *Resource Pack for Industry.* Alcohol Education Centre and Scottish Health Education Unit.

Robinson D. (1976) *From Drinking to Alcoholism: A Sociological Commentary.* London, Wiley.

Shields J. (1977) Genetics and alcoholism. In: Edwards G. and Grant M. (ed.), *Alcoholism: New Knowledge and New Responses.* London, Croom Helm.

Von Wiegand R. A. (1972) Alcoholism in industry. *Br. J. Addiction* **67,** 181.

Wilkins R. (1974) *The Hidden Alcoholic in General Practice.* London, Elek Science.

18. STRESS AND THE INDIVIDUAL

Ann Hollingworth

> 'Everyman expects some miracle – either from his mind or from his body or from someone else or from events.'
>
> *Valéry*

Living consists of a series of events involving the individual and disturbing the homeopathic mechanism of the body. Some of these events will be routine, repeatable daily occurrences. Others are haphazard, unpredictable, dysrhythmic. Each event may have long-term effects or may produce only a passing elation or depression. The sum of these events is life.

Selye (1960) labelled this series of events 'stress', that is, the non-specific responses of the body to any demand made upon it. However 'stress' is surrogate in common use or abuse for the pathological, and at times inappropriate response of the body to life events. I have endeavoured to avoid the semantic dilemma in this chapter by using the word 'stress' as was originally intended by Selye and the terms such as 'strain' and 'distress' to describe pathological responses to stress. The individual response to events results from the interaction of three factors:

1. The event or series of events.
2. The environment in which this event occurs.
3. The individual's coping capacity (perhaps personality).

THE WORK SETTING

Stress and the individual is a broad concept but my intention is to refer solely to stress and the individual in the work setting. Challenge and pride in work are fundamental to man's well-being. Everyone has the right to expect an adequate status, wage and conditions of service. The job should provide some element of personal challenge and the individual should know how well he is performing. He should understand how his job fits with others and there should be some identifiable end product or result. The relationship between the organization and the individual is discussed elsewhere, but a glance at the changing emphasis is relevant here. After three decades of manipulating organizations and management styles, the

Table 18.1. Schedule from Holmes and Rahe (1967).

Life event	Mean value
Death of spouse	100
Divorce	73
Marital separation	65
Jail term	63
Death of close family member	63
Personal injury or illness	53
Marriage	50
Fired at work	47
Marital reconciliation	45
Retirement	45
Change in health of family member	44
Pregnancy	40
Sex difficulties	39
Gain of new family member	39
Business readjustment	39
Change in financial state	38
Death of a close friend	37
Change to different line of work	36
Change in number of arguments with spouse	35
Mortgages over £10 000	31
Foreclosure of mortgage or loan	30
Change in responsibilities at work	29
Son or daughter leaving home	29
Trouble with in-laws	29
Outstanding personal achievement	28
Wife begins or stops work	26
Begin or end college	26
Change in living conditions	25
Revision of personal habits	24
Trouble with boss	23
Change in work hours or conditions	20
Change in residence	20
Change in college	20
Change in recreation	19
Change in church activities	19
Change in social activities	18
Mortgage or loan less than £10 000	17
Change in sleeping habits	16
Change in number of family get-togethers	15
Change in eating habits	15
Vacation	13
Christmas	12
Minor violations of the law	11

philosophy of work is changing. The multidisciplinary approach (for example, line management, medical officers, social psychologists) to the problems of work, which was seen earlier as a clamouring of professionals, has now assumed a more pragmatic stance. The quality of life is seen to be of paramount importance, the quality of working life to be inevitably sub-servient to the demands of the work system. The essential nature of an organization, that is, hierarchy, specialization, continuity, is such that a certain degree of conformity is necessary. Jobs are identified by occupational titles, packaged and offered in such terms with all their positive and negative properties mingled in the package. The fit between an individual and his job therefore requires a certain amount of adaptation on each side. It is neither possible, desirable or necessary for everyone to have fulfilling jobs. It is becoming socially acceptable to earn one's bread in non-hazardous companionable surroundings.

RECOGNIZING THE HAZARD

Prophylaxis is better than therapy; so the aim should be early recognition of pathological responses to stress. It is possible to identify:

1. High risk situations.
2. High risk people.

High risk situations

1. Subjective incongruity and hostility of the environment is discussed in the succeeding chapter, but briefly, overload, rôle ambiguity, restrictions in behaviour and inappropriate career development are problems which within an organization should be avoidable.

Unavoidable potential risk situations are those where the individual is removed from old forms of social support, for example redundancy and retirement. 'Exit counselling' is now well recognized and is discussed later.

2. Life change scale Holmes and Rahe (1967) have attempted to relate life events to health change and questionnaires have been devised (see Table 18.1) in which high scores are associated with the possibility of major health changes. This relationship remains to be proved.

High risk people

1. One of the most interesting theories currently undergoing further research and validation is that relating the Type A personality, stress and coronary heart disease (Rosemann et al., 1966).

A prospective study on coronary heart disease (CHD) was initiated in 1960 among 31 545 men (The Western Collaborative Group Study). All were initially free of CHD and were resurveyed annually. It was shown that in addition to such factors as a family history of CHD, cigarette smoking and hypertension, the exhibition of a specific overt behaviour pattern (Type A) possessed significant prognostic import. Moreover, the exhibition of this behaviour pattern furnished the most important single prognostic entity. The complex thus described is characterised by:

a. A habit of explosively accentuating various key words in ordinary speech and uttering the last few words of sentences far more rapidly than the opening words.
b. A tendency always to move, walk and eat rapidly.
c. An impatience with the rate at which most events take place.
d. An indulgence in polyphasic thought or performance (for example, shaving and eating breakfast).
e. A vague feeling of guilt if periods of relaxation are prolonged.
f. The habit of scheduling more and more things in less and less time.
g. A belief that any success experienced is due in good part to the ability to get things done faster (hurry sickness).
h. A tendency towards hostility and aggression.

Such individuals lack a continuous and basic sense of security, substituting ephemeral periods of security maintained by the successful completion of more and more tasks.

The incidence of CHD in individuals with a Type A behaviour pattern is more than twice that of those with a Type B pattern. The relationship between Type A behaviour and CHD has yet to be verified but it cannot be assumed that it is a causal relationship. Friedman and Rosenman have devised a re-education course for Type A individuals which is discussed below.

2. Burns (private communication) has prognosticated a relationship between the coping capacity of the individual and his susceptibility to abnormal reactions to stress. Questionnaires completed by management personnel indicated nine characteristics which were significantly related to the individual's subjective assessment of his ability to cope. These were the ability to:

a. Recognize the development of a stressful situation and to, at times, prevent a crisis.
b. Control the pace of a stressful situation.
c. Stand back and appraise a stressful situation.
d. Defer thought on a difficult situation until one is ready to deal with it.
e. Relax.
f. Change aspects of one's behaviour.
g. Behave appropriately in a situation regardless of one's personal feelings.
h. Recognize the cause of depressive feelings and to tackle it.
i. Cope with being disliked.

Burns believes that such attributes may be learned responses and has devised a programme, described below, to unlearn or modify a potentially pathological response.

MEASUREMENT OF STRESS

This still defies any simple measurement. A great deal of work has been presented by Lennart Levi and his associates, (Gunderson et al., 1974). It is established that environmental physical stimuli may cause physical disease for a large number of environmental conditions. The physiological effects of extrinsic psychosocial stimuli (that is, those stimuli which originate in social relationships or arrangements) is not so clear. There appears to be a biological programme for each individual; that is, the tendency to react in accordance with a certain pattern when adapting to an environment. This originates from stereotyped phylogenetically old adaptation patterns preparing the organism for fight or flight. Such archaic responses may occur when action is not possible or socially acceptable and may turn inwards to cause pathological changes. The nature and degree of the psychological and physiological reactions evoked by life events depend also on the individual's past experience. Symbols that are gravely threatening to a certain individual may be meaningless to a neutral observer.

Levi (1974) has demonstrated widespread effects on neuroendocrine functions resulting from exposure to a variety of psychosocial stimuli (for example increased catecholamine excretion, raised plasma lipids). In general, deprivation and excess of almost any influence is found to disturb the equilibrium – the greatest disturbance being at the extremes of the stress curve.

MANAGEMENT OF STRESS

There has been an increasing interest in 'stress at work', not only because industry inevitably suffers from manpower wastage and inefficiency, but also because organizations have been held responsible for the induction of stress. There is no clearly defined borderline between constructive and destructive reactions. Where normality ends and disease begins may be merely a question of labelling. Mental health may be simply a slogan permitting new norms to be identified, followed by a demand for them to be met.

There is now greater expectation from the workforce that management should attempt to provide 'healthy' working conditions. In the UK the unions have emphasized physical hazards but psychological hazards have been given scant attention except by more responsible management. For reasons earlier defined, the perfect man/job fit is rare within an organization. With management policy now generally directed towards the maintenance of a fit and therefore efficient workforce, there are now very many methods of protecting against the development of abnormal reactions to stress and of treating 'casualties' early. We have moved a long way from the amateur hand-out to managers shown in Table 18.2.

Table 18.2. Information for men on a management training course of a large corporation.

Keeping the temperature down
People are important to the business – a manager on sick leave is ineffective. Ensure that you stay well.

1. Don't over-react to crises – keep calm.
2. Don't take things too personally.
3. Don't worry about things beyond your control – worry will not alter the situation one iota.
4. Learn to recognize your own tension symptoms – relax when they occur and then come back fighting.
5. If pressures become unbearable have a break but never run away!
6. Discover diversions on the work scene – but remember that the important and probably difficult work must be tackled.
7. Don't over-organize your uncommitted time – use it to think about the major issues.
8. Don't get too bogged down on one problem: leave it for a while and then come back fresh to it. Your subconscious may have solved it for you in the meantime! Or you could try discussing it with a colleague.
9. Give your mind a rest by putting your body to work – sport and the like in your spare time.

The present approach to the management of stress is three-pronged:

1. Rationalizing psychosocial stressors.
2. Training individuals to learn different responses and to adopt potentially less damaging forms of behaviour.
3. Support systems.

The first two differ from the last in that the individual does not have to admit to a problem. To obtain results from support systems such as counselling in the work setting, it is neccessary to develop an organizational atmosphere in which the individual feels able to express his anxieties and ask for help.

Rationalizing psychosocial stresses
This is related to organization and is dealt with elsewhere.

Training individuals to learn different responses and to adopt potentially less damaging forms of behaviour
Personal growth training
This is perhaps a phenomenon of the sixties. 'T'-groups, encounter groups and the like were too readily taken up by management before a scientific appraisal had been made. As a result these have largely fallen into disrepute. A recent survey by Cary Cooper (1977) for the DHSS has done little to favour their continuation; his conclusions were generally that whereas no harmful effects were demonstrated neither were there signifi-

cant long-term beneficial effects. A more moderate and informed management approach to such training might well have been more rewarding.

Behaviour manipulation
This is exemplified in the re-education of Type A personalities; for example the drill against 'hurry sickness':

1. Avoid trying to finish other people's sentences. Never interrupt with such phrases as 'Uh, huh, uh, huh' or 'I see, I see'. (Seek out someone who stutters.)
2. Before speaking ask yourself:
   Do I really have anything important to say?
   Does anyone want to hear it?
   Is this the time to say it?
3. Carry reading matter with you whenever you go somewhere that you may be delayed.
4. Frequent restaurants where you will have to wait.
5. If you speed up to cross the lights at amber, penalize yourself by turning right at the next intersection!
6. Deliberately read books which demand attention and patience, for example Prouşt's *Remembrance of Things Past* – the author needs several chapters to describe an event that most Type A subjects would have handled in a sentence or two.

It should be emphasized that there is, as yet, no evidence that it is possible to modify personality in this way. If such a modification is possible, will this result in a reduction in the incidence of the 'related' CHD?

Modifying learned responses
This work has been recently initiated by Burns. He has identified essential coping characteristics. Individuals are helped to identify their subjective weaknesses in relation to this scale and they receive training to maximize their potential. The results of this work have not been evaluated.

Relaxation techniques
These are philosophically in keeping with today's thinking. The medical profession is well advised to discourage the use of psychotrophic drugs and the associated dependency role, while encouraging the trend towards self help which these techniques exemplify. Ivan Illich might well claim some credit for this philosophical change! Relaxation techniques backed up by biofeedback devices are in the forefront of stress control. Although there is a variety of instrumentation and of approaches to relaxation (yoga, transcendental meditation), the basic principles are the same. The individual learns to relax by use of taped recordings or trigger words (mantra). If this needs to be enchanced, the biofeedback devices which measure skin temperature or resistance are used by the individual to

monitor his response. The ability to raise one's skin temperature consciously, that is, apparently exercising central nervous control over the autonomic system appears to be directly related to relaxation and is a good measure of this. Various audible and visual biofeedback devices are available including one portable audible device for a quick check on one's own stress response. It remains to be seen whether biofeedback devices will become as addictive as other reinforcers such as alcohol and smoking.

Behaviour manipulation and education should make the individual more aware of his psychological and physiological responses and if necessary will indicate when he has reached a stage where he needs help.

Support systems

The most used support system is the primary social group. The greater the expertise which is therefore manifested by all members of society in dealing with distress, the more this group can provide.

Counselling systems take very many forms in industry and this is a time of experimentation with new counselling approaches. There is a growing number of counsellors with varying degrees of training and skills. The clearest use of such systems is in relation to changes in the individual's life-style, for example redundancy or retirement.

Exit counselling

This is now well established in many industries. Redundancy and retirement counselling schemes aim to promote the individual's psychological adaptation to the inevitable change; to exchange information which may be of value to the employer or employee and to stimulate the employee's awareness of his potential outside the current work situation.

The British Steel Corporation have piloted a scheme of peer group counselling to deal with their extensive redundancy problems (Hopson, 1977). Men from the shop floor were selected for counselling training and they then undertook counselling of men who were to be made redundant. The success of the scheme can be measured by the response of the work-force to the voluntary counselling service, which has been consistently between 95 and 98 per cent.

Counselling by professional counsellors

Several organizations employ full-time professional counsellors; others appoint counsellors for short periods, usually to work on a particular project. In the work setting professional counsellors identify several elements in their rôle:

1. To help those already distressed to realize their own resources and grow rather than simply regress to their pre-morbid state.
2. To provide a service for those who recognize strain within themselves and need to elucidate the situation.
3. To demonstrate social dynamics.
4. To act as facilitators and change agents.

Those counsellors who work full-time within an organization have justified a permanent establishment. It remains to be seen whether in the current financial climate other companies will see this as a cost effective exercise.

Peer group counselling

The National Environment Research Council attempted a peer counselling scheme. This had a limited success, possibly through lack of trust arising from by-passing existing organizational structures with a resulting challenge to the traditional role of the manager.

Although peer group counselling and co-counselling are attractive methods of organizing non-dependancy relationships, competition and distrust within commercial organizations is likely to make this a difficult technique to pursue.

Counselling within other roles

This is probably the most acceptable form of counselling within industry, perhaps because the cost is hidden. Line managers, personnel managers, doctors, nurses, trade unionists are all in positions which naturally attract counselling demands. The recent burgeoning of counselling skills courses should help such individuals to perform this ancillary role effectively.

The foregoing challenges earlier concepts about the quality of working life. Increasing technology and complex organization conflicts with personal idiosyncrasy. While work can, and should be, materially rewarding and should have some recognizable result, fulfillment in the work setting is usually related to social support. This may be expressed as a positive effect (liking, admiration and respect) and affirmation (endorsement, agreement with beliefs and perception). But men and women should seek personal fulfillment in the general context of living.

Social psychology is a term which though well born and apparently healthy, seems to have carried deleterious genes. However, it has a rôle in understanding and developing the skills necessary to well-being.

REFERENCES

Cooper C. (1977) *Hurt or Helped.* London, H.M.S.O.

Gunderson E. K. et al. (1974) In: Richard H. (ed.), *Life, Stress and Illness.* Springfield, Ill., Thomas.

Holmes T. H. and Rahe R. H. (1967) Social Readjustment Rating Scale. *J. Psychosom. Res.* **II**, 213–218.

Hopson B. (1977) Setting up a counselling network. *Counselling at Work.* London, Bedford Square Press.

Levi L. (1974) Psychosocial stress and disease; a conceptual model. *Life Stress and Illness.* Springfield, Ill., Thomas.

Rosenman R. N. et al. (1966) Coronary heart disease in the western collaborative group study. *J.A.M.A.* **195**, 2.

Selye H. (1960) The concept of stress in experimental physiology. *Stress and Psychiatric Disorder.* Oxford, Blackwell.

19. STRESS AND THE ORGANIZATION

J. A. Harryman

An industrial organization consists of a number of individuals working alongside each other with a multiplicity of aims. The purpose of my paper is to explore methods by which these aims can be mutualized such that they are not seen to be conflicting. My basic theme is that conflict causes stress and therefore a co-operative approach by the total organization will lead to stress reduction.

Manifestations of stress by individuals has always had a medical interest whether that stress is attributable to the home environment or elsewhere. However, where a large number of individuals are working together in an industrial organization the effects of stress can lead not only to inefficiencies at the individual level, but can also have untold damaging effects upon the total organization. An obvious indication of conflict levels within an organization is the measurement of days lost through industrial strikes. However, this I believe is only the tip of the iceberg and can be looked upon as the blowing of the 'safety valve'. Perhaps just as important are the many instances which are averted at the last moment and which are never publicized. For the individuals within that organization the build-up to such situations can be just as harmful not only to themselves, but also to the long-term efficiency of that organization.

THE UNITARY AND PLURALIST ORGANIZATIONAL MODELS

At this point it may be useful to explore two simple models of an industrial organization; the first being a 'unitary' system where everyone in the organization is striving for the same or similar objectives, the second model being the more traditional 'pluralist' divided organization.

Over a period of time, certainly in the United Kingdom, the pluralist model has been refined and sophisticated but has kept the main features of the Victorian era where the boss of the organization employed workers when they were required in order to produce products as the market dictated. When sales fell, the number of workers was reduced. Similarly, rising sales meant an increase in workers. Thus the concept of buying and selling labour became indistinguishable from the concept of maximizing sales with minimum costs. Although this analysis is very crude and the majority of industrial concerns would decry such a system as even immoral these days, it should be recognized that even sophisticated 'pluralist' organizations have a central theme of 'Them and Us' and tend to treat certain sections of the workforce as enemies of the organization.

Organizations based on this model would have distinguishing characteristics such as 'blue' and 'white' collar divisions: the blue collar workforce would be often highly unionized, with the compensation package decided at the negotiating table, while the white collar, on the other hand, would be treated like civilized citizens and rewarded accordingly. In the same model, the blue collar would be paid weekly and would 'clock in' upon arrival and departure from the workplace, whereas the white collar would be afforded the privilege of monthly payment and could be trusted to put in the appropriate hours necessary to perform their job. Thus a divided organization not only exists but can be seen to exist.

The alternative 'unitary' system is often seen as Utopian and therefore little progress has been made in the United Kingdom to develop a total organization based on this concept. However, when a more detailed analysis of organizations is undertaken it is usual to find sections of that organization working to these principles. The basic concepts behind a 'unitary' approach are that all the individuals are striving for a similar objective – survival and growth of the organization. Once this objective has been accepted wholeheartedly by the individual in the organization the debating arena moves away from the direct conflict over 'why co-operate' into a more profitable arena of 'how to co-operate'. The supporting structures necessary for such a model can then be developed with a clear appreciation of their purpose. The efforts of individuals within the organization can then be harnessed together with a common objective of survival and growth. Individuals within such an organization feel part of the total structure, their input is appreciated, motivation increases, productivity and efficiency rise and, may I hasten to add, stress reduces.

THE DILEMMA FACING INDUSTRY TODAY

If such a simple model not only reduces stress but also creates increased industrial efficiency, why is the system not universal? Throughout Europe, Industrial Democracy in some form or another is already in existence, mainly initiated by legislation. In the United Kingdom the Bullock report was seen as unacceptable by everyone in industry. It would seem to be the old, old situation of different power groups being totally unable to accept a new and dynamic concept due to mistrust of the other side. It is for this reason that I believe we are in a state of revolution and, peaceful though it is at the moment, it is without a doubt the Second Industrial Revolution that is upon us.

Why, therefore, cannot an organization overcome this current dilemma without undergoing self-destruction? The first reason may be that we tend to be status conscious and not accept that every individual within an organization has 'something' to offer. Second, the question of security based upon management prerogative and position within the organization does not lend itself to acceptance that a subordinate may have better abilities and practical application than his supervisor. But third, and most importantly, our education system is geared to criticism and rebuke. How often do we feed back success to an individual? Rarely, I think, and we more often accept a good performance as the norm and therefore only criticize when something goes wrong. One therefore can see that competition 'not through physical stature as in the days of the Iron Age Man' but through verbal distrust has become the norm in modern day society. With this as a backcloth, it is very difficult to accept a 'unitary' approach within an industrial organization.

Co-operation rather than conflict is thus easy to put forward as a concept but much more difficult to practise. Not only do we have to look at organizations in a totally different perspective, but all of us need to learn new skills and then practice them at all times. An organization based on these principles would surely reduce stress; however, it requires training, a new philosophy and a new structure to enable it to develop and thereby become self-generating. Objectives must be clearly defined, but these objectives can only have meaning if all the individuals have been given a voice, have put forward their proposals and if they have not been accepted by that organization they will need to have accepted the logic and reasoning behind the alternative. Individuals need continued success feedback in order to grow within that organization and then start to develop themselves.

Such a system then will reduce conflict, political red-tape may be reduced, and stress within that organization reduced to the odd personality clash. However, I would suggest that to obtain such a position needs faith, the most competent individuals to lead and advise, and a commitment by everyone to make the enterprise a success.

The exact systems required to sustain such an organization can be many and varied, and in order that commitment is universal, need to be developed within the organization. The balance between the democratic voice, and the need to achieve work output is a delicate one. However, with the right training of the total workforce and simple, but well-understood decision making forums, the organization has the capacity for unqualified success.

THE DEVELOPMENT OF MANAGEMENT STYLE

So far I have described the extremes of management style within an organization. In fact, very few industrial companies deliberately work towards either the 'unitary' or 'pluralist' model and therefore an odd combination of styles can be seen to have developed. The reason why a pluralistic approach cannot be pursued in its true form may be due to such things as powerful shop floor unions as well as the legislation that has been placed on our statute books since 1968. Thus it is no longer possible for a company to make large numbers of employees redundant without a lengthy consultative procedure being enacted. Unfair dismissal is another legislative element which ensures that individual employees have industrial rights, but this is only an attempt to redress the balance within a 'pluralist' concept and has no way gone beyond this model. The only legislation so far emanating from the United Kingdom which moves towards a 'unitary' approach is the Health and Safety at Work Act, where employee representatives have a right to be involved in determining the safety policies within an organization. Even talk of a non-political subject such as safety has brought loud cries of alarm from some employers that shop floor democracy will destroy the organization. One would have thought that safety would be a subject where every employee in the organization had similar objectives. Yet it is apparently not, as some shop floor representatives have tried to turn it into a negotiating topic.

The difficulty we now face, therefore, is an organization structure based upon the pluralist model but which has been redressed through legislation and social changes external to the industrial setting. The formal structures, however, are often still centred around the negotiating forum where concessions are made, victories 'won' and accusations of unfair treatment the order of the day. The predominant style, therefore, is generally still one of conflict and issues are often settled not through the logical approach but rather through emotion and threats. The compensation package is still based upon barter and the 'Management' is still seen to give the minimum offer possible at the negotiating table. The unions, on the other hand, are in business to extract the maximum possible in this situation and are often suspicious of company threats of liquidation or bankruptcy. Without a unified aim it is not surprising that this situation develops and often ends in disaster for both parties.

The consultative forum

In order to overcome some of these difficulties many organizations have developed consultative structures of one form or another. These allow a more informal debate to take place at a lower level in the organization. The basis behind this consultative machinery is an attempt to allow some degree of involvement by the workforce. In areas directly linked with the day-to-day operation of the company there can be very significant successes. Information can also be passed down through these forums and it is normal to have a dialogue concerning the company's operation at this level. Also, in many instances, these consultative committees actually start to operate in a low key participation manner. Views and opinions often start to filter up to these forums and positive ideas associated with the running of the enterprise start to come forward. The dilemma then facing the manager responsible for the consultative forum is often whether he has the authority to pursue many of these items. Frustration and stress may well set in, especially if he has seen successes associated with his low key participation 'unitary' approach.

It can be seen, therefore, that although the formal organization structure is most likely to be based upon the 'pluralist' approach, there may well be sections of the same organization operating the 'unitary' approach. If such a situation is not perceived by the participant within the organization, a high stress situation may well develop at the interface which could lead eventually to conflict and to mistrust of the way individuals are actually being treated as a totality. This theme can also be extended into the total area of styles of management within an organization. There are some individuals who naturally display all the characteristics of an open participative management style. If they are working within an organization which is predominantly 'pluralist' in approach they will certainly feel bound by a number of constraints. This also may lead to a high stress level not only for those individuals concerned, but also for the total organization which could lose direction through operating a strange mixture of conflicting styles.

The skill in such situations is for the individuals concerned to be aware of the system within which they are attempting to operate, to ensure that they have clear terms of reference and can identify the constraints under which they operate. Even with all this information totally to hand there may be some individuals still frustrated and confused but, hopefully, they will feel less stress and can work to their optimum efficiency within the guidelines.

The negotiating forum

Let us, therefore, not underestimate the value of the negotiating table if a 'pluralist' situation is the formal company style. It is the formal setting for the reduction of conflict and thus enables individuals within the organization to channel their unresolved problems into the system. Individual stress is therefore reduced but organizational disquiet increases. Grievance procedures and disciplinary procedures are often good examples of formal stress relievers. The system enables individuals within the organization to channel stress away from themselves and back towards the organization. It is then the senior management team who have the job of resolving the issues. Normally this team will be experienced enough to perceive the reality of the situation, but on occasions can itself fail to resolve the issues. Under the 'feudal' system it was always seen to be the deputy manager who bore the brunt of any failures. The same can still be true today in a highly political organization and it can be in many organizations the assistant or deputy manager who is the first to feel the full effects of stress. It is helpful to be aware of this fact, and once again to safeguard against it.

BASIC HYGIENE FACTORS

To date we have looked at conflict and stress as manifested either within the management structure, or between the formal shop floor representative and the company. There is one other section of the organization where stress is manifested and that is at the shop floor level. It is not normal for these individuals to become involved in planning changes to their job pattern until too late in the day. Production lines are built prior to employee consultation, and the only discussion (normally a highly emotional negotiation) is over manning levels. For more than half a century we have been agreeing with the industrial psychologists that motivation requires involvement by people doing the job – but we are still apt to forget such advice. Machines are often built first and then we ask men to operate them – ergonomics is still a very young science. It is the combination of involvement at the earliest stage possible in a project, together with well-studied and evaluated information from experts in ergonomics, that can set such basic 'hygiene' factors at rest.

The size of the organization can also have a bearing on the amount of frustration and stress evident within a company. The larger the organization the more numerous are the levels of management and supervision, and all too often delays occur in decision making. Such delays are a real frustration to the supervisors who often claim that the communication structures within the organization are a deterrent to their completing the job. A successful technique for overcoming such frustration is for the organization to be sub-divided into smaller sections with the necessary authority being afforded to the manager of each section. Decisions can then be taken more rapidly and the employees within that unit tend to develop an affinity or allegiance towards their own group. They can also see the manager responsible rather than feel they are being manipulated by some faceless men heading up the company. The co-ordination of these smaller units into a large company requires skill and a high degree of perception. The smaller units need to be serviced by high level advisers who can balance out not only the needs of the smaller units, but also the generally broader company objectives. For this to take place effectively the company objectives must not only be clear and precise, but also flexible enough to allow the smaller units to manage their own affairs.

All too often companies set out on a decentralization route but in times of crisis revert back to a centralized system in order to tighten up the structure. A decentralization route requires both a high level of skill and expertise in all parts of the company and also a dedicated faith. Individuals within an organization wish to have an input into the running of the enterprise and, if we accept this premise, the communication and decision-making structures will need to be built around this fact. Large, highly centralized structures do not meet this need and tend towards a frustrated demotivated workforce who have little interest in the company they work for.

Most of the routes suggested so far rely on highly skilled supervisors and management, certainly in the field of human relations. Employees holding these posts within a company need not only to be task competent, but also able to develop a spirit of co-operation and effectiveness with their colleagues and subordinates. Such skills are rarely natural, and thus need development and reinforcement on a continual basis. The training needs to be practical in nature rather than theroretical, and back in the workforce it should be developed into natural behaviour.

Such training cannot be confined to management and supervision, but must be extended certainly to employee representatives and, if possible, to the total workforce. Its main theme would be to develop the art of co-operation through the process of inductive learning. The skills would then be acquired at a base level during the training sessions for further development back at the workplace. It has been shown that such training leads to greater efficiency, a higher level of commitment and a reduction in stress.

STRESS REDUCTION THROUGH FORMAL MEANS

In conjunction with the approaches so far suggested which will allow the organization to function more effectively, there are some fundamental points which lead to stress reduction. Policy guidelines for the company need to be clearly defined and on display for everyone in the organization to read. The manner in which they are written should be such that all employees in the company can comprehend them without ambiguity. Procedures should be once again clear and comprehensible to all. They need to be operated fairly and must be seen to be operated fairly. They need to cover all possibilities which may be encountered but at the same time be based upon a simple structure.

Job responsibilities should also be clear and well understood not only by the incumbent, but also by any other employee who has an interface with the job holder. Departmental and divisional meetings should be held on a regular basis to exchange information in a free flowing fashion and also to discuss and influence policy decisions. These mechanisms are all support systems which will enable the organization to operate in an open participative style. Without such structures frustration and stress will be high and the potential of the organization left untapped.

Some stress indicators

I have referred continually to stress reduction in this paper and it may be helpful to touch on some of the indicators of organizational stress. No single indicator can be used but a mixture of the following may be helpful. A high alcoholism rate amongst managers or supervisors and high turnover rates in these categories are indicators. Above-average divorce rates could be looked at, especially where managers are expected to move around the country every three or four years. Absenteeism on crucial days or burning the midnight oil may show instances of stress through the setting of unrealistic targets. But more often it is a case of continual mutterings of discontent that signifies frustration and stress. It is then time to analyse the management styles being operated within the organization and the effects they are having upon its employees.

OUTLOOK FOR THE FUTURE

In summary, therefore, it may be that an organization is forward looking and has taken the truly 'unitary' model to heart in which case further stress reduction will come through practice and hard work. On the other hand if a company operates the traditional 'pluralist' approach you would do better to accept that you are operating within that system. Progress will usually be slow and painful but it can be measured through the small successes that we encounter day by day. When these successes occur hold on to them dearly as they form the hopes of our tomorrow. Look for success and it shall multiply; analyse failure and there should be stress.

20. SHIFT WORK AND HEALTH

J. Malcolm Harrington

Shift work is frequently considered to be a modern practice, consequent upon the mechanization that characterized the industrial revolution. A little thought, however, would reveal that working at odd hours of the day and night has been in use for many centuries. Tending sheep, guarding the castle, patrolling the toll gates or serving inn-dwellers all required people to work outside the 'normal' day. Townspeople for centuries have bought fresh bread in the morning. This means that the bakers must work at night. Ramazzini wrote this of bakers in 1715: '[they] work at night and when other men have finished the day's task and are asleep recruiting their energies, they must work all night and then sleep all day like bats'.

The industrial revolution added a further – and numerically larger – group of workers to the shift working population. This need was to man (or woman or child!) the continuous process machinery in such industries as iron and glassmaking. Modern technology has created newer industries: power supply, oil refining and chemical production. Since 1945, the economic considerations of plant and equipment obsolesence relative to market needs have added to this list of continuous processes such industries as cars, electronic and household equipment ('consumer durables', so called) and computers.

Today, therefore, shift working is required by industrial society for three main reasons: service to society, continuous process industries, and the economic necessity of getting the most out of the equipment before it is outmoded by better machines, newer designs or changing consumer fancy. In developing countries, surplus manpower can be more efficiently used in shift work as this can increase productivity and decrease capital costs.

Although shift working has been deplored by some sections of society as inhuman and socially undesirable, it is, for better or worse, here to stay. Latest estimates (1975) suggest that in Western countries about one in five workers is on shift work. Furthermore, this is not a symptom of rampant capitalism – similar percentages of workers in East-block countries work on shifts. It seems, however, that the rapid rise in such work practices since World War II is now slowing and little further increase is envisaged – except, perhaps, in the service industries.

TYPES OF SHIFT WORK

The term 'shift work' covers a wide variety of working practices in terms of hours worked, time of day and frequency of change of shift. Nevertheless, in broad terms, they can be classified as:

1. 2 or 3 shift
2. Continuous (stabilized or rotating) for 7 days a week
   or
   Discontinuous (alternating or permanent) for 5 days a week.

Continuous shift working affords the greatest opportunity for permutations and combinations especially when it is operated by 3 crews each working 8 hours, the commonest starting times for the shifts being 0600, 1400 and 2200 hours. In this system, workers often rotate from one shift to the next at varying frequencies. For example, the morning shift of 0600 to 1400 hours is followed after a week by the afternoon shift (1400–2200 hours) and then a week later by the night shift (2200–0600 hours). Sometimes the night shift is done entirely by workers on 'permanent nights', while the 'double day' shifts are alternated. Other variations are introduced if the work stops at weekends or is a 7-day-week process. Legislation normally restricts such continuous 3 shifts, 7 days a week systems *in factories* to men; women cannot work such systems at present without special dispensation. Outside factories there are no legal restrictions and it is in health, transport, catering and now computing centres, that most women on shift work can be found.

Shift work for women in factories usually only involves the two 'day' shifts or the 'twilight' shift. The latter usually spans the four to six hours at the end of the normal working day, and is popular with married women who are able to go out to work when their husbands get home and can look after the children.

Recently, there has been a move to introduce rapid rotation of shifts. This usually means replacing the weekly or fortnightly rotation by a system of shift changes every few days. The 'Continental' system involves such rapid changes as (2 X 2 X 3) or the 'metropolitan' (2 X 2 X 2). These cycles, allowing for time off work, may take four to eight weeks before the worker is back to the beginning again. One major disadvantage of the system is that days off rarely coincide with traditional weekends but the rota can be adapted to give the workers larger blocks of time off (3 or 4 days) in compensation for losing his free Saturdays and Sundays.

There has been much argument concerning the pros and cons of different shifts and especially over the merits and demerits of slow or rapid rotation. Unfortunately a lot of the discussion is based on unscientific information and amounts to little more than hot air. Strongly held views on shift systems frequently reflect the political bias of the proponents rather than an opinion based on scientific evidence.

Notwithstanding, there is some good evidence to suggest, at least subjectively, that workers do not like the 1400–2200 hours shift. It is socially paralysing and leaves the worker with little time to indulge his extramural interests. The morning shift 0600–1400 hours at least provides the workers with a long afternoon and evening to do other things, even if he does have to get up early in the morning. It is, however, the night shift that provokes the greatest discussion and most heated argument. It is unphysiological (as Ramazzini noted) and, so the argument goes, must be bad for the workers' health. It can also disrupt sexual relations. Considering how many workers are employed on such shifts and how long such working practices have been in use, one would think that the health effects would have been well documented by now. Unfortunately this is not so. The arguments for and against night work continue and are frequently discussed on the basis of emotion and conjecture. For example, it used to be argued that the longer the worker stayed on a given shift (especially the night shift) the better he would adapt to the abnormal sleep/awake patterns. The flaw in this argument is that the worker does not stay on nights every night for weeks at a time! On his nights off, he reverts to the normal sleep/awake routine and therefore nullifies his adaptation. In view of this, many physiologists now feel that as real adaptation in such a slow rotation is impossible, then perhaps it would be better to rotate the shifts so rapidly that any adaptation is precluded. By this method, at least the worker does not have to endure disagreeable shifts for very long. The 2 X 2 X 2 system is such an example.

One final point regarding shift working is worth considering before we move on to look at the evidence for health effects of such practices, namely, 'moonlighting'. Shift work is more amenable to providing the worker with opportunities to do another job than the nine to five routine. Figures are hard to come by regarding the prevalence of moonlighting – frequently because it is work for cash and therefore involves tax evasion! What data are available suggest that up to one-third of all shift workers do other jobs at some time or other (Maurice, 1975). This will provide an extra burden to the worker which could influence his health. Such effects might then be misconstrued as due to the shift work and it is difficult to prove or disprove this when the worker denies extramural earnings.

GENERAL HEALTH EFFECTS

'Health' is a difficult concept to define. It is not just the absence of disease though, in practice, much of the research on shift work and health has interpreted it as such. Furthermore, many of the studies of the health of shift workers are based on the worker's own conception of what shift working is doing to him. For example, if the worker thinks his hours of employment are unnatural he may assume, *ergo,* that his health will be affected. He then interprets the investigator's questions from the preconceived notion that he must be less fit than the day workers. The results of such researches then demonstrate that shift workers are not healthy!

I recently reviewed the world literature on shift work and health (Harrington, 1978) and after reading two hundred references came to the surprising, and disappointing, conclusion that much of the evidence cited for ill effects of such work was of dubious validity. Some was astonishingly unscientific, some very good. In order to spare the reader a boring catalogue of cited studies, the references quoted will be those which either have the greatest merit or the greatest influence on opinion. These two attributes are not necessarily synonymous! Some employees, and their politically orientated supporters contend that, as shift work is 'unnatural' it must be unhealthy. Some employers and their supporters cite workers who died in their eighties and nineties after working shifts all their life and argue that it causes no problems. Both views are erroneous. The truth, as is so often the case, lies between the two extremes. Studies cited later will show that while shift work disturbs physiological, social and sexual equilibria, it seems to produce remarkably little ill-health.

Mortality studies
Considering that death can be frequently construed as the end product of ill-health, it is surprising that only one mortality study of shift workers appears to have been undertaken. Taylor and Pocock (1972) analysed 1578 deaths occurring in a 13-year period in a population of 8603 male manual workers employed with 10 organizations. Their study was done meticulously but revealed virtually no evidence that shift workers had excessive death rates compared with day workers. Ex-shift workers did seem to be slightly worse off than current shift workers and this might imply some selecting out of the less fit men from shift working, leaving only the fitter men to cope with the 'abnormal' working hours.

Sickness absence
This subject is covered in depth in Chapter 21 of this book but there is little evidence to suggest that shift workers are more frequently absent from work due to sickness than day workers. On the contrary, most evidence shows that they are less frequently absent. This may be due to a greater *ésprit de corps* among such groups, higher pay or fitter people selecting themselves into such jobs.

Aanonsen (1964) felt that the lower rates of absence among shift workers may mask an effect of their work, as they appeared to have more severe illnesses (longer absences) when they were off work. He is also one of the few researchers to look at the health patterns of ex-shift workers. These men in his study of Norwegian electro-chemical industry workers had more absences than current shift workers or day workers. It is not clear, however, which came first, the ill-health or the desire to leave shift work. Taylor (1967) also found lower sickness absence rates in his shift workers and in a later study Taylor et al. (1972) compared absence records of 965 matched pairs of men from 29 organizations over a 2-year period. Shift workers were consistently less often absent – certificated and uncertificated sickness as well as non-medical absenteeism. Drop-outs from shift work tend to occur in the first 4 years and Thiis-Evensen (1963) noted a twofold excess of digestive tract ulcers in shift workers compared with day workers. Half of these men, however, had their ulcers before they worked shifts and after the first 4 years, the remaining shift workers had 20 per cent less absence from work than other workers.

So far as different shifts are concerned, sickness absence rates suggest that the afternoon shift rota produces the least absence. The night shift is associated with more absences than the two day shifts but the spells are frequently of short duration. Absences on the morning shift may be unpremeditated (Shepherd and Walker, 1956) – the result, presumably, of over sleeping! The new rapid rotating shifts have not usually caused more absence than the slower rotations, but evidence so far is conflicting.

Circadian rhythms

Circadian rhythms were a concept developed in the late 1950s and described the rhythmicity observed in various bodily functions over the 24 hour cycle. This periodicity applies not only to the more obvious cycles: sleep/awake, body temperature, bowel function, but also to virtually all biochemical and physiological parameters measurable in the body. The rhythm in man seems to be affected by exogenous social factors as well as by climatic and light/dark phases. These external influences (*Zeitgebers*) then modify an inherent free running periodicity of between 23 and 25 hours. Anyone who has flown on intercontinental air liners, especially in an eastward direction, or stayed up all night, will be aware that it takes several days to get back into a normal rhythm again. Some biochemical cycles, such as urinary excretion of inorganic salts and plasma cortisol levels can take weeks to revert to normal. Body temperature is an easy way of measuring such circadian rhythm functions and temperature curves consistent with normal day/night cycles take several weeks to 'invert' when the day/night, awake/sleep phase is shifted by 12 hours. Early evidence of this change is the flattening of the temperature curve which is evident within a few days of changing the phases. Colquhoun and his colleagues have done much of the pioneer work in this field and his results have been succinctly summarized recently (Rentos and Shepherd, 1976).

These and other studies have clearly demonstrated that shift work, and particularly night work, causes considerable disruption of circadian rhythms. Temperature curves 're-entrain' to some extent but other physiological parameters do so less easily. Individuals differ greatly in the speed at which they can adapt and this may have an important bearing on adaptability to shift work in general.

Sleep

Sleep is clearly disrupted by night work, and, to a lesser extent, by the other shifts. Unfortunately there is little objective evidence to support the contention in some circles that the sleep of night shift workers is not only shorter but of inferior quality to normal night time sleep. Wilkinson (1971) has undertaken objective studies of the sleep of subjects whose day/night cycle has been shifted out of phase. Nevertheless, it is still far from clear how good or bad is the night workers' sleep. Certainly, on his days off, the night shift worker sleeps longer and therefore makes up for the deficit accrued whilst working. Whether this correction of the hours lost is all that is required or whether he is still deficient in 'good' sleep is not known.

The other important factor leading to poor sleep for the night worker is his home environment. His shorter sleep may be due more to living in a noisy neighbourhood going about its business during the day, whilst he tries to sleep in a poorly sound-proofed bedroom, than to phase shifting of his rhythm.

Performance, output and accidents

This area of shift work sequelae is particularly poorly studied. Many published reports use ill-defined measures of performance, output or accident rates and frequently such studies cannot be compared with others. The subject is well reviewed by Colquhoun et al. (1972) and Rutenfranz et al. (1977). Some consensus has been achieved, however, in five areas:

1. Performance is worst for long stints of repetitive work and best for cognitive work with high motivation.
2. Loss of sleep effects are greatest on the night shift and least on the afternoon shift.
3. Fatigue can increase errors and diminish performance but this can be offset if the motivation is great and breaks in the work are feasible.
4. Short cycle shift working minimizes temperature adaptation and probably prevents performance adaptation as well.
5. Individual differences in performance are often much greater than group differences.

SPECIFIC HEALTH EFFECTS

Physicians concerned with the health of shift workers frequently cite two main sources of potential health risk: disruption of sleeping patterns and variations in eating habits. Worker complaints are centred on nervous disorders, gastro-intestinal disturbances, fatigue, poor housing and inadequate facilities at work during the night shift.

Gastro-intestinal illness

Ramazzini was the first to cite this in his treatise on the health of learned men! He felt that burning the midnight oil would cause '. . .a diversion of the spirits to other organs (and) cause their stomachs to abound in the acid of undigested food. . .'. Written 250 years ago there is more evidence today for peptic ulceration in shift workers than most other diseases purported to be related to such work. A more recent reference to peptic ulcers – but also couched in outdated terminology – appears in a monograph on night work published by the International Labour Office, '. . .ulcers are a common somatic manifestation of a dysfunction of the central nervous system and particularly the hypothalamus, which is the organ of fatigue' (Carpentier and Cazamian, 1977). It is curious statements like this that add to the confusion over the ill effects of shift work.

More objective scientific evidence, however, does exist and although there is conflict of opinion, the epidemiological evidence available does suggest that rotating shift work may play a part in either inducing gastro-duodenal ulceration or at least exacerbating latent or pre-existent disease. Shift working with its irregular hours and disordered meal times is not conducive to ulcer management. Improvement in catering facilities at work, especially at night and greater awareness by workers of their need for careful dietary control could conceivably diminish gastro-intestinal morbidity.

Cardiovascular disease

Despite the fact that some people feel that the 'strain' of shift working will be detrimental to the cardiac well-being of workers, no evidence exists to show this to be true.

Neurological and psychiatric disorders

Too often vague terms like 'fatigue', 'malaise' and 'nervousness' are bandied about with reference to shift workers, implying that such work will produce these neuropsychiatric syndromes. No evidence exists to suggest that shift workers suffer unduly from disabling or serious psychoneurotic disorders, neither do they appear to suffer excess absence attributed to sickness or death from neurological disease. Fatigue and diminished work performance can undoubtedly occur, especially on the night shift, but the tiredness appears to be self limiting in view of the lack of objective evidence of associated morbidity or mortality.

Other related factors

Age is a factor related to morbidity but it does not, of itself, lead to more disease in shift workers compared with day workers when matched for age. *Sex* is difficult to assess as so few women work shifts and hardly any research has included them. It is conceivable that women with children might be subject to greater social and familial disruption if they worked nights but there is no evidence whatsoever to suggest that sex, *per se,* is a factor in determining ill health in shift workers. It would be interesting to study the behaviour of children whose mothers are on shift work. Little is known about the effects of *temperature, drugs* or *pre-existing morbidity* but it is likely that these factors could initiate or exacerbate ill-health in shift workers due to the variable hours of work consequent upon the job. One factor frequently overlooked is that an agreement to work rotating shifts could produce considerable problems for certain workers, who, by virtue of their *race* or *religion* are precluded from working on certain days or certain times of the day. An extension of shift working to developing countries will eventually cause this conflict between wage earning and adherance to certain moral or religious beliefs.

FAMILY AND SOCIAL LIFE

Adjustment to shift work, particularly night work, is frequently greatest with regard to family and social commitments. Young people, whose desire to earn money may be great, dislike the social privations imposed by shift work – particularly the afternoon and night shifts. Workers with young families have, perhaps, the greatest incentive to earn more money but shift work (which may pay the best rates) means that they see less of their growing family, can help least with their education and care, and frequently leave their spouse alone at night or in the evenings. Mott et al. (1965), Sergean (1971), Walker (1978) have all reviewed the social and familial consequences of shift work in some depth.

Once again the attitudes of the workers to their job plays a crucial role in whether they tolerate it. If the worker has a stable home environment with a spouse who actively supports the job practices of his or her partner then discord in the home is minimized. If one adds to this, a shift worker who enjoys solitary pastimes, like gardening, rather than group activities like playing (or watching) football, and who enjoys a family-orientated life rather than a community-orientated one, then conflict is further diminished. By contrast, shift work could prove very stressful for the man thinking of working shifts who was an active Church goer, local councillor, amateur football player, lived in an apartment overlooking a main road, and had a wife who enjoys nights out on the town. Most of these problems are less if the shift work either does not include nights or if there is no rotation of shifts.

Divorce is alleged to be more common among shift workers but such cause-and-effect statements are difficult to confirm due to the multi-factorial nature of marital discord. Outside the family, shift workers seem to make and possess fewer friends. It is perhaps ironic that as industrialization progresses and more emphasis is placed on leisure time and less emphasis on work, shift workers – a product of that increased mechanization – are the ones least able to benefit from it. Studies of workers' attitudes suggest that approximately 20 per cent of those who commence shift work, abandon it, the majority tolerate it and a few, around 10 per cent, actually like it.

THE IDEAL SHIFT SYSTEM

The first thing to be said in this context is that there is no system which will suit everyone all of the time. Nevertheless, considerable improvements in the present system of working practices could be made which would make life a lot more tolerable for shift workers and considerably lessen the chances of ill-health if they do exist.

What should be clear from the preceding pages is that shift work cannot just be abolished because it might be bad for people – even if the evidence for such ill effects was incontrovertible, which it certainly is not.

The asbestos, lead and coal industries are all undertakings well recognized as carrying risks of disease and death among the workers in those industries, but the continuing need for these materials implies that solutions have to be found to the problems of worker exposure. This is no less valid for shift working in general. There are two aspects of shift working which need to be considered in discussing optimal systems: the shift rotation itself, and the appropriate preventive health measures.

Shift scheduling

Management frequently gives little consideration to the implications of introducing shift work; neither do they experiment enough with different systems. The rigid adherance to the three shifts at 0600, 1400 and 2200 hours is unphysiological in many ways. Many physiologists feel that, in addition to selecting suitable persons for shift work, more attention might be paid to changes in the timing of the shifts: for example 0400–1200–2000 hours or 0800–1600–0000 hours. These rotas might lessen the social unacceptability of the morning or night shifts.

There are good scientific grounds for exchanging slow rotational shifts for rapid rotating ones and no epidemiological evidence to suggest that the latter is more detrimental to the worker than the former. Such schemes can result in 48 hours off every week for 3 weeks and 72 hours off every fourth week. As night work seems to cause the most problems, the hours worked at night might be reduced or each night on could be followed by 24 hours off. Several physiologists and psychologists subscribe to the view that if sufficient volunteers could be found to work permanent nights (and apparently this is feasible in many instances) then the other workers could rotate on rapidly alternating morning/afternoon shifts. A wider use of flexible timing and a greater participation of workers in shift practices decisions could alleviate a lot of the current difficulties.

Preventive health measures

Where shift systems including night work are unavoidable, then work at night should be made as palatable as possible. Working conditions at night are usually the least adequate. Better meals, improved health care, transportation and recreational facilities would make work at night less unattractive. Employees should be screened for their suitability to such routines and those with serious disease excluded. Such conditions as insulin-dependent diabetes, epilepsy, severe coronary artery disease, active gastro-duodenal ulceration and probably also those with a high neuroticism index would be well advised to eschew shift work. If women eventually undertake more shift work, employers or local authorities will have to contemplate providing facilities for child care.

In short, more consideration is needed. Thoughtful collaboration – and compromise – between employer and employee should aim towards an ideal system.

CONCLUSIONS

Shift work is an integral part of modern industrial society, and current trends suggest that one-fifth of the work force will continue to be so employed. Scientific experiments involving subjects exposed to varying degrees of circadian rhythm disturbance have demonstrated clearly that biological rhythms can be upset markedly by such phase shifts. Night workers' sleep is shorter than day workers' and greatly exacerbated by poor housing conditions. Work performance and output can be diminished by such circadian rhythm changes but the evidence that accidents are greater or more severe at night is inconclusive. Such performance effects can be largely eliminated if the work is made more interesting, less repetitive and adequately interspersed with short rest periods. Individual responses to such fatigue can overshadow any group effects.

Given this background of well-documented physiological effects of shift working, there is a remarkable dearth of objective ill effects on health. Whilst this may be due in part to poor epidemiological investigation, it is most unlikely that major health effects have been overlooked. There is, for example, no evidence for excess mortality in shift workers, and little evidence for increased morbidity, excepting the ex-shift workers. This latter group may be 'poor adaptors' in some ways and there is a need to try and establish ways of identifying these poor adaptors as early as possible – preferably at a screening examination before starting shift work. The only specific illness that seems to be related to shift work is gastro-duodenal ulceration and even here it is difficult to judge whether shift work initiates the disease or exacerbates latent or pre-existent disease. Moreover poor catering facilities at work – especially at night, may play a part in the aetiology of peptic ulceration in this situation.

Different shift schedules produce differing degrees of physiological disturbance. Night work seems to be the worst – particularly with regard to sleep deprivation, decreased work performance and fatigue. Improved arrangements for night workers both at home and at work could greatly diminish these effects.

The present prohibition of women from many shift work schedules has no scientific or physiological foundation. Sex seems to play no part in determining the level of 'ill effects' from shift work. The continuation of such legislation is much more likely to be maintained through male workers' dislike for change – particularly as shift work pay rates are frequently higher than for day work.

Attitudes also play a major role in some of the confusion over whether shift work is detrimental to health. Only the minority of shift workers positively like it; the greatest dislike occurs in relation to the night shift but much of this is probably motivated by the social and marital privations that are consequent on working such hours. Greater use of volunteers for night work would diminish this dissatisfaction, leaving the remainder of the work force to alternate rapidly between morning and afternoon shifts.

Greater attention needs to be paid to collaborative shift schedules with greater flexibility of hours worked out jointly between management and workers. This could alleviate a lot of the *angst* that presently surrounds shift working in some industries. Optimal shift schedules could then be established for a given work force.

For the future, it is clear that more detailed long-term health studies are needed to answer the many remaining questions concerning this subject. The medical literature is replete with ill-conceived, poorly executed studies often with frankly biased conclusions. There are notable exceptions, but even reviews of the subject frequently contain misleading information which may be based on either misconstrued data or coloured by politically motivated preconceptions. Definitive studies would help to clarify the true picture. On present evidence, there are no grounds for believing that shift work is a major health hazard.

REFERENCES

Aanonsen A. (1964) *Shift Work and Health.* Oslo, Universitetsforlaget.

Carpentier J. and Cazamian P. (1977) *Night Work.* Geneva, International Labour Office.

Colquhoun W. P. (ed.) (1972) *Aspects of Human Efficiency.* London, English Universities Press.

Harrington J. M. (1978) *Shift Work and Health: A Critical Review of the Literature.* Health and Safety Executive (EMAS) London, HMSO.

Maurice M. (1975) *Shift Work.* Geneva, International Labour Office.

Mott F. E., Mann F. C., McLoughlin Q. et al. (1965) *Shift Work – The Social, Psychological and Physical Consequences.* Ann Arbor, University of Michigan Press.

Rentos P. G. and Shepherd R. D. (1976) *Shift Work and Health: A Symposium.* HEW Publication No. (NIOSH) 76–203. Washington DC, US Govt. Printing Office.

Rutenfranz J., Colquhoun W. P., Knauth P. et al. (1977) Biomedical and psychosocial aspects of shift work. *Scand. J. Work Environ. Health* **3**, 165–182.

Sergean R. (1971) Managing shift work. *Industrial Society.* London, Gower.

Shepherd R. D. and Walker J. (1956) Three-shift working and the distribution of absence. *Occup. Psychol.* **30,** 105–111.

Taylor P. J. (1967) Shift and day work: a comparison of sickness absence, lateness, and other absence behaviour at an oil refinery from 1962–1965. *Br. J. Ind. Med.* **24,** 93–102.

Taylor P. J. and Pocock S. J. (1972) Mortality of shift and day workers 1956 to 1968. *Br. J. Ind. Med.* **29,** 201–207.

Taylor P. J., Pocock S. J. and Sergean R. (1972) Absenteeism of shift and day workers. *Br. J. Ind. Med.* **29,** 208–213.

Thiis-Evensen E. (1958) Shift work and health. *Ind. Med. Surg.* **28**, 493–497.
Walker J. (1978) *The Human Aspects of Shift Work.* London, Institute of Personnel Management.
Wilkinson R. T. (1971) Hours of work and the 24 hour cycle of rest and activity. In: Warr P. B. (ed.), *Psychology at Work.* Harmondsworth, Penguin, pp. 31–54.

21. ASPECTS OF SICKNESS ABSENCE

Peter Taylor

Absence from work for one reason or another must surely be as old as labour itself. An ancient Egyptian papyrus classified the three main reasons as 'sick, lazy, and placating the Gods'. Today, despite various elaborate and occasionally confusing classifications used by some organizations, I would suggest that the triad might be altered only in the description of the third type since sports matches, especially football, seem, for the modern worker, to have replaced the devotional excuses of his Egyptian predecessor. By far and away the most important cause of absence from work is however that *attributed to incapacity,* and this term is a great deal more accurate than 'sickness absence'. Modern industrial societies, usually with universal social security, all seem to have found that rates of absence attributed to sickness or injury have been increasing, and this chapter reviews the problem and indicates the wide range of factors which have been shown to influence rates of absence. The literature is now very extensive and a comprehensive bibliography prepared by Froggatt has recently been updated by Taylor for the reprinted proceedings of a symposium edited by Gardner (1977).

It is necessary to emphasize at the outset that sickness absence must never be considered synonymous with morbidity. Many people seem to assume that high or low rates of absence attributed to incapacity indicate more or less disease, but this is not necessarily so. Those who seldom or never take time off work are not *ipso facto* perfectly fit. There is evidence to show that such people may often have signs of physical or psychological disease (Taylor, 1968a; Smith, 1970; Rhoads, 1977). It is a common experience of doctors and nurses practising in industry that many high-frequency 'sick' absentees have no demonstrable signs of ill health. Medical conditions are but one of the many causes of absence attributed to incapacity, and most cases fall into that large grey area between absolute incapacity on the one hand and complete fitness for work on the other. An extensive list of factors which have been demonstrated to influence sickness absence can be culled from the literature and a selection of these is set out in Table 21.1. As may be seen, only two of the factors listed (epidemics and medical conditions) are strictly concerned with ill-health, and the phenomenon is clearly governed by the interplay of numerous factors, in other words of multifactorial aetiology.

Sickness absence is, of course, costly, not merely to the state – and thus to the taxpayer – as shown by the ever increasing expenditure on social security benefits – but is also costly to employers, in sick pay, in overheads and in payments to others to cover the work normally done by the absentee. An estimate of the cost of sickness absence to the British national economy (Office of Health Economics, 1971) produced a sum very similar to the entire annual revenue expenditure on the National Health Service. The cost to companies was presented in a booklet by the British Institute of Management (1961), and a recent (1976) calculation in one large organization showed that the daily cost of absence of a semi-

Table 21.1. Some factors influencing sickness absence.

Country	Organization	Personal
Region	Nature	Occupation
Climate	Size	Sex and age
Race	Personnel policy	Hours of work
Economy	Quality of supervision	Job satisfaction
Pension age	Sick pay	Commuting journey
Social security	Labour turnover	Family responsibility
Health services	Working conditions	Personality
Epidemics	Occupational health service	Medical conditions

skilled worker, excluding sick pay, was at least £10. Apart from these economic reasons there are important social and medical consequences which also account for the concern that the subject produces. Since the underlying trend is rising in many if not all industrialized countries, whatever their ideology, it is scarcely surprising that the subject seems to encourage sweeping and ill-informed statements from many quarters. Unfortunately these do little to clarify the problem, still less to solve it.

Assertions that 'It's all because. . .' may frequently be heard from these armchair or tap room critics as they variously attribute the rise in sickness absence rates to causes such as malingering, exploitation, alienation or a poor quality of working life (much depends upon the speaker's own attitudes!). The medical profession provides a convenient scapegoat with the accusation that doctors sign sick notes without good cause. There are many doctors who have been trying, without success, to abolish their statutory obligation to certify incapacity for work.

THE MEASUREMENT OF ABSENCE

In contrast to the relative simplicity of births or deaths which, by definition, must be singular occurrences, sickness absence is a repetitive phenomenon. An individual may be away from work for any number of occasions. The duration of each spell of absence can range from a single day to several months. That being so, it follows that it is not possible to use a single index or measurement to describe the situation. Similar considerations apply, of course, to the measurement of safety performance. In this area it has long been accepted that both frequency and severity rates must be used. It is therefore a constant source of surprise that many organizations which maintain adequate safety records still attempt to measure absence by one rate only, usually the lost-time percentage (defined below), and take no account of frequency.

The search for an agreed set of standards by which absence shall be measured has been almost like that for the Holy Grail. The literature is full of pleas for agreed standards. Thus the Health of Munitions Workers Committee in 1918, its peacetime successor the Industrial Fatigue Research Board in 1923 and Newbold in 1925 all proposed the adoption of standard methods. More recently the problem was the main topic discussed at the First International Conference on Sickness Absence in 1957. The proposals were set out once more by the Subcommittee on Absenteeism of the Permanent Commission on Occupational Health in 1973. For various reasons, some of which might be cynically described as 'original thought' or alternatively as 'reactionary individualism', some organizations insist on producing figures which seem to be unique, while some others refuse to believe that anything other than an overall lost-time percentage is of any relevance. Slowly, however, more and more seem to be accepting the need for uniformity of measurement. A current survey by one university, however, has found that very few large companies produce figures which permit direct comparisons to be made. Many firms in the private sector of industry, in contrast to those in the nationalized sector, are reluctant to reveal their absence rates, perhaps because they are ashamed to do so.

There are three main types of measure that can be used:

1. *Frequency rates*, mostly calculated as the average number of spells of absence per person at risk per year, sometimes called spell inception rate.
2. *Severity rates*, either calculated as the average annual days of absence per person at risk, or alternatively as the percentage of potential normal working time, lost due to absence.
3. *Prevalence rates*, usually the percentage of employees away on a particular day.

These three measures are quite distinct and should not be confused, even though the use of a percentage to measure time lost and also to measure the proportion of people away can and often does just this.

The prevalence rate is undoubtedly the easiest measure to make. It has some value in manpower planning on a daily number basis but it gives absolutely no indication of whether those absent are off for one day only or for long periods. It is also seldom used in the research literature. Problems can also arise in the units used to measure severity; the annual duration in days per person may be measured in working days (or shifts) or in calendar days. Calendar days are most frequently quoted in the occupational medicine literature, and working days in personnel or industrial psychology journals. A third measure, which often adds to the confusion, is used for National Insurance purposes in the UK, and is based on a 6-day week, 312-day year. Even the lost-time percentage is not immune from problems. Despite international agreement that it should be based on the total amount of normal working time which would have been obtained, without overtime, if all employees had attended, some firms do include overtime, others count actual time worked, and so on. The lesson from all this is clear; if asked to comment upon an absence rate, always insist upon knowing precisely how it was calculated. All organizations do indeed keep some form of record about absence of individual employees, if only because tax laws and social security benefit rules make it obligatory. It is at the stage of collection and preliminary analysis of this information that matters can get out of hand.

COMPARISONS WITH NATIONAL RATES

Most practising occupational health doctors will have been asked at some stage how the sickness absence level in their own organization compares with 'national figures'. To the best of my knowledge it is not possible to answer this question in precise and reliable terms. Social security figures in each country are governed by their own, often idiosyncratic, rules relating to benefit payment and entitlement due to sickness or to industrial injury. These seldom if ever equate completely with sickness absence from work.

In the UK for example, apart from the 312-day year already mentioned, national insurance statistics usually exclude absences lasting for less than 4 days, include 312 days each year for those permanently sick or disabled under pension age, most of whom are not employed at all, and exclude the absences of all civil servants, Post Office employees and members of the Armed Forces. Furthermore a majority of employed married women are also excluded because they have chosen not to insure for sickness benefit, even though they must by law be insured for industrial injuries. Social security figures are of course of considerable value for monitoring trends over time, but they cannot be directly compared with figures from industry. One attempt has been made to compare the social security sickness absence rates from eight countries (Taylor, 1972), but this required a number of assumptions. Of the eight, four used a 365-day year, two a 312-day, one a 300-day and one a 260-day year. Six included short spells while two did not, and so on. The estimated calendar days of absence attributed to incapacity per person for the year 1968 were: Netherlands 21, Sweden 18, Czechoslovakia 16, Great Britain, West Germany and Poland 15, Italy 14 and Yugoslavia 12. Sickness absence rates in all these countries, and also in the USA, had shown substantial rises between 1955 and 1969, and there is anecdotal evidence of similar trends from many other industrialized countries.

Fortunately there are other sources of national information about absence from work attributed to incapacity, but these also have their limitations. In the United States for example, the Bureau of Labor Statistics collects weekly prevalence data as part of their monthly surveys of the labour force, while the National Health Survey records from sample household interviews details of days of work limitation and other information on illnesses on behalf of the Department of Health, Education and Welfare. The figures from these two sources are not, however, comparable. In Britain, the General Household Survey which has been running since 1971 provides information from a carefully selected sample of over 10 000 households on matters such as health, work, housing and so on. Although the first report (Office of Population Censuses and Surveys, 1973) included estimates of working days lost attributed to ill-health in various occupations, subsequent reports have merely included prevalence rates of people absent in a one or two week period. Finally the Earnings Survey undertaken on a 1 per cent sample of employees for the month of April each year by the Department of Employment, provides information on the number whose pay was affected by absence, but here too the resulting figures are in the form of prevalence rates. These problems can be somewhat frustrating for occupational health staff, since managers find it hard to accept that national figures are not of direct comparability.

For those organizations that have kept sickness absence statistics for several years, one way around this problem is to compare the secular trend with that of the national statistics or indeed with similar rates obtained from other companies. The Post Office, for example, has maintained records of absence for very many years and a comparison since 1953 when the first national rates were calculated can be informative (Fig. 21.1). Note that the ordinate is labelled 'reported days per person' since the Post Office records calendar days while the National Insurance rate is based on a 312-day year. Before the last war, Post Office rates were about 9 calendar days per person and they rose sharply between 1948 and 1950 in the first year of the National Health Service and universal Social Security system. Since the early 1960s, however, Post Office rates have remained steady – apart from fluctuations associated with influenza epidemics – whereas national figures have shown a gradual rise. Most industrial organizations can be shown to have experienced quite substantial rises in this period.

COMPARISONS WITH OTHER ORGANIZATIONS

Here one may be on firmer ground, for many companies now keep figures of some sort, if only of crude overall rates in the form of lost-time percentages. Unfortunately the number undertaking separate analyses for men and for women, for the main grades or status groups of employee – white or blue collar and so on – and also for different age groups, are comparatively few and far between. Pitfalls also exist for the unwary unless the details of measuring severity are known, not only because working or calendar days may be used but because some companies count only absences lasting more than a couple of days or so up to 3 or 6 months, whilst others may include a full year for an individual absent throughout the period. Most information published from companies in the

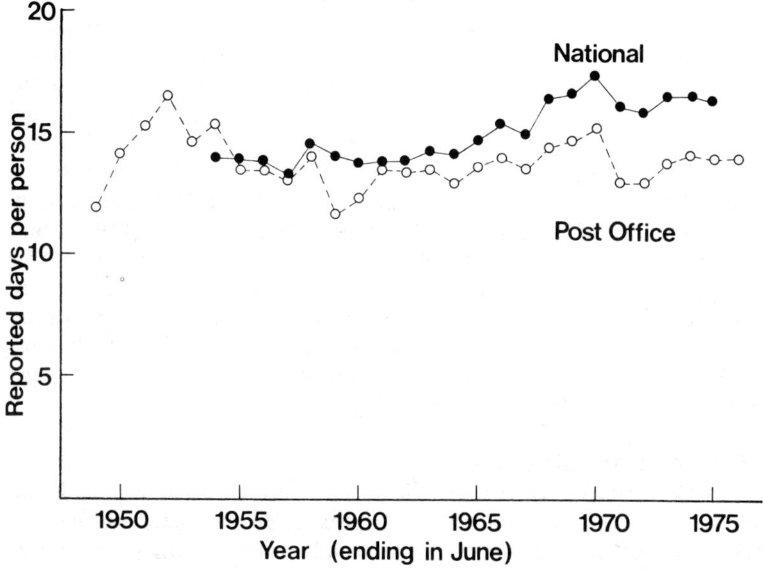

Fig. 21.1 National Insurance and Post Office sickness rates.

USA, for example, *excludes* brief absences of less than a week. This too can be misleading to anyone in the habit of considering absences of all durations.

Absence rates from quite a large number of companies may be found in the published literature, often used as background information in analytical studies of absence (for example, Behrend and Pocock, 1976). Perhaps the most widely known organization in the UK to publish its absence statistics in a form that can be easily be used by others is London Transport. Starting with a book over twenty years ago (London Transport Executive, 1956), a second publication has described the interesting and substantial changes that have been recorded since the early 1950s (Ager and Raffle, 1973). The Rubber Manufacturing Employers Association (1966) also produced a comprehensive book of statistics on similar lines, while copies of annual reports on sickness absence may often be obtained by *bona fide* enquirers from the Chief Medical Officers of some large organizations, mostly those in the public sector. Some selected lost-time percentage statistics from industry can be found in the booklet from the Office of Health Economics (1971) although sadly there is no central source in the UK from which this information can be obtained. This is in contrast to the situation in Holland where the Institute for Preventive Medicine in Leyden has collected, since 1947, standardized sickness absence and injury statistics from many companies all over the country.

Just as the cobbler's children were reputedly the last to have shoes, occupational health services are only now starting to be set up to meet the needs of those who work in hospitals. This development has resulted in a number of papers about the (relatively high) rates of absence amongst various grades of hospital staff. Apart from the most informative annual reports from the experimental service set up some years ago in Bedford, recent papers on this subject include: Barr (1960), Bendall (1965), Brown (1968), Butler and Hay (1977), Clark (1975), Franks (1972), Kearney (1977) Kleish and Wheeler (1969), Lunn (1975), Pounds (1974) and Rushworth (1975). This is a field in which many problems still await analytical study and it is likely that useful and constructive research may be forthcoming. In this, and in any other inter- or even intra-organization comparison, it is absolutely essential to consider, and if necessary allow for any differences in the fundamental demographic factors such as sex, age and status or job, in the two groups being compared.

REGIONAL COMPARISONS

Most organizations with branches in various parts of a country find that their rates of sickness absence show appreciable and consistent differences even if the branches are similar in size and nature of activity. This may cause some concern unless it is pointed out that national social security and other sources of information always show substantial differences, not merely in the UK but also for example in Eire (O'Muircheartaigh, 1975), in Finland (Harni, 1975), Italy (*Annuario Statistico*, 1969) and presumably also in most other countries. Such regional differences are not of course restricted to sickness absence but are found in a wide range of health, economic and social indices.

Within the UK the differences between the regional National Insurance sickness absence rates are very substantial. In the year 1972/73 for example, men in Wales had almost exactly three times as many days of certified incapacity as men in the South East of England (32 days and 10·5 days). Rates above the national average are also regularly found for Northern Ireland, the northern half of England and for Scotland. More disturbing, however, is that compared with regional rates twenty years before the differences have become more exaggerated. Thus in 1953/54 the rates for men were: Wales 20 days and the South East (then combined with East Anglia) 10 days. There has as yet been no conclusive explanation for this increased disparity although a number of possibilities spring to mind. The first and most obvious is in the type of industry in the regions. The usual annual statistics cannot help as they take no account of this, but in a special study in Great Britain (but not Northern Ireland) for the year ending in June 1962, a 5 per cent sample of all employed men and a 2·5 per cent sample of women was fully analysed in relation to occupation and place of residence. The report (Ministry of Pensions and National Insurance, 1965) is a unique and valuable contribution to our knowledge of sickness absence. In this context it showed that regional differences of a similar magnitude applied to those living in rural areas as well as in the towns and that differences were found in nine main occupational groups. This shows that the regional pattern applied to all, not merely to coal-mining or other special industrial groups. Agricultural workers in Britain for example had an age standardized rate of 5·5 days per man. In Wales it was 7·5 days and in the South East it was 5 days. Unfortunately this fascinating study was not repeated around the 1971 census and it remains the only national study of employed people in Britain.

The Post Office records now allow comparisons to be made between various parts of the UK taking occupation as well as age and sex into account. Postmen, telephone technicians and so on do the same sort of work all over the country and thus the study of regional differences can be taken one stage further. The results for the two years 1975/77 are set out in Table 21.2. Rates are standardized for age and for occupation to the

Table 21.2. Regional sickness absence among Post Office men and women 1975/77. (Severity rates in calendar days per annum standardized for age and occupation.)

Region	Men		Women	
	Cal. days/yr	Ratio	Cal. days/yr	Ratio
Northern Ireland	18·8	143	19·2	113
North West	15·7	119	19·6	115
Wales and Marches	14·9	113	17·3	102
North East	13·9	106	18·2	107
Scotland	13·4	102	17·7	104
London	13·2	100	18·0	106
South West	13·2	100	16·0	94
Midlands	12·8	97	14·6	86
South East	11·6	88	14·6	86
Eastern	9·9	75	13·6	80
All Post Office	13·2	100	17·0	100

total population of the entire Post Office. Substantial regional differences can be seen but not to the same degree as are found in the crude National Insurance figures, and it is notable that Post Office men in Wales have a rate only 13 per cent above the national average. The Post Office regional boundaries are, however, not always the same as those of the standard regions used for government statistics. Although Northern Ireland and

Scotland are exactly the same, the main differences apply to 'Wales and the Marches' which includes Hereford, Shropshire and the western half of Cheshire, and to the 'North East' which includes the standard Yorkshire and Humber region and the eastern half of the standard Northern region.

Here too is another aspect of absence attributed to sickness that requires more study. It seems likely from the results of other work into regional rates of death and disease that climatic, economic, and demographic factors may all be involved, but they would probably not explain the increasing disparity over the past twenty years.

Another aspect of regional differences which may be of relevance in some countries is the relationship with ethnic or genetic factors. Collins (1962) showed that of the employees in the Singapore dockyard, the Malays had the lowest rates of sickness absences, the Indians the highest and the Chinese were intermediate. Other evidence has come from the USA where Zborowski (1952) demonstrated major differences in attitudes towards pain and disease between Jews, the Irish, the Italians and the 'Old Americans'. There have also been some internal reports from large companies in Sweden and West Germany concerning sickness absence in various categories of immigrant workers. There is no published evidence available in the UK, possibly because of an inhibition as a result of race relations legislation.

COMPARISONS OVER TIME

Although most of the studies reported about sickness absence have been cross-sectional in that they relate to periods of a year or so, longitudinal – or secular – investigations over periods of several years are sometimes more useful, particularly because the pattern of absence has changed quite considerably in the past two or three decades. In my experience many companies are still operating absence control procedures which were set up to meet the problems of the 1950s but which are now less appropriate because the problems themselves have changed.

The underlying rising trend in absence attributed to sickness has already been mentioned since it applies throughout the world. In the UK for example Morris (1965) was one of the first to draw attention to this and the matter was further discussed by Whitehead (1971). Rises in the USA and Canada were the subject of a symposium of the Industrial Hygiene Foundation (1969) and the changes in national statistics from nine countries between 1950 and 1968 were described by Taylor (1969). Some common problems have been noted from these and other studies, the most obvious of which is that the rise in severity has been less marked than that of frequency, implying that spells of absence have become on average shorter in length. This increase has been most obvious amongst younger people in whom high frequency short duration absence is now the greatest problem. The pattern of diagnoses has also changed quite appreciably over the past 20 years. Tuberculosis and other infections have become much less important – even though influenza in an epidemic year can still be the most important single cause – and substantial falls have also been recorded in peptic ulcers and septic conditions. On the other hand minor injuries and ailments, together with cardiovascular disease, have all increased very substantially (Taylor, 1974). Similar changes in diagnostic pattern have been found in other countries.

Here there is the paradox of absence attributed to incapacity – a growing trend despite improved standards of health care, of living, of education and of longevity. The explanation may be summarized from the factors set out in Table 21.1 since only two out of the twenty four factors listed are strictly related to ill-health.

The other aspect in which time trend studies have been of help relates to the matter of the *prediction of absence*. Innumerable medical man-hours must still be wasted all over the world by the performance of recruitment medical examinations conducted at the request of managers because they believe that this will enable the doctor to advise them about the candidate's future sickness absence. There is no evidence to support this myth, even though there can be other perfectly valid reasons to undertake such examinations on applicants for certain jobs such as driving and so on. The presence or absence of a medical condition must not be taken to imply that the individual will or will not take time off work with it; some of the 'never sick' men described in Taylor's (1968a) paper had quite seriously limiting chronic conditions. The weight of evidence available shows that the only reliable predictor of absence is previous absence and although even this is not always accurate, it applies best to groups. The paper by Hinkle and Plummer (1952) about women employees, and its successor about men in the same telephone company (Hinkle et al., 1956) are among the classics in this field. More recently, the matter has been studied using more sophisticated statistical techniques by Froggatt (1970) in relation to one and two day absences, and by Pocock's (1973) detailed study of the records of 454 manual workers over the first five years of employment which showed that prediction of absence amongst individuals, based upon their record in the first year of service, was a good deal more reliable for frequency than it was for severity. This concept has been further developed by Behrend and Pocock (1976) using the records from an engineering factory in Glasgow. The subject of absence prediction is of course closely allied in statistical theory with that of accident proneness about which there have been numerous and often conflicting views expressed in the past 60 years.

In summary therefore, the whole pattern of absence attributed to incapacity has changed over the past three decades and there is no reason to believe that the gradual increase in rate is likely to reverse its trend. In parenthesis it is worth noting that the commonly held view that absence and unemployment have an inverse relationship was not confirmed by Taylor and Pocock (1969), nor have recent experiences confirmed it either. This change in level of absence, which has been accompanied by substantial changes in the diagnostic pattern, has been most marked in the younger age groups and the evidence from secular studies of individuals suggests that they are likely to persist in their own pattern of absence behaviour. The outlook is therefore that absence attributed to incapacity will increase still further in the future.

SEX, AGE AND OCCUPATION

The necessity to take adequate account of these three factors before attempting any comparison of absence rates cannot be over-emphasized, whether considering severity, frequency or prevalence rates. Although it is clearly preferable to obtain such basic information about every individual at risk as well as all those who have been absent, so as to enable rates to be calculated for each sex, by age and by main job or status groups, it may often be impracticable in the field situation to obtain all these data. In most inter-departmental or inter-factory comparisons of overall lost-time rates it is usually possible to establish whether the proportions of the two sexes, the proportion of older employees and the proportion of white and blue collar staff are reasonably comparable. Without such information any comparison of absence would be pointless and could be grossly misleading.

Recognition that these three factors are of fundamental importance is far from being new. Froggatt's (1967) description of the actuarial studies of friendly society records refers to 'Price's Law of Sickness' in 1769 which stated that 'sickness amongst females is considerably greater than among males' and states that the Rev. Dr Price produced point prevalence fractions for 'a state of incapacitation from illness or accidents' which rose from 1/48 under the age of 32 to 1/24 between the ages of 58 and 64 years. Point prevalence rates of between 2 per cent and 4 per cent would only be found today in well-motivated non-manual workers. By the mid nineteenth century the sickness insurance schemes of the friendly societies were providing cover for millions of workers and Finlaison set out his 'Laws' in 1854:

1. Females have more incapacity than males, even excluding pregnancy.
2. Sickness rates rise with age (he was referring to severity).
3. The duration of spell is inversely proportional to the inception rate and the product of the two is a constant for each age throughout the country.
4. The quantum of sickness annually falling to the lot of man is in direct proportion to the demands on his muscular power.

These statements, at least in general terms, still hold good today and it is salutary to reflect that many of the observations that one may make in this field are merely repeating the studies done over a century ago.

Interest in sickness absence among women has recently become greater, largely because legislation on equal opportunities and pay has now been adopted in several countries. A few years ago it was not uncommon to hear from managers that although women took much more time off work than men, this was not of great concern because they were usually paid less. Now that equal pay is a statutory requirement in the UK and, even more important, it is forbidden to discriminate against the employment of women simply because they will take more time off work, the matter has become of greater interest. To what extent is the premise about excess female absence really justified? The overall national figures are not particularly useful since, given that manual work incurs more absence, and given that a high proportion of women are employed in non-manual jobs, the similarity of overall absence rates for men and women recorded in the social security, the earnings and the household surveys is of little relevance. Comparisons between the sexes in terms of occupational status, however, does reveal higher absence rates for women, particularly for married women with families or other dependent relatives.

In one of the authoritative reviews on the subject, Isambert-Jamati (1962) suggested that such differences were largely artificial because women tended to be employed in jobs of lower pay and status which provided less job satisfaction, and that there would be little difference in the rates of absence attributed to incapacity when jobs were truly equivalent. She also observed that many women were faced with a 'conflict of obligations' towards work and family. One section of a Department of Employment booklet (1975) was concerned with this subject and concludes with the following (somewhat misleading) sentence: 'On absence, however, the evidence quoted shows little difference between men and women generally'.

Table 21.3. Sickness absence severity rate ratios for women and men in certain occupations.

Occupation	Reference	Ratio of severity rate Women	:	Men
Teachers	Simpson, 1962	1·5	:	1
Nurses	Ministry of Pensions, 1965	2·0–1·1	:	1
Teachers	Ministry of Pensions, 1965	1·5–1·6	:	1
Clerks	Ministry of Pensions, 1965	1·4–1·1	:	1
Bus conductors	Ager and Raffle, 1973	2·0–1·5	:	1
Clerical and technical	Ager and Raffle, 1973	1·9–1·8	:	1
Airline cabin crew	Preston, 1977	1·7	:	1
Postal clerical	Post Office, 1975–77	1·6	:	1
Telephone clerical	Post Office, 1975–77	1·3	:	1
Postmen/women	Post Office, 1975–77	1·2	:	1

There are some jobs in which men and women work on equal terms, and the available evidence on absence rates in these occupations does show that women take more time away from work attributed to incapacity than men. A selection of ten such occupations are set out in Table 21.3. To avoid complexities arising from different ways of measuring severity, the comparisons between rates are presented in the form of ratios based on male rates of unity. Where two figures are given for women, the first refers to married and the second to single, or, as the social security statistics describe them, 'other' women.

Thus the belief that women have more absence than men has been confirmed in spite of some misunderstandings in the review literature. This leads to another paradox, for it is incontrovertible that women's rates of mortality are considerably more favourable at all ages than those of men. Yet objective evidence of disabling disease shows that the rates in both sexes are similar. Consultation rates for women with their general practitioners do, however, exceed those for men, particularly between the ages of 15 and 44 years. Lewis and Lewis (1977) have recently reviewed these issues and quote evidence to show that women tend to demonstrate a greater interest in health than men from childhood and indeed they influence the health behaviour of men. Single men and widowers for example get ill more quickly and die earlier than men who have a woman at home. They conclude by posing the question: 'What is the better measure of equality – for women to die like men, or for men to live (a little bit) like women?'

OTHER PERSONAL FACTORS

The list of factors set out in Table 21.1 under the heading 'Personal', covers a wide range of situations and it is not possible in this chapter to consider each one of them in depth. The term 'hours of work' for example covers not merely the length of the working day or week but also overtime and shift work. Whilst shift work has been extensively studied and relevant information can be found in Chapter 20, the length of the working day or week and overtime have, perhaps surprisingly, been studied scarcely at all in recent years. Work during world wars showed that when compulsory weekly hours exceeded 60, rates of sickness and accidents rose while those of output fell (Health of Munitions Workers Committee, 1918). The lack of recent papers might perhaps be taken to infer that basic weekly hours well below this have little if any effect, but one might expect studies to show whether the 10- or 12-hour day for a 4-day week, which some now advocate, has any noticeable effect on absence. Flexible working hours have been alleged to reduce absence but I am not aware of any scientifically controlled investigations to support this. Overtime too has apparently been little studied although Lokander (1962) showed no relationship in a large Swedish engineering company. An (unpublished) study that I have undertaken showed that annual overtime, expressed as average hours per week available at work, showed an inverted shallow U-shape relationship with absence; that is, men doing the smallest and the largest amounts of overtime had less absence than those doing a moderate amount. Further studies would be helpful, particularly since many managers believe that high overtime is in itself a cause of absenteeism.

Motivation to attend for work despite the presence of a mild or even moderate ailment is strongly influenced by personality, the social work ethics of the individual and of his working group, and also by the extent to which he obtains 'job satisfaction'. These factors influence not merely the decision to take a day off with a minor ailment but also the decision on how speedily to return to work after a longer absence with a more serious medical condition. The rôle of job satisfaction was reviewed by Taylor (1974) and by Nicholson et al., (1976) and it is clear that the term is an imprecise one which covers a variety of attitudes to a wide range of factors relating to work. Personality, as measured by standard psychological tests, has also been found to influence behaviour (Cooper and Payne, 1967; Taylor, 1968b; Howell and Crown, 1971). Extroverts who need more stimulation and easily become bored have been shown to form the majority of those who take excessive high frequency, short duration absences; strong neurotic features have been found amongst those who have had long absences and to a lesser extent also among the high frequency absence group. Alcoholism, or less emotively 'problem drinking', is an additional important factor in frequent absentees and also in some of those with longer spells of absence (Lokander, 1962; Pell and D'Alonzo, 1970; Ferguson, 1972).

There is no doubt at all that in the overwhelming majority of cases of absence attributed to incapacity, whether certified by a doctor or not, it is the individual himself who really determines whether or not he goes off sick and at what stage he will return to work. This message formed a central part of the British Medical Association's evidence which was accepted by the Fisher Committee on the Abuse of Social Security Benefits (1973). Underlying this, and distinct from the influence of job satisfaction, is the individual's attitude towards adopting the 'sick rôle'. There is now a considerable body of literature, much of it from the pens of sociologists, on this subject. The review by Mechanic (1969) included 33 references. Other relevant papers include those by Kasl and Cobb (1966), Suchman (1970) and, in a more strictly medical context, Ferguson (1973). Linked to this concept has been the assessment of life changes and personal stress as predisposing factors (Rahe, 1968; Rubin, et al. 1971; and Theorell, 1976). In summary then it seems clear that, with the exception of the most disabling of medical conditions, and these are by definition relatively uncommon in a working population, the presence of a mild or moderate condition alone does not necessarily mean that the affected person will take time off work. Only when this is combined with other factors, either in relation to the work, or more importantly in the individual himself, will absence attributed to the condition ensue.

CONCLUSION

This review of the complex problem of absence attributed to incapacity is manifestly incomplete, but it has attempted to indicate and assess some of the more important problems which are likely to face those working in occupational health who become involved, willingly or unwillingly, in this subject. When I started to undertake some research in this area, some occupational health doctors of my acquaintance expressed surprise that anyone should want to study 'such a dull subject'. I can only hope that this chapter will explain why I do not subscribe to this view.

REFERENCES

Ager J. E. and Raffle P. A. B. (1973) *Patterns in Sickness Absence: Experience of London Transport over Two Decades.* London, London Transport Executive.

Annuario Statistico (1969) Napoli, Istituto Nazionale per Assicurazione contro le Malattie.

Barr A. (1960) Sickness absence amongst hospital nurses. *Br. J. Prev. Soc. Med.* **14,** 89–98.

Behrend H. and Pocock S. J. (1976) Absence and the individual, a six year study in one organization. *Int. Lab. Rev.* **114,** 311–327.

Bendall E. R. D. (1965) Wastage, sickness and allocation. *Nurs. Times* **61,** 760–763.

British Institute of Management (1961) *Absence from Work: Incidence Cost and Control.* London, B.I.M.

Brown I. M. (1968) Hospital staff sickness absence. *The Hospital,* March 94–98.

Butler E. A. and Hay B. J. (1977) The passionate statistician: a computerised record of nursing sickness and absence. *Nurs. Times* **73,** 149–155.

Clark J. (1975) *Time Out? A Study of Absenteeism among Nurses.* London, Royal College of Nursing.

Collins C. P. (1962) Sickness absence in the three principal ethnic divisions of Singapore. *Br. J. Ind. Med.* **19,** 116–121.

*Committee on Abuse of Social Security Benefits (*1973) (Fisher Committee) Cmnd. 5228. London, HMSO.

Cooper R. and Payne R. (1967) Extroversion and some aspects of work behaviour. *Personnel Psychol.* **20,** 45–57.

Department of Employment (1975) *Women and Work: A Review.* Manpower Paper No. 11. London, HMSO.

Ferguson D. (1972) Some characteristics of repeated sickness absence. *Br. J. Ind. Med.* **29,** 420–431.

Ferguson D. (1973) A study of neurosis and occupation. *Br. J. Ind. Med.* **30,** 187–198.

Franks G. L. (1972) Off sick: Who? Where and Why? *Nurs. Times* **68,** 1596–1597.

Froggatt P. (1967) Ph. D. Thesis. Belfast, Queen's University.

Froggatt P. (1970) Short term absence from industry. *Br. J. Ind. Med.* **27,** 199–210.

Gardner A. W. (ed.) (1977) *Proceedings of a Symposium into Absence from Work attributed to Sickness.* Updated edition. London, Society of Occupational Medicine.

Harni A-L. (1975) Regional variation in the development of illness in Finland. *Br. J. Prev. Soc. Med.* **29,** 249–257.

Health of Munitions Workers Committee (1918) *Final Report.* Cmnd. 9065. London, HMSO.

Hinkle L. E. and Plummer N. (1952) Life stress and industrial absenteeism. *Ind. Med. Surg.* **21,** 363–375.

Hinkle L. E., Pinsky R. H., Bross I. D. J. et al. (1956) The distribution of sickness disability in a homogeneous group of 'healthy adult men'. *Am. J. Hyg.* **64,** 220–242.

Howell R. W. and Crown S. (1971) Sickness absence levels and personality inventory scores. *Br. J. Ind. Med.* **28,** 126–130.

Industrial Fatigue Research Board (1923) *Third Annual Report.* London, HMSO.

Industrial Hygiene Foundation of America (1969) *Current Concepts of Biostatistical Services for Industry.* Medical Series Bulletin No. 15. Pittsburgh, Pa., IHFA.

Isambert-Jamati V. (1962) Absenteeism among women workers in industry. *Int. Lab. Rev.* **85,** 249–261.

Kasl S. V. and Cobb S. (1966) Health behaviour, illness behaviour and sick role behaviour. *Arch. Environ. Health* **12,** 246–266.

Kearney J. M. (1977) Sickness patterns in hospital staff. *Occup. Health* **29,** 162–165.

Kleish W. F. and Wheeler M. K. (1969) A hospital health service evaluation of absentee control. *Ind. Med. Surg.* **38,** 46–49.

Lewis C. E. and Lewis M. A. (1977) The potential impact of sexual equality on health. *N. Engl. J. Med.* **297,** 863–869.

Lokander S. (1962) Sick absence in a Swedish company, a socio-medical study. *Acta Med. Scand.* Suppl. 377.

London Transport Executive (1956) *Health in Industry.* London, Butterworth.

Lunn J. E. (1975) Absenteeism: an occupational hazard. *Nursing Mirror.* May 22, 65–66.

Mechanic D. (1969) Response factors in illness: the study of illness behaviour. In: Baker F., McEwan P. and Sheldon A. (ed.), *Industrial Organisation and Health.* London, Tavistock, pp. 192–214.

Ministry of Pensions and National Insurance (1965) *Report on an Enquiry into the Incidence of Incapacity for Work.* Part II. London, HMSO.

Morris J. N. (1965) Capacity and incapacity for work: some recent history. *Proc. R. Soc. Med.* **58,** 821–825.

Newbold E. M. (1925) Industrial sickness statistics. In: Industrial Fatigue Research Board, *Fifth Annual Report.* London, HMSO. pp. 46–52.

Nicholson N,. Brown C. A. and Chadwick-Jones J. K. (1976) Absence from work and job satisfaction. *J. Appl. Psychol.* **61,** 728–737.

Office of Health Economics (1971) *Off Sick.* London, OHE.

Office of Population Censuses and Surveys (1973) *The General Household Survey: Introductory Report.* London, HMSO.

O'Muircheartaigh C. A. (1975) *Absenteeism in Irish Industry.* Study No. 12. Dublin, Irish Productivity Centre.

Pell S. and D'Alonzo C. A. (1970) Sickness absenteeism of alcoholics. *J. Occup. Med.* **12,** 198–210.

Permament Commission and International Association on Occupational Health (1973) Sub-committee on absenteeism: draft recommendations. *Br. J. Ind. Med.* **30,** 402–403.

Pocock S. J. (1973) Relationship between sickness absence and length of service. *Br. J. Ind. Med.* **30,** 64–70.

Post Office (1977) Report of Chief Medical Officer on sickness absence and medical wastage. London, Post Office. (Obtainable on request from C.M.O).

Pounds F. J. (1974) *The Sick Nurse.* A review of the years 1969 to 1973 in the King's College Hospital Group. London, Pounds.

Preston F. S. (1977) The health of female air cabin crew. In: *Health of Women at Work.* London, Society of Occupational Medicine, pp. 11–22.

Rahe R. H. (1968) Life change measurement as a predictor of illness. *Proc. R. Soc. Med.* **61,** 1124–1125.

Rhoads J. M. (1977) Overwork. *J. Am. Med. Ass.* **237,** 2615–2618.

Rubber Manufacturing Employers Association (1966) *Health in the Rubber Industry: A Pilot Study*. Cambridge, RMEA.

Rubin R. T., Gunderson E. K. E. and Arthur R. J. (1971) Life stress and illness patterns in the US Navy. *J. Psychosom. Res.* **15**, 89–94.

Rushworth V. (1975) Not in today. *Nurs. Times* **71**, 121–124.

Simpson J. (1962) Sick absence in teachers. *Br. J. Ind. Med.* **19**, 110–115.

Smith D. J. (1970) Absenteeism and 'presenteeism' in industry. *Arch. Environ. Health* **21**, 670–677.

Suchman E. A. (1970) Health attitudes and behaviour. *Arch. Environ. Health.* **20**, 105–110.

Taylor P. J. (1968a) Sickness absence resistance. *Trans. Soc. Occup. Med.* **18**, 96–100.

Taylor P. J. (1968b) Personal factors associated with sickness absence. *Br. J. Ind. Med.* **25**, 106–118.

Taylor P. J. (1969) Some international trends in sickness absence 1950–68. *Br. Med. J.* **4**, 705–707.

Taylor P. J. (1972) International comparisons of sickness absence. *Proc. R. Soc. Med.* **65**, 577–580.

Taylor P. J. (1974) Sickness absence: facts and misconceptions. *J. R. Coll. Physicians Lond.* **8**, 315–333.

Taylor P. J. and Pocock S. J. (1969) Post war trends in sickness absence and unemployment. *Lancet* 1120–1123.

Theorell T. (1976) Selected illnesses and somatic factors in relation to two psychosocial stress indices. *J. Psychosom. Res.* **20**, 7–20.

Whitehead F. E. (1971) Trends in certificated sickness absence. In: *Social Trends No. 2.* London, HMSO. pp. 13–23.

Zborowski M. (1952) Cultural components in responses to pain. *J. Soc. Issues* **8**, 16–20.

22. SCREENING FOR ALL: EXCELLENCE OR EXTRAVAGANCE

Michael D'Souza

INTRODUCTION

In 1977 the Annual General Meeting of the TUC passed a resolution urging the British government to bring in general health check-ups for all workers. In the same year two new screening centres opened in the north of England similar to the now famous BUPA centre in London which sells health check-ups mainly to visiting Arabs and British managers and executives. The time is then perhaps right to review the scientific basis for advocating more widespread use of such screening in British industry. The substance of this chapter will therefore be to attempt a serious appraisal of the value of the general health check-up in occupational medicine.

Historical review

The idea of using the medical examination on the apparently healthy probably originated in the late nineteenth century as a by-product of producing sufficiently fit men to serve in the armed forces.

The occupation of the common soldier has throughout history been both miserable and hazardous and the notion that only fit men should undergo the risks of being decimated in the trenches was perhaps a bit ironic. This army screening often resulted in some quaint reasons for rejecting men such as the notorious 'flat feet', but perhaps more seriously it sometimes damaged fit men's opinions of their own health. The most famous instance of this is given in the anecdote of the man who was told in his army medical prior to the Great War that he had a serious heart condition. This poor unfortunate spent the next 20 years as a bed-bound invalid until another doctor revealed to him that his heart murmur was in fact completely innocent.

Notwithstanding this report, and doubtless others like it, the army medical almost certainly saved many sick and enfeebled human beings from having to face the horrors of war in addition to their other burdens and as such was both useful and humane.

Insurance companies were not slow to see a potential commercial value in screening the apparently healthy. Poor-risk lives were clearly poor business unless the insurance premiums could be suitably loaded by the calculations of actuaries. The insurance medical, either by clinical examination or by self-administered questionnaire soon after the turn of this century, become established business practice. However to this day there seems little clear scientific reasoning being applied to the question of precisely what tests should be included in the insurance medical or to establish its precise value in economic terms to the business of insurance.

The use of screening in the more general context of providing the public with a regular screening service first commenced in Peckham in 1926. The Peckham Pioneer Health Centre, which although surviving and indeed thriving until the Second World War, failed to remain economically viable when it re-opened after the war. This Centre aimed at providing what was later to become a W.H.O. ideal, namely physical, mental and social health. The screening it undertook was also directed at obtaining research information about the biology of urban man. The screening uncovered a great deal of ill-health and minor ailments. Indeed in their work published in 1943 Pearse and Crocker revealed that 86 per cent of their male population and 95·7 per cent of their female population had some abnormality found on screening. They remarked that 'nothing short of periodic health overhaul on a national scale can lead to the national application of medical science for the elimination of disease' (Pearse and Crocker, 1943).

When the National Health Service was established in 1948 the lessons learned from the Peckham experiment were largely ignored. Indeed even now, 50 years after the beginning of the Peckham Centre, no comparable complete community service which combines both disease care and the promotion of the wider aspects of health in a personal community setting has been attempted.

In modern times the workplace has become separated from the home and is, in its own right, a very important community. Thus the notion of undertaking screening at work rather than in general practice has gained favour.

Modern approaches

In America in 1942 the Kaiser Foundation began a small scale health service plan which later included screening as part of its services. In 1964 a controlled trial within this plan was introduced and was the first planned evaluation of screening ever to be undertaken. Since this time, it is the United States that has pioneered the development of screening and the bulk of the modern literature has originated from that country. Technical advances such as mass miniature radiography, biochemical auto-analysers and computer data handling have each been exploited by those planning screening programmes and the majority of the reports centred around such technical ways in which screening could be accomplished, rather than any evaluation of their effectiveness in achieving better health – indeed this is often assumed to be a self-evident outcome of earlier diagnosis. The changing pattern of morbidity in the developed countries, with chronic degenerative diseases replacing the acute infections as the major health problems, has encouraged many to believe that screening could produce considerable benefits.

At the time of writing, Australia, Canada, Ireland, Israel, Italy, Sweden, France, Germany, Japan, New Zealand, Norway, South Africa, Scotland, England and the United States have all contributed to an ever-growing body of information on screening. The characteristic of most of these contributions is that they are nearly always enthusiastic in the belief that screening represents a major advance in medical philosophy and technology. The other, perhaps most significant, factor is that nearly all these reports originate in wealthy developed countries where there has been a blind acceptance that expenditure on welfare items such as health care and education are automatically good ways of spending surplus monies. In fact there are now hardly any rich countries which do not provide extensive screening facilities.

DEBATES AND DEFINITIONS

Despite this enthusiasm, or possibly because of it, there has been a strong wave of criticism of too hasty an acceptance of screening, particularly screening for degenerative disease in the middle aged. The objectives of screening have been examined more thoroughly and distinctions drawn between different programmes that utilize screening tests. Wilson and Jungner (1968) produced a lucid and comprehensive review of screening throughout the world and enunciated 10 common-sense criteria that should be applied before it could be considered that it was worth screening for a particular disease.

These criteria are:

1. The condition sought should be an important health problem.
2. There should be an accepted treatment for patients with recognized disease.
3. Facilities for diagnosis and treatment should be available.
4. There should be a recognizable latent or early symptomatic stage.
5. There should be a suitable test or examination.
6. The test should be acceptable to the population.
7. The natural history of the condition, including development from latent to declared disease, should be adequately understood.
8. There should be an agreed policy on whom to treat as patients.
9. The cost of case-finding (including diagnosis and treatment of patients diagnosed) should be economically balanced in relation to possible expenditure on medical care as a whole.
10. Case-finding should be a continuing process and not a 'once and for all' project.

In 1968 too, the Nuffield Provincial Hospital Trust produced a book which dealt with the current state of the art in screening for a number of chosen conditions and again the general tone of this book was less enthusiastic than the literature of the preceding decade. Recently Hart (1975) has edited a work specifically devoted to screening in the context of British general practice. In it the flame of enthusiasm appears to have been fanned, unfortunately not on account of any new evidence.

A series of articles in *The Lancet* (1975) was generally more critical of screening and it emerged that most of the good evidence in favour of screening being of use centred around pregnancy and early childhood. Following this series of articles, letters to *The Lancet* revealed elements both of confusion and messianic zeal in the debate on whether public health services should increase their involvement with screening. Sackett and Holland (1975), characterizing the opposing teams as 'snails' and 'evangelists', produced a cogent explanation of the main elements in the debate. They observed that the key to much of the argument lay in confusion over the use of terms, particularly what was meant by 'screening'.

Although this term has a multitude of applications, far removed from the medical context, numerous attempts have been made to define its medical use precisely. The World Health Organisation Regional Committee for Europe accepted the definition of the US Commission on Chronic Illness (1957) that screening is 'the presumptive identification of unrecognized disease or defect by the application of tests, examinations, or other procedures which can be applied rapidly. Screening tests sort out the apparently well persons who probably have a disease from those who probably have not. A screening test is not intended to be diagnostic. Persons with positive or suspicious findings must be referred to their physicians for diagnosis and necessary treatment'.

Since then a more elegant definition has been drafted by McKeown (Nuffield Provincial Hospital Trust, 1968) who suggested that the term should be applied to any 'medical investigation which does not arise from a patient's request for advice for specific complaints'. Despite such efforts at semantic draughtsmanship, there is still no universally accepted definition, and most doctors simply look upon screening as the use of any sort of test to identify possible disease. It is, therefore, perhaps wiser not to try to pontificate on any universal use of the term but merely to make it clear whenever it is used, what precisely is being done, by whom, for what reason and in what context.

Sackett and Holland did this in their attempt to clarify the issues. They described three quite distinct programmes or activities which all use screening tests but which have quite different ethical and cost implications. The first activity they termed 'case-finding', which was an unfortunate choice of words because other people have used the term in a much more general sense (cf. Wilson and Jungers' use). However, in Sackett and Holland's usage, case-finding implies the identification of disease by medical workers such as general practitioners using screening tests on patients who have already consulted them for unrelated symptoms. Coope (1975) gave a classical instance of this when he related how he found a case of hypertension by measuring the blood pressure of a man who attended to have his ears syringed. Next they referred to 'screening' proper. This implies approaching a defined group of people, be it an at-risk group or a total population, and offering them screening. This screening might be one test (monophasic) such as mass X-rays, or it might be many tests (multiphasic), but the essential difference between screening and case-finding is that in the former the population has been approached by the doctor rather than vice versa. Thus the ethical implications of screening are much more serious; for when the doctor approaches the patient he implies he has a benefit to offer. Should he produce any harm by his screening (such as incorrectly labelling a fit man as diseased) he cannot claim the defence of the clinical case-finder, namely that he was merely responding as best he could to the patient's request for help.

The method and style of approach is the main thing that distinguishes screening from the third activity, namely survey-work. In surveys one attempts to get information from the whole of a defined population. The quality of the survey must in part be judged by how much of the population it has failed to cover. So, whereas in screening one can talk of response rates, almost as a measure of how interested the population was in receiving the service, in survey work all those failing to respond to simple invitations should properly be further persuaded to participate, often by direct person-to-person contact. In surveys both the ethical considerations discussed above and the costs assume an even greater significance than in screening.

THE MOTIVES FOR SCREENING

Much discussion as to the motives of screening has also appeared in the literature. Sackett (1973) talked of four reasons for doing screening: *first* to influence the gamble of life insurance, *second* to protect people other than the patient as in industrial and public health screening, *third* to obtain clinical base-lines and *fourth* to do the patient some good – so-called prescriptive screening. Clearly, there are other motives to screening such as financial reward, biological research, satisfying public and medical demand and gaining information for administrative purposes. Often an amalgam of these objectives is achieved as a spin-off from the activity rather than as a result of any specific design. Certainly most of the debate surrounding screening has been to do with Sackett's last category, namely prescriptive screening. The general aim of prescriptive screening for doing good might encompass several separate medical goals. Most often the notion of secondary prevention is considered in this context of screening, early diagnosis being seen as postponing death or preventing disability.

But in the context of infectious disease such as tuberculosis, a public health dimension to the prevention is also added by screening which may result in removing the patient from where he would continue to act as a focus of infection. Furthermore, tuberculosis screening also provides the opportunity to cure the patient of the disease, so cure and prevention were clearly definable goals. In more recent times interest has refocused on caring as opposed to curing, particularly on the care of the elderly and disabled. The notion of using screening for identifying people in need, or indeed in itself providing a form of care, is receiving increasing attention. Lowther et al. (1970) and Anderson (1976) have provided both evidence and opinion in favour of this.

Methods and techniques

Largely from the United States has come a debate of a wholly different character. This concerns the method by which screening should be carried out. Distinctions were drawn up not on the basis of the approach to populations since population-based medicine is still far from established in that country. Rather it concerned the merits of periodic health examination by a physician as against multiple automated testing by technicians. As early as 1951 Smillie was condemning the impersonal approach of multiphasic screening in screening clinics on the grounds that it was 'inferior medicine', and instead he advocated regular physician check-ups. Broadbent must have seemed like a voice crying in the wilderness when in 1963 he expressed the opinion that even such regular physician check-ups were a waste of time which he would prefer to devote to his symptomatic patients. Nevertheless, the strongest argument put forward for multiphasic screening by technicians was that it provided perhaps the only means by which some indigent patients could get access to any form of medical service. Unfortunately, such reasoning easily leads to the situation where the extension of personal medical services to the needy is delayed.

In recent years the phrase 'Automated Multiphasic Health Testing' (AMHT) has featured increasingly in the American literature. The basis of this new term is the sophisticated use of the computer as an integral part of the screening operation. Much work has been done on cutting costs and producing quicker results by such devices as the mechanized administration of branching questionnaires by on-line computers. The improvement of the repeatability and reliability of tests has also been attempted, and the financial and epidemiological implications of a test's sensitivity (ability to identify true positives) and specificity (ability to exclude true negatives) have been extensively discussed and mathematically explored. It is perhaps ironic, however, that despite all this undoubted technical ingenuity, very few American authors have devoted time to evaluating seriously the health benefits to their patients of such prescriptive screening.

THE EVALUATION OF PRESCRIPTIVE SCREENING

One of the earliest attempts to evaluate the effects of screening originated with the insurance use of screening. In 1921 Knight produced evidence that such screening might be effective in saving lives. He reported over a 5-year period only 217 deaths had occurred where 303 would have been expected in an uninsured population of 6000 having periodic health examination, a mortality '28 per cent less than expected'. A similar study was reported by Roberts et al. (1969) on a population of 20 648 men who were having 'employer-sponsored' periodic health examinations. These authors reported a favourable ratio of actual to expected deaths, but were more cautious in their interpretation and recommended well-controlled prospective studies on the question.

Caution is of course appropriate, for such studies can rarely be considered satisfactory because they are so dependent on the suitability of the comparison groups used to calculate the 'expected mortality'.

In fact, the assessment of screening is beset with difficulties. Feinleib and Zelen (1969) and more recently Sackett (1973) have pointed to at least three ways in which false conclusions can be reached. *First,* regression towards the mean, or the natural tendency for high or low readings at one occasion subsequently to be nearer their mean level, may easily be interpreted erroneously as clinical improvement in longitudinal screening follow-up studies. *Second,* the increased survival of, say, a cancer patient after detection by screening might be interpreted as benefit of early diagnosis, but in fact be merely a reflection of the so-called lead-time, that is that the total duration of the disease process has itself remained unchanged but since the diagnosis has been made earlier the patient appears to survive longer from the time of diagnosis. *Third,* there is the danger that the net of any screening process will tend to select out the more chronic and least severe diseases which would, by definition, have a more favourable clinical course, again tending to suggest falsely that screening was beneficial.

Careful controlled trials should be able to overcome many of these difficulties. Indeed, taking these issues into consideration, Shapiro (1973), in a huge controlled trial appears to have demonstrated successfully that it is possible to reduce the mortality from carcinoma of the breast in women aged 50–59 years by a mass screening programme. However, the capital and manpower used to achieve this success are beyond the resources of most countries.

In the field of multiphasic screening five controlled trials have so far been attempted, one in Yugoslavia, one in Great Britain, two in the United States and one in Sweden. The Yugoslavian study which is the only trial in which final results are not yet published will be of great interest as it has been undertaken on a random sample of the town of Titograd where initial results of screening have revealed a relatively high prevalence of tuberculosis. Although this might mean that its results will have less relevance to more developed countries it should reveal whether screening does help in regions of high TB prevalence (Thorner et al., 1973).

American trials

The first real evaluation of screening to be attempted was started in the Kaiser Permanente scheme in California. The study design was that of an approximate control trial. Some 10 000 people were chosen at random from the 46 000 who were Plan members in 1964 and these 10 000 were then randomly divided equally into control and treatment groups. The 'treatment' consisted of urging those in the treatment group to attend for screening and approximately 60–70 per cent did respond every year. Unfortunately, being Plan members, the control group were also entitled to screening and some 20 per cent of these were also screened annually. The screening itself was multiphasic and covered all organ systems. It consisted of questionnaires, laboratory and clinical tests and physical examinations (Cutler et al., 1973).

In 1973 the first 7 years of the study were evaluated and control treatment comparison made on a variety of morbidity and mortality criteria (Ramcharan et al., 1973; Dales et al., 1973; and Collen et al., 1973).

The overall death rates during this period were not significantly lower in the screening population. However, certain specific causes of mortality in particular age groups did appear to be significantly improved in the screening group, notably carcinoma of the colon. However some 60 significance tests were performed on these mortality data and only three were reported as significant: two in favour of screening and one against it. This is approximately the same outcome that one would expect purely by chance. It is a pity therefore that the authors failed to make this point more clearly in their discussion of the results. For instance, it could just as readily be argued that screening caused deaths through accidents, violence and suicide since these were significantly higher in the screening group than in the controls. It seems much more likely however that this programme had no important impact either on death rates or on the pattern of mortality.

The overall picture emerging from this first large study was that even if some benefit could be achieved by such elaborate screening it would certainly not be very impressive.

The second study coming from America was reported by Olsen et al. (1976). This was a controlled study of morbidity and health service workload and was of much shorter duration. It failed to find any measurable effect from screening except an increase in the screening group of the number of nights spent in hospital. Most importantly, however, it observed that following screening there was very little intervention by the doctors. It seemed that finding diseases was not as big a problem as having something useful to offer to diseased patients revealed by screening.

The Swedish study

An important epidemiological study investigating the effects of screening was begun in Malmö in Sweden in 1970. This was a very well-designed random controlled trial carried out on all men born in 1914, residing in the town of Malmö.

This cohort of men were randomly divided into screening and control groups. After screening, these investigators concentrated on treating blood pressures ⩾ 165/110 and smoking (using a quit-smoking project). The overall death rates after 4 years showed no statistical differences between the screening and control groups but very interestingly there was a significant shift in the causes of death. Twice as many people died of cardiovascular disease in the control group as in the screening group. Unfortunately this was offset by a significantly higher death rate in the screening group from cancer and other causes. Furthermore the authors did not provide any evidence that they had lowered the blood pressure or the smoking levels in their screening population, so it might well be that the observed difference in cardiovascular deaths was due to chance rather than to the screening; certainly no-one would seriously suggest that screening increases the rate of cancer death which could be just as well argued from their findings. (Lannerstad et al., 1977).

The British study

This study, the most comprehensive evaluation of screening so far published, was a 10-year controlled trial carried out in two South London group practices (South East London Screening Study Group, 1977).

The general plan of this study is shown in Fig. 22.1. The tests used in the study are shown in Table 22.1. Similar to the Peckham study nearly 40 years earlier, a large amount of illness was detected at screening; on average 2·3 diseases per person screened. Furthermore over 90 per cent of the population had some diagnosis made after screening (*see* Table 22.2).

Similar to findings in the Olsen study, despite detecting a lot of illness there was very little new treatment initiated by the doctors except that all smokers were encouraged to stop and those with anaemia and hypertension were frequently treated (D'Souza et al., 1976).

The main results of this study are shown in Tables 22.3 to 22.6. As can be seen the population offered screening showed no measurable improvement over the controls in terms of mortality or morbidity. Extensive and detailed multivariate analyses were undertaken to make quite sure that these negative results were not due to hidden bias and the general conclusion of the research was that in view of their manifest failure to produce any health benefits such general health check-ups do not warrant any expenditure of scarce resources.

It is of real interest to inquire why there was little or no benefit observed in these studies. The whole truth is still uncertain. However, I feel that there are three clear reasons that can be discussed which go a long way to explain why what has seemed common-sense truth to so many people has been confounded. *First,* screening is not very good at picking up the major life-threatening diseases. In one study in America, over half

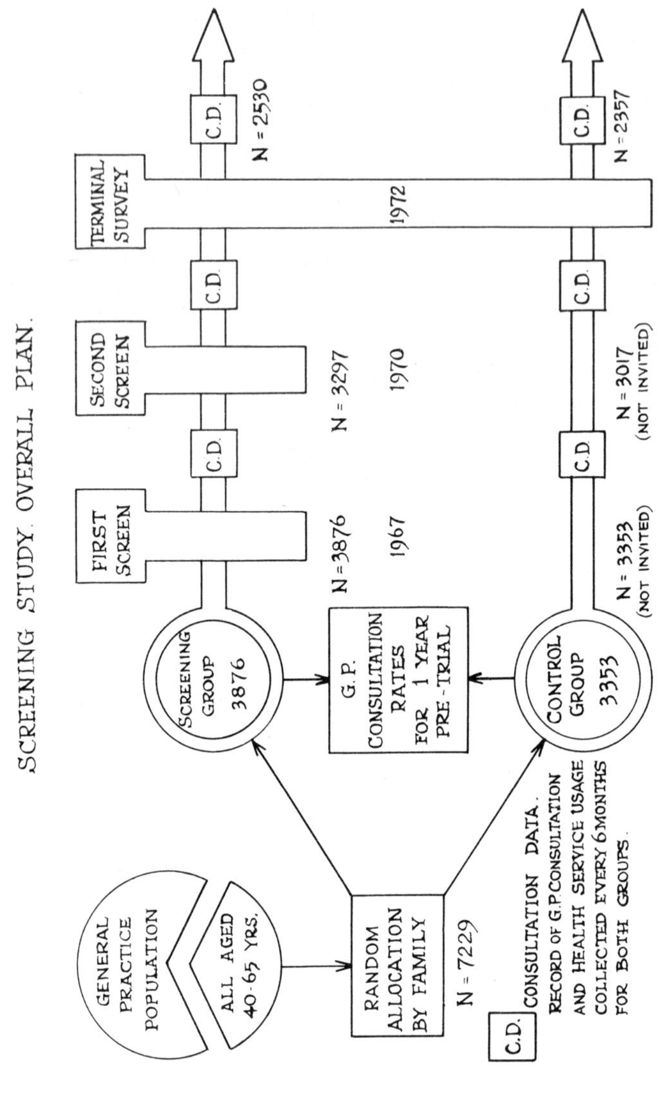

Fig. 22.1

the people dying of cancer and heart attacks had been declared completely fit at their previous annual check-up (Schor et al., 1964).

Second, when many diseases are discovered on screening, doctors do not believe there is much useful medical aid to be offered, and, *third,* even for those conditions such as raised blood pressure for which useful treatments do exist, many patients find that sticking to treatment over long periods of time is more than they can stand and they often seem to prefer to take their chances with fate.

However, irrespective of any reasons why these trials have failed to show much success, I feel that the results speak for themselves. The paucity of real medical benefit derived from such a huge outlay in human effort is to say the least disappointing. It supports those doctors who feel that most screening in adults is not yet sufficiently advanced for them to spend time usefully on it. It supports health administrators who feel that the benefits to be derived from such screening do not match the costs. Thus, if decisions have to be made for committing public or private money or indeed medical time to such screening activities, then this evidence should weigh heavily against any such commitment. It is important to recognize, however, that since new screening methods and treatment are being developed each year, the position will require periodic review by further trials.

The general screening methods used in all these studies have not yet been superseded in any significant way and were their protocols to have been written now, no important changes would be made.

Table 22.1. Test used in multiphasic screening procedure.

1. Self-administered symptoms questionnaire*
2. Interviewer-administered questions on occupational data
3. Anthropometry – height, weight, skinfold thickness
4. Visual testing – near, distant, visual fields*
5. Audiometry
6. Chest X-ray
7. Lung function tests – peak expiratory flow rate, FEV_1, FVC
8. Electrocardiogram – 12 leads
9. Blood pressure
10. Blood tests – Hb, PCV, blood urea, random blood sugar, protein-bound iodine, serum cholesterol, serum uric acid
11. Stool for occult blood†
12. Basic physician examination‡ – skin, mouth, teeth, joints, abdomen for herniae, legs for varicose veins, breast and pelvic examination

* Bennett A. C. and Ritchie K. (1975) *Questionnaires in Medicine.* Nuffield Provincial Hospitals Trust

† Only carried out at first screening

‡ Not carried out at terminal survey

Philosophical considerations

A much more difficult issue to consider, is whether such screening should be judged only on its success in improving health. Clearly there is considerable public demand for screening. The question arises as to whether doctors and governments and firms should satisfy such demands, irrespective of the results of controlled trials. (Certainly it cannot be claimed, for example, that our existing social services have much established scientific support for their effectiveness.)

Table 22.2. Proportion of those examined at screening 1967/8 found to have some definable abnormality.

Men			
Age group	*Number examined*	*Number abnormal*	*Percentage*
40–	253	197	77·9
45–	288	264	91·7
50–	212	193	91·0
55–	217	207	95·4
60+	167	164	98·2
Totals	1137	1025	90·1
Women			
Age group	*Number examined*	*Number abnormal*	*Percentage*
40–	337	294	87·2
45–	332	289	89·8
50–	240	224	93·3
55–	224	206	91·9
60+	160	153	95·6
Totals	1283	1166	90·9

Arguments in favour of this viewpoint look upon medicine as a business which provides a consumer service – a service that is part essential and part luxury. Screening can be viewed within such a service as a useful source of reassurance which should be evaluated only in terms of its market appeal. Apart from the fact that there is no strong evidence to support the idea that screening allays more anxiety than it causes (for example, terrifying women who have only benign breast lumps) such an argument must be seen both as retrogressive and also as out of keeping with the spirit of informed medical concern. While it can be readily observed that the predominantly urban societies of the developed world exhibit high levels of anxiety for which they often seek technological solace, the provision of impersonal screening clinics would at best be merely palliative and at worst distinctly meddlesome. It would seem much more sensible to try to prevent such anxiety by searching for ways of creating more self-supporting personal communities within our cities, similar to that attempted by the Peckham experiment. Meanwhile, until evidence can be found for its medical usefulness, such screening should assume the status of a low priority superfluous service.

CONCLUSIONS

My conclusions are, therefore, that there is now insufficient evidence that general health screening by industry will benefit anyone. There is evidence that screening may well, at least temporarily, increase absences and for a few unfortunate people generate unnecessary anxiety. There is also the dangerous potential of screening for invading privacy.

Table 22.3 Some measures of morbidity – screening v. control groups at the concluding health survey in 1972/73 five years after the initial screening.

	Percentage			
	Control group N = 1950 (MAX)*	Screened 1967/68 N = 1651 (MAX)	Refused screening N = 327 (MAX)*	Total screening N = 1978 (MAX)*
A. *Questionnaire measures of general health*				
1. Percentage claiming to have good or excellent health in the fortnight preceding the survey	56·5	53·2	56·7	53·6
2. Percentage admitting to any major disability e.g. inability to dress or undress themselves	1·8	2·0	5·0	2·5
3. Percentage showing downward social mobility, i.e. a fall in social class over the preceding 5 years	27·4	27·4	27·1	27·4
B. *Cardiovascular disease*				
1. Percentage with evidence of angina on questionnaire†	22·4	21·9	21·4	21·9
2. Percentage with raised diastolic blood pressure ⩾ 105 mm Hg (Ph V)	3·1	2·7	2·4	2·8
3. Percentage with ischaemic changes on ECG‡	16·6	17·6	21·0	17·9
C. *Respiratory disease*				
1. Percentage still smoking	50·8	51·5	56·2	52·3
2. Percentage complaining of any bronchitic symptoms (MRC, 1966)	30·6	28·4	34·9	29·0

* Maximum means that this was the largest of the denominators used to derive the percentages below. These denominators varied according to the information available for the multifactor analysis.
† Rose G. A. (1962) *Bull. WHO* 27, 64[illegible].
‡ Rose G. A. and Blackburn H. (1968) *WHO Monogr. Ser.* No. 56.

Table 22.4 Average annual G.P. consultation rates for subjects in

Totals: C = 2730 S = 2844
Consultation rate by diagnostic group (ICD, 1957)
Overall consultation rate
Neoplasms ICD codes: 140–229 with 519.2 except 149, 166–169, 182–189 and 208–209
Selected endocrine and metabolic diseases ICD codes: 250–254, 260, 287–289.2, 786.4
Mental, psychoneurotic diseases ICD codes: 300–318.3, 320–326, 780.7, 781.9, 786.2
Central nervous system diseases ICD codes: 330–398 with 780–781.7 except 335–339, 346–349 and 358–359
Cardiovascular diseases ICD codes: 400–468 with 782.0–785.3 except 417–419, 423–429, 435–449, 454–459
Respiratory disease ICD codes: 003.1 and 241, 470–527, with 782.3–783.7 except 476–479, 484–489, 494–499, 503–506, 508–509 and 527.1
Digestive disease ICD codes: 530–545, 560–561, 570–578, 580–587, 782.8 and 784–785.
Skin diseases ICD codes: 690–698, 700–716, 788.2
Diseases of bones and organs of movement ICD codes: 720–727, 730–738, 740–749
Accidents, poisoning and violence ICD codes: N800–N822, N824–N848, N850–N856, N860–N936, N940–N963, N967–N999.3
All others

*NB. Since we have restricted this table to those who were in the study for more than one year, the numbers are smaller than in Table 22.1

the study for more than one year; control v. screening.

	Men		**Women**	
	Control	*Screening*	*Control*	*Screening*
	N = 1244*	N = 1321*	N = 1486*	N = 1523*
	3·1 (S.E. = 0·09)	3·2 (S.E. = 0·09)	3·8 (S.E. = 0·09)	4·0 (S.E. = 0·09)
	0·07	0·08	0·06	0·06
	0·03	0·04	0·07	0·09
	0·22	0·27	0·49	0·52
	0·21	0·20	0·21	0·22
	0·13	0·14	0·12	0·08
	0·51	0·52	0·42	0·43
	0·19	0·20	0·15	0·16
	0·14	0·12	0·14	0·17
	0·39	0·31	0·31	0·30
	0·13	0·15	0·11	0·12
	0·21	0·21	0·50	0·50

Table 22.5 Hospital admissions control v. screening 1967–1976.

	Control group (N = 3132)
Number of PEOPLE admitted once or more 1967–1976	862
Rate per 100 man/yrs at risk +	49·6
Total number of ADMISSIONS + per 100 man/yrs at risk	70·7

Hospital admissions by some of the principal diagnoses

	Control group	
Principal diagnosis at admission ICD (1957)	Persons admitted once or more	Admission rate* per 1000 man/yrs at risk
Neoplasms ICD codes: 140–229 with 519.2 except 149, 166–169, 182–189 and 208–209	185	9·1
Central nervous system ICD codes: 330–398 with 780–781.7 except 335–339, 346–349 and 358–359	88	4·3
Cardiovascular disease ICD codes: 400–468 with 782.0–785.3 except 417–419, 423–429, 435–449, 454–459. and 784	192	9·5
Respiratory disease ICD codes 003.1 and 241, 470–527, with 782.3–783.7 except 476–479, 484–489, 494–499, 503–506, 508–509 and 527.1	79	3·8
Digestive disease ICD codes: 530–545, 560–561, 570–578, 580–587, 782.8 and 784–785	174	8·6
All other diagnoses	415	21·3

*NB. These rates have been calculated using different times at risk, because once a particular event occurs the individual is no longer at risk for that event. This means that the time the individual will be at

I I

Screening group (N = 3292)

944

50·7

73·4

Hospital admissions by some of the principal diagnoses

Screening group	
Persons admitted once or more	Admission rate* per 1000 man/yrs at risk
217	10·0
92	4·2
210	9·6
71	3·2
195	9·0
396	18·8

risk depends on the event in question; obviously for total admissions the individual is at risk until he dies or is lost to observation.

Table 22.6 Death rates by cause control v. screening 1967–1975.

Cause of death (First certified) I.C.D. (1957)	Control group (N = 3132) Total time at risk = 18404·4 man/yrs		Screening group (N = 3292) Total time at risk = 19672·3 man/yrs	
	No. died	Death rate per 1000 man/yrs at risk	No. died	Death rate per 1000 man/yrs at risk
Neoplasms ICD codes: 140–229 with 519.2 except 143, 166–169, 182–189 and 208–209	47	2·6	50	2·5
Central nervous system ICD codes: 330–398 with 780–781.7 except 335–339, 345–349 and 358–359	13	0·7	17	0·9
Cardiovascular disease ICD codes: 400–468 with 782.0–785.3 except 417–419, 423–429, 435–449, 454–459, and 784	52	2·8	84	4·3
Respiratory disease ICD codes: 603.1 and 241, 470–527, with 782.3–783.7 except 476–479, 484–489, 494–499, 503–506, 508–509 and 527.1	37	2·0	28	1·4
All other causes	20	1·1	17	0·9
Total deaths (all causes)	169	9·2	196	10·0

*N.B. Time at risk is less than for previous analyses due to delays in ascertaining cause of death

Screening is, however, a developing technology, and research must go ahead. The development of new methods for improving the monitoring of health and safety at work is obviously of great importance. However, any new methods so developed must be rigorously tested by controlled trials before being extensively and expensively applied to our workforce, on the whim or enthusiasm of the well meaning.

The use of the controlled trial in this context is in my opinion perhaps our most important advance in technology and is at present the best way of evaluating such areas of concern. Despite the fact that these trials are difficult and costly to perform they do provide evidence of a far more reliable quality than can be obtained in any other way. Indeed one wonders why they are not applied more generally in other areas of political controversy. When, as now, we have the results from controlled trials we should not be too hesitant to act upon them. This implies that existing programmes for general health screening in industry should certainly not be extended and that active consideration should be given to cutting back those already in use. Thereafter, all new ventures in this area should be, by design, quite deliberately experimental.

REFERENCES

Anderson F. (1976) The effect of screening on the quality of life over seventy. *J. R. Coll. Physicians Lond.* **10,** 161–169.

Broadbent R. V. (1963) Annual check-ups are a waste of time. *Med. Economics* **40,** 245–256.

Collen M. F. et al. (1973) Multiphasic check-up evaluation study 4. *Prev. Med.* **2,** 236–246.

Commission on chronic illness (1957) *Chronic Illness in the United States* Vol. I. Cambridge, Mass. Harvard University Press.

Coope J. (1975) Controversy in the detection of disease. *Lancet* **2,** 454.

Cutler J., Ramcharan S., Fieldman R. et al. (1973) Multiphasic check-up evaluation study, 1. *Prev. Med.* **2,** 197–206.

Dales L. G. et al. (1973) Multiphasic check-up evaluation 3. *Prev. Med.* **2,** 221–235.

D'Souza M. F. et al. (1976) Screening for hypertension in general practice: The results of a long term controlled trial. *Lancet* **1,** 1228–1232.

Feinleib M. and Zelen M. (1969) Some pitfalls in the evaluation of screening programmes. *Arch. Environ. Health* **19,** 412–415.

Hart C. R. (1975) *Screening in General Practice.* Edinburgh, Churchill Livingstone.

Knight A. S. (1921) Value of periodic medical examination. *Statist. Bull. Metrop. Life Insur. Co.* **2,** 1.

Lannerstad O. et al. (1977) *Scand. J. Soc. Med.* **5,** 137–140.

Lowther C. P. et al. (1970) Evaluation of early diagnostic services for the elderly. *Br. Med. J.* **3,** 275.

Nuffield Provincial Hospitals Trust (1968) *Screening in Medical Care.* London, Oxford University Press.

Olsen D. M. et al. (1976) A controlled trial of multiphasic screening. *N. Engl. J. Med.* **294,** 925–930.

Pearse I. and Crocker L. (1943) *The Peckham Experiment.* London, Allen & Unwin.

Ramcharan S. et al. (1973) Multiphasic check-up evaluation 2. *Prev. Med.* **2,** 207–220.

Roberts N. J. et al. (1969) Mortality among males in periodic-health-examination programs. *N. Engl. J. Med.* **281,** 20.

Sackett D. (1973) Periodic health examinations and multiphasic screening. *Can. Med. Ass. J.* **109**, 1124.

Sackett D. and Holland W. W. (1975) Controversy in the detection of disease. *Lancet* **2**, 357–359.

Schor S. S. et al. (1964) *Ann. Intern. Med.* **61**, 999.

Shapiro S. et al. (1973) *Proc. 7th Nat. Cancer Conf.* Philadelphia. p, 663.

Smillie W. G. (1951) 'Multiphasic' screening tests. *J.A.M.A.* **145**, 1254–1256.

The South-East London Screening Group (1977) *Int. J. Epidemiol.* **6**, 357.

Thorner R. M. et al. (1973) A study to evaluate the effectiveness of multiphasic screening in Yugoslavia. *Prev. Med.* **2**, 295–301.

Whitby L. G. (1974) Screening for Disease: Definitions and Criteria. *Lancet* **2**, 819–821.

Wilson J. M. G. and Jungner G. (1968) *Principles and Practice of Screening for Disease. W.H.O. Public Health Paper.* Geneva, World Health Organisation.

Index